REACHING THE UNDERSERVED

Volume 3, Sage Annual Reviews of Community Mental Health

EDITORIAL BOARD

Sage Annual Reviews of Community Mental Health

Co-Editors: **Richard H. Price**
Community Psychology Program
University of Michigan

John Monahan
School of Law
University of Virginia

C. Clifford Attkisson
Dept. of Psychiatry
Langley Porter Institute
University of California
San Francisco

Morton Bard
Center for Social Research
City University of New York

Bernard L. Bloom
Dept. of Psychology
University of Colorado

Stanley L. Brodsky
Dept. of Psychology
University of Alabama

Anthony Broskowski
Northside Community Mental
Health Center, Inc.
Tampa, Florida

Saul Cooper
Washtenaw County
Community Mental Health Center
Ann Arbor, Michigan

Emory L. Cowen
Dept. of Psychology
University of Rochester

Barbara Dohrenwend
Division of Sociomedical Sciences
School of Public Health
Columbia University

Kenneth Heller
Dept. of Psychology
Indiana University
Bloomington

Murray Levine
Dept. of Psychology
State University of New York
Buffalo

Ricardo F. Muñoz
Social & Community Psychiatry Program
University of California, San Francisco &
San Francisco General Hospital

Frank M. Ochberg
Dept. of Mental Health
State of Michigan
Lansing

Amado M. Padilla
Dept. of Psychology
University of California
Los Angeles

Thomas F.A. Plaut
National Institute of Mental Health

N. Dickon Reppucci
Dept. of Psychology
University of Virginia

Stanley Sue
Dept. of Psychology
University of California
Los Angeles

Carolyn F. Swift
National Council of Community
Mental Health Centers &
Southwest CMHC, Columbus, Ohio

Edison J. Trickett
Dept. of Psychology
University of Maryland

Volume 3
SAGE Annual Reviews of Community Mental Health

REACHING
the
UNDERSERVED
Mental Health Needs
of
Neglected Populations

edited by
Lonnie R. Snowden

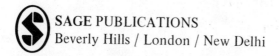

SAGE PUBLICATIONS
Beverly Hills / London / New Delhi

Randall Library UNC-W

Copyright © 1982 by Sage Publications, Inc.

All rights reserved. No part of this book may be reproduced or utilized
in any form or by any means, electronic or mechanical, including photo-
copying, recording, or by any information storage and retrieval system,
without permission in writing from the publisher.

For information address:

SAGE Publications, Inc.
275 South Beverly Drive
Beverly Hills, California 90212

SAGE Publications India Pvt. Ltd.
C-236 Defence Colony
New Delhi 110 024, India

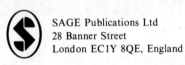

SAGE Publications Ltd
28 Banner Street
London EC1Y 8QE, England

Printed in the United States of America

Library of Congress Cataloging in Publication Data

Main entry under title:

Reaching the underserved.

    (Sage annual reviews of community mental health ;
v. 3).
    Bibliography: p.
    1. Mental health services—United States.
2. Minorities—Mental health services—United States.
3. Poor—Mental health services—United States.
I. Snowden, Lonnie R., 1947-   II. Series.
[DNLM: 1. Community mental health services. 2. Ethnic
groups. 3. Medically underserved areas.
4. Socioeconomic factors. W1 SA125TC v.3. WA 305 M5483]
RA790.6.R418 1982   362.2'042'0973   82-10722
ISBN 0-8039-1856-9
ISBN 0-8039-1857-7 (pbk.)

FIRST PRINTING

RA790
.6
.R418
1982

Contents

235361

Series Editors' Foreword

In this third volume of the Sage Annual Reviews of Community Mental Health, the volume editor, Lonnie Snowden, and his contributors draw our attention to the development and delivery of services for those in our society whose needs may be greatest and least acknowledged. Seldom is it clearer what is at stake in community mental health than when we consider the circumstances of the elderly, children, chronic mental patients, the rural poor, Blacks, Native Americans, Pacific Americans, Asian Americans, and Raza populations.

Even if we pause only for a moment to think about the well-being of these groups, we recognize that, as Snowden suggests in his introductory chapter, the debate about services to the underserved is really a debate about society and how we will meet our individual and collective responsibilities for social problems and their solutions. Wisely, Snowden reminds us that in thinking about these issues we must focus at the same time on the unique themes, requirements, and cultural concerns of various groups in our society and on the universal—those needs, concerns, fears, and hopes that we share with all of our fellow citizens. It is only in understanding the balance of universals and particularities that we can begin to think humanely and intelligently about these issues.

This is both a book of criticism and a book of new ideas. In some ways it reflects the fruits of twenty years of serious thought by many mental health professionals and citizens about the mental health needs of all of our citizens. It may be something of a shock to recognize that the community mental health movement is now more than two decades old. After two decades of experimentation yielding both reforms and reversals, we are now in a time of political and economic retrenchment. Because these times demand even more courage and ingenuity, we are fortunate that Snowden and his colleagues have been able to identify the gains of the last two decades and to chart directions for future efforts. This volume will be a valuable source of understanding to policymakers, researchers, and practitioners who will play a role in designing future mental health services that are responsive to both our unique qualities and our universal needs.

-Richard H. Price
John Monahan

1

Services to the Underserved

An Overview of Contemporary Issues

Lonnie R. Snowden

University of California, Berkeley

An unmistakable and increasingly troubling aspect of mental health services has been that of restricted access to these services based on social standing. Until some two decades ago, this state of affairs aroused little more than resignation. Minorities and those who were poor, rural, chronic mental patients, or too young or too old were poorly served, it was admitted, but for sound and inescapable reasons. Because of their lack of adequate intellect and psychological sophistication, their distance created by overwhelming "reality" factors, and their location away from metropolitan centers, certain groups in society were considered beyond the reach of conventional mental health practice. These positions were taken with an eye on certain "reality" factors affecting the professional: Working with members of outgroups was held to provide little challenge, prestige, or income.

The passage of time has brought a climate in which such callousness is no longer considered acceptable. An official change in stance has taken place, affecting mental health services more strongly in word than in deed, but significantly in both. As service delivery has become sponsored by the public sector, the prospect of only an elite clientele has been rejected, leading to efforts to respond effectively to the mental health needs of the underserved.

Changes in views about underservice have taken place as part of larger social changes. Within the field of mental health, conceptions of boundaries, methods, and institutions have undergone genuine revision, given greatest expression in the community mental health movement. As critics have noted, some of this has been illusion; the reality of change falls short of the appearance (Snow & Newton, 1976). It is also true, however, that in considering mental health, a role for social, cultural, and economic forces has become more accepted and the need for flexible, diversified programs of service is better recognized.

Beyond the field of mental health, currents moving within society at large have influenced perceptions of mental health underservice. Until very recently, the burden of responsibility for services had been shifting away from those in need and toward society and the mental health establishment. Such developments are expressions of a larger debate over the fundamental character of society, calling into question equity in the distribution of power and resources, and individual and collective burdens of responsibility for social problems.

The history of public responsibility for the provision of mental health services accessible to all may be traced in a record of federal action. In 1963, Congress enacted the Community Mental Health Centers Act, authorizing a network of community mental health centers, each with a defined region of responsibility. The act struck directly at the formerly exclusive character of mental health services in its provisions barring discrimination and its attempt to minimize denial of care because of inability to pay. In subsequent federally directed evaluation of community mental health centers, one standard of accountability was proportional representation of minorities within agency caseloads. Later, a presidential commission was appointed to examine the state of mental health in America. Its report took special note of underserved groups in society, documenting the extent of their need and the limitations imposed by obstacles to effective service delivery (President's Commission on Mental Health, 1978).

The struggle with underservice has now continued for two decades. Although no one would claim that the issues of concern have been laid to rest, or are even fully understood, constructive steps have been taken: New settings and service providers have been enlisted, diagnostic and treatment procedures have been revised, and ties to communities have been forged. In a time of social reaction and economic retrenchment such as the present, it is wise to review these efforts in order to consolidate past gains and suggest a focus for future development. Such a review is the purpose of the present volume.

Within the body of the volume, specific topics related to underservice are reviewed in detail by contributors who bring special qualifications to the preparation of reviews. At a broader level, certain themes are suggested by the literature that require a general overview to be perceived clearly. As an orientation to the volume, certain of these general issues are outlined in the following sections.

Identifying the Underserved

At one time it was possible to designate certain social groups as underserved in mental health without controversy. Overt racial prejudice, unsubsidized, prohibitive cost, and direct acknowledgment that certain people were "untreatable" made it apparent that services were systematically unavailable to some.

However, recent history has witnessed a growing awareness by many social groups that appropriate care for their mental health problems has been neglected. Their appeals have sought important practical advantages from federal policymakers, who have assigned priority status to meeting the mental health needs of those inadequately served. In keeping with this commitment, federal support has become more readily available for training and service to underserved groups. Thus certain incentives now exist for being designated as underserved and, predictably, the number of claims to this status has mounted. Some observers have commented wryly that everyone now seems to be underserved.

In point of fact, everyone *is* underserved. There is considerable evidence that available services and existing problems are separated by an immense gap (Kiesler, 1980). It is also true, however, that some are more underserved than others. Because of their financial and social circumstances, members of certain societal groups find existing services particularly inhospitable and ineffective and are limited to fewer options in their quest for alternatives.

As a practical rule of thumb, the groups that have been considered underserved are those that encounter special problems related to mental health: racism and stigma, poverty and powerlessness, immigration and cultural divergence, underrepresentation and dropping out of treatment. This kind of general standard has been useful for focusing attention and resources on problems in need of rectification. However, it is worth examining in greater detail the basis for making such judgments. This closer look brings to light an interplay of science, social values, and politics.

Certain questions about underservice are empirical in nature. It is important to gather data describing psychological and social problems and their distribution among social categories and geographical regions. The well-known and reliable relationship between socioeconomic standing and mental illness is perhaps the best established of such findings. Studies of this kind conducted within the field of psychiatric epidemiology provide an important body of empirical findings.

Along with problems, it is necessary to take account of mental health resources and their availability and utilization by those in need. The study of mental health resources has largely examined formally designated professional mental health practice. Studies have shown, for example, that rural communities have proportionally few mental health professionals, a factor important to consider in evaluating their mental health needs (Richards & Gottfredson, 1978). The widespread and successful use of other mental health resources, including self-help, social support, and indigenous healers, has received greater attention recently (Veroff, Kulka, & Couvan, 1981). Still, little is known about this active and universal system of underground care, and additional research should be conducted to provide a complete picture of practices that solve mental health problems.

It is tempting to view underservice in mental health as strictly an empirical problem—a calculation of the discrepancy between measured problems and resources. However attractive the seeming rigor of such an approach, it must be kept in mind that certain issues in judging underservice simply cannot be rendered in objective terms. Data can be collected to describe problems and resources, but not to indicate which problems are taken into account, how each is defined, and how heavily each is weighed. To answer questions such as these is to define a perspective reflecting social objectives, priorities, and values (Sullivan & Snowden, 1981). In this realm, alternatives are best chosen in the process of developing a comprehensive and explicit social policy.

Indeed, there is broad intent behind much of what is now associated with being designated as underserved. This status has become a means to focus attention on the mental health needs of particular groups and to suggest that money and actions out of the ordinary may be in order for those so designated. Thus a community that presents little psychopathology at present, but is known to be at high risk to do so, might justifiably command special attention. Past discrimination that resulted in denial of mental health services might be offset through special attention in the present. Movement toward self-determination may be legitimized and supported by special attention to a group's mental health condition. These and other social purposes are expressed in society's response to the mental health needs of underserved groups.

Similarities and Differences
in Psychological Functioning

An important focus in services to the underserved has been to devise interventions attuned to unique ethnic, regional, and age-defined needs. Simply to make available services intended for mainstream clientele as a remedy for underservice, critics have repeatedly stressed, is an inadequate solution. A crucial assumption of this position is one of pluralism: Significant behavioral differences underlie demographic and regional diversity, it is maintained, and are represented in how psychological problems originate, are expressed, and can be cured.

In part, pluralism is a reaction to an unbounded universalism that has long dominated psychological thought. The universalist's assumption is that, apart from individual variation, human functioning is largely governed by uniform processes and modes of expression. Pluralism has arisen to suggest that group-related differences exist and must be taken into account.

But pluralism itself must have limits. To completely partition the population into categories defined by combinations of race, region, age, class, and other major social divisions creates an unwieldy number of categories. Must we make a fresh start in addressing the mental health needs of each household? Clearly, even allowing for diversity, important uniformities exist also, and must be recognized in psychological practice.

To paraphrase an old truism, everyone is like all other people, like some other people, and like no other person. The Chicana or Navajo or rural white is not only a member of an underserved group, but also a human and an individual. To say this is not to endorse vapid eclecticism, but to suggest a complicated task of unraveling what is generally true from what is true in particular.

This sorting out has occurred most in the area of direct clinical practice with ethnic minorities. Padilla (1981), for example, emphasizes core features of effective psychotherapy that apply to Hispanics as much as to anyone else. Among these are sensitivity and concern, explanation of the problem, and increased hope and expectations for improvement. On the other hand, distinctive cultural norms relating to familialism and authority suggest that other therapeutic tactics are most effective with many Hispanics when modified from standard clinical procedures.

The capacity to draw distinctions between the general and the specific is central to effective work of all kinds, with all underserved populations.

No less than therapy, intervention seeking to restructure environments and enhance support must struggle with universals and variations, and with problems of distinguishing between the two. No less than ethnic minorities, the experiences and outlooks of people who are rural, elderly, or chronically mentally ill are both similar to those of everyone else and different in ways that must be recognized and taken into account.

Level and Scope of Intervention

A remarkable feature of proposals for services to the underserved has been the broad spectrum over which needed changes have been identified. Demands have been directed at levels ranging from the broadest institutions of government, economics, and mass media to the face-to-face therapeutic encounter. At times, tension has arisen between the two most contrasting perspectives (Jones & Korchin, 1982). On the one hand, proponents of broad social change have condemned efforts to work with individuals as misguided, distracting, and supportive of the very oppression that must be overthrown. On the other hand, proponents of better strategies for improved individual functioning have condemned social activists for too readily sacrificing the certain and immediate benefits of personal improvement in favor of a greater good that is very long range and quite uncertain.

Such polarization of views is ill founded. Origins of mental health problems and needed interventions may be found at both levels of analysis, as well as many places in between. Recent views of the origin and course of psychopathology and the nature of mental health (see Dohrenwend, 1978) implicate a broad range of psychological and social factors and suggest constructive action directed toward large societal structures, mediating structures, and individuals.

A systematic view of this diversity may be gained by outlining possible goals for services to the underserved related to mental health. One category of goals pertains to freedom from excessive social stressors. Racism, economic marginality, poor physical health, language barriers, and recent immigration are examples of major pressures that bear particularly on those groups that have traditionally received the least help in handling their greater need. In many cases, the sources of these stressors lie within major social institutions, and it is to them that attempts at constructive change would be directed most effectively.

The second category of goals is associated with personal resources for coping—skills for effective social performance and for maintaining freedom from crippling thoughts and feelings. The target of intervention to achieve these goals is typically an individual suffering from psychological problems, who is treated with one of the various forms of psychotherapy or training in personal coping responses. If help is effective, the person treated emerges with a strengthened capacity to engage the environment in a satisfying and effective fashion.

A third category of goals is made up of those that share a concern with provision of access to social roles and opportunities for meaningful social integration. This category is like the first in emphasizing environmental determinants of mental health. It differs from the first, however, in a concern with opportunities for positive experiences, rather than with freedom from negative experiences. To live effective and satisfying lives, members of underserved groups, like others, must have meaningful opportunities for self-expression and social reward. Interventions designed to create these opportunities will have an important impact on mental health. Efforts to support economic, cultural, and political institutions within the local community, and to create additional opportunities within society at large, are carried out in the service of these ends.

There are indeed many services needed by the underserved. In the literature this theme is expressed repeatedly, and in various forms: Services must be comprehensive; problems do not respect disciplinary boundaries; it is impossible to separate psychological functioning from physical and social functioning; coordination of diverse programmatic efforts must be maintained. Whoever would improve services to the underserved must be prepared to work on many fronts and in many ways.

Overview of the Volume

This volume is a review of mental health services to the underserved. In its twelve contributed chapters the underserved are described and considered with respect to their problems and the interventions, settings, and policies that have been debated as solutions. The purposes of this review are several and include consolidation of gains already achieved, clarification of directions for future work, and renewal of our commitment to promote mental health for those with particular and special needs, or those found near the bottom of the social order.

Underservice by Age, Region, and Chronicity

Those in society with certain statuses are underserved, particularly the old and the young, rural residents, and the chronically mentally ill.

Clearly, there is remarkable diversity within these groups, as well as considerable overlap among them and with other social categories of the underserved defined by race, culture, and socioeconomic standing. This correlation among statuses makes it difficult at times to distinguish which factor is the primary reason for a person's receiving inadequate services. However, for a great many people the primary and major barrier is associated unmistakably with age, rural residence, and being chronically mentally ill.

Chapter 2 is by Barbara Felton, who reviews services to the aged. Felton notes that the biological facts of aging, expectations and concerns of the aged, and stereotypes about the condition of old age all conspire to undermine effective service delivery. Felton further observes that despite aging being a universal experience, the mental health system has never seriously come to grips with its consequences, and has too often responded either with complete neglect or with excessive, incapacitating confinement.

Another era of development that has been poorly served in mental health is childhood. In Chapter 3, Sheila Namir and Rhona Weinstein review the status of this neglect, setting it in historical context and making recommendations for public policy that would rectify it. They cite this nation's record of erratic attention to childhood problems, directed to single areas of concern viewed in isolation, as a major obstacle to a rational system of services. Namir and Weinstein note that at present, childhood problems are assigned to separate bureaucracies; if mental health services are to avoid becoming yet another competing territorial interest, they must become integrated within a unified system of care.

One group finding itself with fewer mental health services than it needs is that of residents of rural America. In Chapter 4, Richard Blouch documents this condition of underservice, and identifies geographical and social factors that perpetuate it. Blouch makes it clear that rural communities are not simply smaller versions of urban communities, but are distinctive in their institutions, norms, and development. Among the most promising attempts to increase delivery to rural areas, according to Blouch, are those that reorient professionals in their conception of practice and augment natural helpers and social structures.

Historically, the mental health system badly served a large group of clientele, the chronically mentally ill. In recognition of this, a strong movement arose discouraging hospital-based services and stressing community mental health. In Chapter 5, Steven Segal and Jim Baumohl consider the outcome of these efforts. They report disappointing results. Partly because of poor planning, but largely because of inadequate funding, community service and life-sustaining functions formerly performed within the mental hospital have come to be neglected. According to Segal and Baumohl, a system of community care has arisen that is haphazard and incomplete, transforming the condition of the chronically mentally ill from being destructively served to being destructively unserved.

Underservice by Race and Culture

Much raising of professional and public consciousness about problems of underservice has been accomplished by groups representing racial and cultural minorities. The middle four chapters in this volume are devoted to underservice as it affects four such groups: La Raza, Asian and Pacific Americans, Native Americans, and Black Americans. Like those populations considered in the first four chapters, these groups are marked by considerable diversity; however, use of broad designations remains the prevailing convention.

La Raza is a term applied to a large, diverse group of people linked by the Spanish language and Hispanic culture. In Chapter 6, Manuel Barrera, Jr., reviews mental health service delivery to this group. Barrera finds that the literature supports viewing this group as indeed underserved, pointing out that two alternative hypotheses to underutilization of services—reliance on social support and nonprofessional healers apply also to the mainstream population. Some reforms in service delivery have produced encouraging results. However, as he looks to the future, Barrera wonders about efficient use of scarce resources, and whether it is better to further upgrade direct mental health services or to improve jobs, education, and general conditions of life.

American Indians and Alaskan natives are two of the few populations for whom the federal government takes considerable direct responsibility. However, as reviewed by Spero Manson and Joseph Trimble in Chapter 7, the system created fails to provide mental health care that is demonstrably appropriate or effective. Manson and Trimble report many gaps in information, making it difficult to know the true nature of mental health problems and service delivery. From the evidence available, there appear to be many obstacles to utilization of existing services, and only preliminary groundwork for efforts at preventive mental health.

For Black Americans, according to Thom Moore in Chapter 8, mental health should not be considered without first considering the social forces that control it. Moore takes note of an inclination pervading psychology to focus on Black people themselves, and not the conditions they confront, in seeking the source of mental health problems. Moore examines conditions of life for Blacks in statistics on income, health, and education, demonstrating that any picture of progress made in absolute terms dissolves when the point of comparison is progress made by whites.

In Chapter 9, Herbert Wong reviews the state of mental health service delivery to Asian and Pacific Americans. Comprising some 32 distinct and fast-growing subgroups, Asian and Pacific Americans have mental health problems seen by Wong as requiring a comprehensive service program. Wong concludes that cultural beliefs, immigration, community institutions and resources, and financial factors must all be taken into account by those seeking to design effective services for this group.

Toward Better Therapies, Organizations, and Policies

A strong tradition has arisen of considering problems of underservice by focusing on separate underserved populations, as is done in the first eight chapters of the present volume. However, one consequence of this scheme can be an unfortunate fragmentation, by which similar lessons continually must be rediscovered and developed without benefit of a broader perspective that allows for population comparisons.

The final four chapters of this volume follow a thematic approach. Each chapter is concerned with a topic suggesting promising directions for effective service delivery that cut across boundaries of underserved populations. Bringing to light common threads helps to unify the knowledge base for services to the underserved.

Chapter 10, by Enrico Jones and David Matsumoto, reviews the literature on psychotherapy with the underserved, particularly those with the lowest socioeconomic standing. Jones and Matsumoto emphasize the continuing importance of psychotherapy, and view it as neither incompatible with nor preempted by the need for social change. They go on to question whether certain assumptions long held about lower-class clients continue to apply—particularly the notion that with the poor, traditional psychotherapy is difficult to implement and of negligible benefit. The most fair and productive course of action, in the view of Jones and Matsumoto, is to focus directly on attitudes and dispositions that bar effective therapeutic work; these will be found throughout the socioeconomic hierarchy.

Psychotherapy and other direct services to clients are influenced by the organizational contexts in which they occur. Chapter 11, by Nolan Zane, Stanley Sue, Felipe Castro, and William George, reviews the literature on designing systems of service delivery especially for ethnic minority clientele. Zane, Sue, Castro, and George find a set of service system features mentioned repeatedly, including: achieving a good match between services and client problems and cultural patterns; taking an active stance to promote mental health in the community and to encourage service utilization; deploying a comprehensive range of services and coordinating them; encouraging community control; and developing and disseminating knowledge about effective service systems. The time has come, according to these authors, for a commitment to implement these recognized principles on a widespread basis.

An early response to underservice encouraged by federal policy was recruitment and training of a cadre of community-grounded paraprofessional workers. In Chapter 12, Yvette Flores-Ortiz reviews the history of the paraprofessional movement, with particular attention to indigenous and minority paraprofessionals and their involvement with minority communities. Flores-Ortiz observes that despite marginal status, and training and assignments that are too often confused, indigenous paraprofessionals appear to be a genuine asset. However, a competitive job market, perceptions of paraprofessionals as second-class service providers, and poor understanding of the means to achieve effective paraprofessional utilization all conspire to make the future for these workers appear bleak.

In Chapter 13, Lonnie Snowden, William Collinge, and Cecilia Runkle set mental health service delivery in its context of ongoing behavior in the community. Snowden, Collinge, and Runkle review the literature related to help seeking—that is, processes of recognizing a need and identifying and using health care resources, both formal and informal. Timing and expectations at entry into the mental health services must be understood within larger help-seeking patterns, according to these authors; these patterns themselves are molded by individual psychology, reference-group culture, and larger society. The authors of Chapter 13 suggest that the true significance of appearance or failure to appear at a mental health agency cannot be grasped without an understanding of the nature of processes related to help seeking.

References

Dohrenwend, B. S. Social stress and community psychology. *American Journal of Community Psychology*, 1978, 6(1), 1-14.

Jones, E. E., & Korchin, S. J. Minority mental health perspectives. In E. E. Jones & S. J. Korchin (Eds.), *Minority mental health*. New York: Praeger, 1982.

Kiesler, D. A. Mental health policy as a field of inquiry for psychology. *American Psychologist*, 1980, 35(12), 1966-1980.

Padilla, A. M. Pluralistic counseling and psychotherapy for Hispanic Americans. In A. J. Marsella & P. B. Pedersen (Eds.), *Cross-cultural counseling and Psychotherapy.* Elmsford, NY: Pergamon, 1981.

President's Commission on Mental Health. *Report to the president of the President's Commission on Mental Health.* Washington, DC: Government Printing Office, 1978.

Richards, J. M., & Gottfredson, G. D. Geographic distribution of U.S. psychologists. *American Psychologist,* 1978, 33, 1-9.

Snow, D. L., & Newton, P. M. Task, social structure, and social process in the community mental health center movement. *American Psychologist,* 1976, 31(8), 582-593.

Sullivan, J. M., & Snowden, L. R. Monitoring frequency of client problems: Comparison of four methods. *Evaluation Review,* 1981, 5(6), 822-833.

Veroff, J., Kulka, R. A., & Douvan, E. *Mental health in America: Patterns of help-seeking from 1957-1976.* New York: Basic Books, 1981.

PART I

UNDERSERVED POPULATIONS

2

The Aged

Settings, Services, and Needs
Barbara J. Felton
New York University

Despite the fact that biological and social factors of late life put older people more at risk for mental health problems than people of other age groups in our society, older people are notoriously poorly and only intermittently assisted by our mental health service delivery system. Mental illnesses of late life go undetected, reversible brain syndromes persist unreversed, older people are exposed unnecessarily to the secondary consequences of institutionalization because they are disproportionately allocated to inpatient treatment, and preventable traumas due to life crises that can be anticipated result in unnecessary anguish to older people themselves and to those whose material and emotional lives depend upon the well-being of those older people.

The prospect of attempting to rectify this situation is an awesome task. On the one hand, we have evidence of glaring need, of vast neglect, or, in some cases, of inappropriate and consequently harmful treatment. The intersection between the mental health system and the lives of older people describes a relatively small area, and one not riddled with "successful" encounters. It is difficult *not* to feel moved to act to increase the quantity and quality of care available to older people.

On the other hand, the same factors that seem to account for the less-than-perfect fit between older people and the mental health service delivery system are those that are likely to mar our efforts at change. We can be reasonably sure that older people, like the other groups excluded from mental health treatment, have not been randomly selected for neglect. Pervasive agism in attitudes, entrenched status differentials between older and younger people, professional reward systems that provide incentives for delivering some types of service and not others, a sparse and skewed knowledge base replete with untested assumptions about what kinds of problems are tractable, and an inability to "converse" with older people in mental health terms have all been cited as explanations for our failure, and all suggest that relatively fundamental changes must occur in order for us to be able to assist the aged.

The labeling of a group as in need of mental health services has consequences for the members of that group that suggest caution in planning. To the extent that older people are more vulnerable than others to mental health problems because of biological and social factors, it is reasonable to be particularly concerned about the consequences of our treatments: The risks of failure are higher where people are more susceptible. On the other hand, to the extent that older people are not more vulnerable but are simply perceived as such, targeting them for special service attention introduces the risks of inducing a status differential, of reinforcing socially based expectations of deficiency, and of instituting dependency on the part of older people.

This chapter begins with the premises that many older people have mental health problems that require currently unavailable services from mental health professionals and that the process of delivering services and the institutions involved in their delivery exert powerful influences on service recipients that, despite our best intentions, cannot be assumed to be benign. It examines the nature of the mental health needs of older people as we know them and examines the current meshing of older people and mental health systems for clues about the pitfalls and possibilities available to us in our attempt to provide for the elderly constructively and ethically.

The Mental Health of the Aged

The Nature of Mental Health Problems Among the Aged

Describing the mental status of the aged, a reasonable first step in defining what the mental health system ought to be doing for older people, is a task that severely taxes currently available knowledge. Epidemiological data on the age distribution of mental illness come from studies that use varying criteria for evaluating mental health and thus result in considerably different estimates of the prevalence of mental disorder (Gurland, 1976; Zarit, 1980).

Reliance on data derived from service utilization patterns is tempting (see Redick, Kramer, & Taube, 1973), though marred by the strong biases that account for differential usage of services. Institutional policies clearly affect usage: McDonald's (1973) study of the age distribution of a sample of first admissions to public hospitals in England and Wales led him to conclude that the age curve reflects "simply an overall reluctance to admit young and old people to hospital" (quoted in Gurland, 1976, p. 786). In addition to age-based differentials in admission policies, we have fairly solid evidence that the older person's risk for institutionalization is strongly related to the individual's own social supports (see Lawton, 1981; Shanas & Maddox, 1976; Tobin & Kulys, 1981): Being married and having more rather than fewer or no children make institutionalization far less likely to occur. This social support bias in the use of institutions by older people is so great that several studies have now demonstrated that for every impaired aged person in a long-term care facility, there are three others with comparable levels of disability living in the community (Gurland, Bennett, & Wilder, 1981). Nonetheless, the facts that institutional policies and social supports determine the likelihood of institutionalization and that objective level of functional impairment is so weakly related to institutional status underline the importance of community surveys for estimating the prevalence of mental disorder among the aged.

Differences in the nature of the samples studied in community surveys compound the difficulties in summarizing findings produced by differences in the methodologies and criteria for evaluating mental disorder used. Wide variations in results ensue, but give us some basis for considering what is needed in the way of mental health services.

When all types of mental disorder are considered, estimates of their prevalence among people aged 65 and over living in the community tend to range from 10 percent to 20 percent (Palmore, 1973; Redick et al., 1973; Zarit, 1980). One of the more carefully controlled studies, which included in its sample both community resident and institutionalized older people in the English city of Newcastle-Upon-Tyne, determined that 26 percent of the aged had psychiatric disorders (Kay, Beamish, & Roth, 1964). Summarizing results from several northern European epidemiological surveys, Juel-Nielsen (1975) concludes that the total prevalence rates for mental disorders in old age range from 25 percent to 40 percent.

In contrast to the rates for less severe mental disorders, the most severe mental disorders are, across the life span, less prevalent, and rates for older people tend to be more closely comparable to those among younger people. Estimates of the prevalence rates for all psychoses among older people range from 4 percent to 8 percent (Juel-Nielsen, 1975; Riley &

Foner, 1968; Shanas & Maddox, 1976), reflecting both the late-life onset of mental disorders and the aging of long-term chronically mentally ill adults.

Organic brain syndromes predominate among the severe mental disorders of late life. Palmore (1973, p. 46) concluded from community prevalence surveys that "more than half of the psychotic persons over 65 have primarily organic psychosis (acute or chronic brain syndromes including cerebral arteriosclerosis and senile brain disease)," though he cautioned that diagnoses tend to be unreliable and, at times, arbitrary. About 43 percent of all of the aged who were institutionalized in psychiatric facilities in 1969 were diagnosed as having organic brain syndrome, and a similar proportion of nursing home residents had diagnoses of chronic brain syndrome (Redick et al., 1973). Kay (1972) reports that among new admissions of people aged 65 to 74 to state and county mental hospitals, about 75 percent present this problem; 90 percent of all such mental hospital admissions of people over age 75 are diagnosed as chronic brain syndrome cases. Shanas and Maddox (1976) summarize cross-national data and find roughly comparable rates in several industrialized countries.

While organic brain syndromes are by far the most prevalent of the severe mental disorders in late life, older people experience the full range of psychotic diseases. The second most prevalent diagnosis among elderly psychiatric inpatients in Kramer, Taube, and Redick's (1973) study was schizophrenia. The 35 percent prevalence rate for schizophrenia among inpatient residents contrasts sharply with the 4 percent rate of schizophrenia among new admissions to psychiatric facilities by elderly clients (Kramer et al., 1973). This differential presumably reflects the aging of schizophrenics in psychiatric institutions and points to the need to consider the two groups among the severely mentally ill aged: those whose mental problems have emerged in late life, and those with chronic mental problems who have grown old.

Definitional criteria for the milder forms of mental illness vary even more widely than those used for diagnosing severe mental disorders; thus estimates of the rate of psychoneurotic disorders are even more variable. Palmore (1973) cites estimates of the prevalence of the milder forms of mental illness, which range from a low of 7 percent (Pasamanick, 1962) to a high of 50 percent (Leighton, Harding, & Macklin, 1963). Busse, Dovenmuehle, and Brown's (1960) study of elderly volunteers, a group that the authors describe as "reasonably well-adjusted" found that at least 25 percent suffered from neuroses and an additional 20 percent had a mixture of neurotic and psychotic difficulties.

In the absence of clearly defined objective criteria for evaluating mental status, self-reports of distress would seem to be a valuable index for service planning. Currently, however, there is little reason to put a great deal of confidence in subjective reports of problems. Carp and Carp (1981) effectively demonstrate the influence of question format on the reporting of problems; their work, coupled with the work of others who have documented the tendency of older people to describe their "objective" circumstances with an apparently unwarranted degree of optimism (see Campbell, Converse, & Rodgers, 1976; Nydeggar, 1977), strongly suggests that current cohorts of older people are biased toward underestimating the presence of problems. Estimates of the prevalence of "mild" mental disorders, consequently, are very likely to underestimate the numbers of older people contending with emotional and psychological problems of a magnitude that shields them from contact with mental health professionals.

Despite varying estimates of the prevalence of neuroses, it is clear that depression, in forms ranging from psychotic affective states to transient depressive reactions, is by far the most frequently experienced mental health problem of the aged (Butler & Lewis, 1977; Gatz, Smyer, & Lawton, 1980; Zarit, 1980). Among people over age 55, the incidence of depression alone has been found to be as high as 10 percent (Gurland, 1976). The prevalence of depression-related problems, including, most significantly, suicide rates, reiterates age curves for depression and shows the elderly to be the group, next to adolescents, with the highest rate of suicide. Alcoholism, most prevalent among adults aged 45 to 55, persists for many as a late-life mental health problem and presents itself for the first time as a problem for many others (Gatz et al., 1980).

The social conditions of late life undoubtedly contribute to the frequency of mental health problems among the aged, and the nature of many of the mental disorders characteristic of the aged can be traced to the types of losses and stresses that tend to accompany aging. Palmore (1973) includes in his list of psychological and social factors contributing to mental disorder among the aged socioeconomic status, marital status, and community disintegration, as well as the age-specific stresses resulting from loss of income, loss of role and status, bereavement, isolation through disability, and loss of cognitive functioning. The combinations of these stresses, coupled with organic deterioration, have been fairly clearly linked to higher rates of severe mental illness found among the aged (Palmore, 1973). Considering the factors predisposing the aged to the experience of depression, Jarvik (1976, p. 326) writes: "Perhaps the most important unanswered question may be: Given these biological changes, the rising frequency of somatic illness, physiological decline, physical debilities, malnutrition, overmedication (iatrogenic or self-induced), sensory deficits, reduction in mental agility, economic deprivations, social losses, and the increasing proximity of death, all of which are associated with advancing chronological age, why is not every old person in a profound state of depression?" Part of the answer undoubtedly lies in the large individual variations in competence among older people and in the strengths that accumulate over the life span, but little is actually known about the development of mental health resources and deficits over the life span.

Limitations of the Current Knowledge Base

Overall, the quality of information available for evaluating the mental status of the aged is poor. Both methodological problems and the conceptual dilemmas of assessment hamper our efforts to document the range and nature of mental disorders in late life and make it all but impossible to learn about age differences in mental health problems from the currently available information.

Definitive classification systems for the mental disorders of late life are virtually absent. Ambiguities in diagnosing mental disorders have been increased rather than clarified by the most recent *Diagnostic and Statistical Manual,* according to Butler and Lewis (1977), who find "age prejudicial and invalid statements" in descriptions of such late-life disorders as senile dementia.

Fundamental etiological and nosological questions remain unsolved; controversy surrounds the question of whether senile brain disease consists of a quantitative increase in a normal developmental process or whether it is a qualitatively different entity. The existence of a late-life schizophrenia the etiology of which is linked to aging processes and the manifestation of which is different from schizophrenias of earlier adult life is still debated. The causes of senile brain disease are virtually unknown.

Not surprising, in view of the above, is that diagnoses of mental illness among the aged tend to be unreliable and, in many cases, arbitrary (Palmore, 1973). Use of the term "senility" has now been largely discarded as pejorative and insufficiently precise; the chronic brain syndromes that produce the confusion, disorientation, and memory loss that characterize what is colloquially known as senility, however, are difficult to distinguish on the basis of current diagnostic criteria. The inadequacy of available assessment techniques is most painfully obvious in textbooks' reliance on pathological evidence as the basis for differential diagnoses (for example, see Butler & Lewis, 1977; Ciliberto, Levin, & Arluke, 1981; Zarit, 1980).

Diagnostic confusion is also evident in the tendency of treatment professionals to diagnose acute brain syndromes as chronic conditions (Busse & Pfeiffer, 1973; Butler, 1975). Many acute conditions are induced by reactions to transient psychological losses, and many are consequences of physical illnesses (Nowlin, 1973). Congestive heart failure, malnutrition, infection, drugs and alcohol, diabetic acidosis, liver failure, uremia, emphysema, and blindfolding during eye surgery are a few of the many physical conditions that can induce brain syndromes and lead to an erroneous diagnosis of chronic brain disorder (Butler & Lewis, 1977). The fact that our knowledge is limited by what has been tried means that, in the absence of efforts to "reverse" syndromes, they become, by default, irreversible.

In addition to diagnostic error and ambiguities in diagnostic categories, inadequacies of theory limit our capacity to describe the mental health problems of the aged. Critical questions about age changes and age differences in mental disorders cannot be answered without precise age-based epidemiological data on the incidence and prevalence of disorders, and inadequacies of theory make it difficult to identify "comparable" diagnoses among young and old. In its current state, life-span developmental theory provides no clues about expectable developmental variations and consistencies in the forms of mental health problems. Thus counts of the incidence of mental disorders, which require information about whether a given episode of illness is a new disorder or a recurrence of a preexisting condition, are of unknown reliability. In the absence of knowledge of the forms of "normal" aging, stereotypes assume an inappropriately influential role in interpreting behavior. Several authors have suggested that the prevalence of depression among the aged is grossly underestimated because the symptoms of depression mimic our stereotypic images of older people (Epstein, 1976). Without age-based norms for assessment techniques used with the aged, and without developmental theory that identifies and predicts changes in the forms of psychological functioning over the life span, our knowledge of the mental health status of the aged will remain ambiguous.

Knowledge of life-span mental health from a developmental perspective is hampered by the absence of longitudinal studies. Cross-sectional studies of mental health differences with age have limited value in efforts to develop a life-span developmental understanding of mental health, and contain biases that can actually impair our understanding of adult development.

"Selective attrition" is one bias that creates problems in interpreting data on age differences in mental health. When cross-sectional data are used, age-based estimates of the prevalence of mental disorder become increasingly skewed with age due to differential survivorship. Low socio-economic status, ethnic minority membership, social isolation, and other factors that put people at risk for mental illness (Dohrenwend & Dohrenwend, 1969; Srole, Langnes, Michael, Kirkpatrick, Opler, & Rennie, 1975) also tend to reduce longevity. In addition, many mental health problems, such as alcoholism, impair health and directly reduce longevity. Differential mortality rates for adults with mental health problems may result in prevalence rates for older people that are smaller than they would be if all those young and middle-aged adults with mental health problems were to survive into late life. Thus the fact that mental disorders do not become more prevalent with age (Zarit, 1980) is hollow assurance that the mental health needs of adults are being met.

That the elderly are those who have survived into old age has profound implications for those planning mental health services. Reversible but untreated problems in middle age may well make people more vulnerable to the stresses that attend late life (Maas & Kuypers, 1975). Late life, in fact, may not be the most fruitful point at which to intervene to rectify "late-life" mental problems (Fozard & Popkin, 1978).

Older people constitute a group that is continually changing in its characteristics. Average life expectancies mean that approximately one-third of the people who are aged 65 and over are replaced by others every five years. Successive cohorts of older people represent groups of people whose lives have been shaped by different sets of historical events. The contexts of their lives are seldom directly knowable to current cohorts of professionals, and the senses of well-being, illness behavior, and help-seeking behavior that result from those early and subsequent socialization experiences are frequently at variance with contemporary styles. The apparent strength of cohort effects (Schaie, 1970) emphasizes the importance of understanding adult psychology at all stages of the life span.

We can conclude that older people have mental health problems in need of professional treatment. Whether or not mental health problems themselves have been proven more prevalent among the aged than among younger age groups, it is certainly true that many of the conditions that produce mental disorders are more common among the aged. The gaps in our knowledge suggest a major agenda for conceptual and empirical work, and some caution in planning services. Before considering needed services, however, it is useful to consider recent and current interactions between older people and the mental health system.

The Interface Between Older People and the Mental Health System

Older Clients and Mental Health Services

Mental health treatment of the aged takes place, by and large, in institutional settings. The extensive analysis of patient care episodes undertaken by Kramer et al. (1973) revealed that, in 1968, 85 percent of all mental health treatment of the aged occurred in institutions of one type or another, including state and county mental hospitals, nursing homes, and inpatient psychiatric units of general hospitals.

The "institutional bias" (Gatz et al., 1980) in the mental health treatment of the aged is also evident in utilization rates for outpatient services. Kramer et al.'s (1973) analysis details that patients under age 18 accounted for 33 percent of the patient load in outpatient clinics in 1968; adults aged 18 to 44 accounted for another 51 percent, patients aged 45 to 64 for 14 percent, and patients aged 65 and over, for 2 percent. Similar utilization rates appear in community mental health centers, where approximately 4 percent of the patient load in 1968 was aged 65 or over.

Given that 52.7 percent of all patient episodes (for patients of all ages) were in outpatient settings, the 15 percent figure for older patients represents a substantial differential in the locus of treatment for older and younger people. Older people constituted about 10 percent of the total population in 1968, and, given that we have no basis for believing that mental disorders are less prevalent among the aged than among younger people, outpatient service utilization rates of 2 percent to 4 percent for older people represents an underutilization of community services by this age group compared to younger age groups.

Perhaps even more disconcerting is the evidence that suggests that even within outpatient services, there is a bias toward more custodial treatment for the aged. Reporting on the distribution of community mental health services in 1971 for the caseload of patients over age 65, Kahn (1975) points out that older patients accounted for 7 percent of the inpatient population, 2 percent of the partial-hospitalization services, and 3 percent of the outpatient services.

In addition to being more likely than younger mental patients to reside in institutions, older mental patients are far more likely to reside in nonpsychiatric institutions. Kahn's (1975) study of the treatment locations of older mental patients revealed that, in 1969, fully 75 percent of the institutionalized aged mentally ill were residents of nursing homes.

Historically, the increased use of nursing homes rather than mental hospitals as the residences for the elderly mentally ill can be traced to the "deinstitutionalization" movement. Increases in the number of nursing home beds prior to 1963 meant that, in that year, nursing homes had become "a resource for the care of the aged mentally ill second only to the State mental hospital" (Kramer et al., 1973, p. 450). The "mental health revolution," which took the form of drastic reductions in the numbers of mentally ill people treated in mental hospitals, resulted in the replacement of the mental hospital by the nursing home as the primary locus of care for the aged with mental disorders. Mental patients over age 65 were the first, and the largest, group of mental hospital residents to be moved out of mental hospitals (Lerman, 1980; Moroney & Kurtz, 1975; Sherwood, 1975; Vladeck, 1980). In fact, since older people account for the vast majority of patients moved out of mental hospitals in the mid-1960s, much of the "success" of deinstitutionalization efforts can be attributed to the availability of nursing home beds.

Analyses of the reasons for the preferential move of the older, rather than younger, mental patient away from mental hospitals, although not out of institutions, have pointed to the locus of funding: Lerman (1980) and Vladeck (1980) propose that the availability of federal funds for the treatment of the aged mentally ill in nonpsychiatric settings allowed state administrators to empty their mental hospitals at federal expense. The net result was that, despite the fact that mental health professionals deemed community treatment to be the "treatment of choice" during this time period (Shinn & Felton, 1981), only younger mental patients were relocated to the noninstitutional community.

The location of treatment is important for a variety of reasons: Some settings are more desirable than others, and evidence of bias is present in reports of where older mental patients are to be found. Kahn (1975, p. 26), on the basis of the historical analysis of treatment locations for older and younger patients, claims: "It is obvious that the elderly are being neglected by the mental health establishment." Evidence of bias can be found in microlevel analyses of decision making about treatment as well as in these macrolevel analyses: Sue (1976) reports that, after ethnicity, age is the best predictor of outpatient treatment referral practices: Regardless of diagnosis, older people are more frequently referred to group rather than to individual treatment. That "older people" are, in many cases, members of minority groups as well as old, does not make these findings any more reassuring. Evidence of age-based differences in treatment for depression shows that older people are more likely than younger people to be referred for electric shock treatment and drug therapy (Klerman, 1976). Gatz et al. (1980, p. 6) conclude from a similar survey that older people clearly receive a "biased sample of the range of services available."

In addition to indicating the presence of age bias in treatment practices, information about the location of treatment provides us with partial information about the quality of treatment given. While we lack evidence that, across the board, institutional care of the elderly mentally ill is less effective than community-based treatment (Dellario & Anthony, 1981; Test & Stein, 1978), it is fairly clear that when community care is sufficiently comprehensive and long term, it is decidedly more beneficial for the chronically mentally ill than institution-based treatment (Test, 1981). Though the process of being institutionalized is not universally deleterious for older people, as early studies seemed to indicate, relocation to institutions does seem to pose additional risks of mortality and morbidity for those older people with serious health problems (Palmore, 1973).

Treatment location does seem to have clearer implications for the well-being of the elderly when the choice between medical versus psychiatric institutions is considered. Nowlin (1973) describes the problems posed by what he calls the "physician's frame of reference": He cites studies showing that, in decisions about whether older patients should be assigned to psychiatric or medical units, retrospective assessments reveal that up to 16 percent of elderly patients are misassigned. Beyond that fact, these findings suggest tremendous ambiguity in diagnostic processes; they take on added significance in light of study results that show that those inappropriately assigned have higher death rates than those properly assigned (Kidd, 1962).

Given such ambiguities in diagnoses, it is perhaps not too surprising that, at times, the setting itself determines the nature of the diagnoses given to individual problems. Serious but undiagnosed medical problems, according to a study by Agate (1970) of new admissions of older people to psychiatric units, occur in as many as 52 percent of cases. The difficulties encountered by those attempting to estimate the prevalence of psychiatric impairment among nursing home residents suggest that many mental disorders go undetected in medical settings. It may well be that Lawton's (1977) hypothesis about the increased influence of the environment on behavior under conditions of lowered competence, which he originally posited as a description of person-environment relations among the aged, may apply to treatment professionals as well: "Environmental docility" may well describe the tendency of professionals under conditions of ignorance about late-life mental health to use, by default, the environment as the basis for diagnosis.

Overall, we have evidence that institutional placement, from a historical perspective, is better explained by funding shifts and institutional policies than by treatment-based knowledge or by the mental health system's convictions about what forms of treatment are best for its clients. At an individual level, treatment placement is better explained by social-network factors than by level of impairment, suggesting that, where possible, institutionalization is avoided through reliance on family members. That treatment placement is affected by factors other than treatment considerations is cause for worry in view of evidence that inappropriate assignment may lead to premature death, that settings determine the range of problems diagnosed as needing treatment, and that settings constrain the range of services offered. All of this suggests that the treatment bias exhibited by the mental health profession toward older people in the past years has not been in the best interests of older people themselves.

Older People's Perspectives on Mental Health Services

The above describes the interface between older people and the mental health system once older people have come into contact with mental health professionals. Epidemiological data suggest that many older people who have problems that make them candidates for mental health service never make contact with the mental health system. Explanations for this underutilization of mental health services by the aged point to the biased attitudes of treatment personnel as well as to the inaccessibility and the inappropriateness of the services offered (Gatz et al., 1980). Many of the factors that make older people particularly vulnerable to mental health problems describe conditions that form barriers to the use of mental health services: chronic illness and its attendant impairments, poverty and loss of income, losses of critical social supports such as occur through widowhood and deaths of friends, and ethnic minority membership, which entails cultural and, frequently, language differences that discourage service use. For many older people, the demands of "being served" exceed their social resources and personal capabilities.

The inappropriateness of many of the services offered is reflected in older people's orally and behaviorally expressed preferences for services. Estes (1979) points out that the formally provided services that older people want consist of "basic services": housing, meals, and income assistance, for example. In contrast, what professionals prefer to provide

are "life-enhancing" services: socialization experiences, cultural development, and recreational programs. Because of the ideological rationales
needed to justify their professional status, and because of the kinds of
incentives for individual advancement within professions, professionals
themselves are unlikely candidates for providing the services that older
people see themselves as needing (Caro, 1974).

Consistent with their voiced preferences, and, perhaps, their capabilities, current cohorts of older people are, overall, less likely than younger
people to seek help from professionals and formal agencies. While this
general pattern is less characteristic of older people's use of medical
services (Haug, 1981), it is particularly pronounced for adults' use of
psychiatric and psychological services (Veroff, Kulka, & Douvan, 1981).
Kulka and Tamir's (1978) analysis of the help-seeking patterns of
American adults of all ages in 1957 and in 1976 indicates that older
cohorts are less likely to define problems they have had as relevant for
help. Among those who define problems as such, older people are equally
as likely as younger people to seek help. Since adults' readiness to define
their problems in mental health terms has increased over the past 20 years
(Veroff et al., 1981), it is likely that future cohorts of older people will
more readily seek help from mental health services than current ones.

Even if future cohorts of older people contain larger numbers of people
more willing to seek out mental health professionals than has been true so
far, the mental health system's ability to serve the mental health needs of
the aged will continue to depend on its ability to recognize critical mental
health problems and address them with services that are effective independent of personal initiatives. What follows is an overview of some of the
directions in which mental health efforts are likely to be made, as well as a
consideration of some of the pitfalls that may accompany these paths
(Gatz et al., 1980) and some of the characteristics of treatment and
training organizations that are likely to affect our success.

Needed Considerations in Planning
for the Mental Health Needs
of the Aged

Prospects for Future Services

The number of older people in the population is steadily increasing.
Recent demographic trends suggest that, in addition to an overall increase

in the proportion of older people in the population, increases will occur among those groups of older people most at risk for mental health problems. The proportion of older people over the age of 75, for example, is increasing more rapidly than the proportion of older people in general; the risk of chronic physical illness, of senile dementia, and of suicide all increase significantly in these upper age groups. The numbers of minority aged are increasing more rapidly than the numbers of white aged, despite the lowered life expectancy of minority aged. All indicators point to increasing mental health needs among the elderly.

Societal responses to this increasing need can be expected to be colored by the prevailing atmosphere of economic retrenchment, in which all large-scale social programs are viewed with pessimism, if not disdain. Smyer's (1981, p.1) recent overview of the future of mental health services for the aged used the theme formulated by Pennsylvania's Governor Edmund Thornburgh to describe the current governmental stance toward services for the aged: "Do more with less."

Within this general atmosphere of austerity, it seems likely that the thrust of service provision will follow the trends in professional thinking that have been emerging over the past few years. Using as their prospectus the *Report to the President of the President's Commission on Mental Health* (1978), Gatz et al. (1980) anticipate that the future mental health system will feature: community-based services, decentralization, planning and coordination, social support systems and "linkage," targeting services to the most vulnerable, and prevention. Certainly these emphases reflect "state of the art" thinking in human service delivery and thus represent the best of what we know how to provide. Nonetheless, our past experiences with services built on these emphases suggest effort be directed at forestalling some of the unintended but possible side effects of these emphases.

The continued focus on community services, according to Gatz et al. (1980), has the potential of leading to neglect of institution-based services. The need for intensive, specialized nursing care is unlikely to diminish over the next decade (Sherwood, 1975; Vladeck, 1980), and psychologists must be prepared to provide direct and indirect services in traditional institutional settings as well as in newly emerging community settings. Recent research suggests that the contrast between community-based and institution-based care may not be a fruitful one for service delivery or policy planning: Community-based alternatives to institutions are not unequivocally superior to services provided in institutional settings, either in the quality of care or in cost effectiveness (Gurland, Bennett, & Wilder, 1981).

Research on the effects of housing and on the role of environmental factors in the sustenance of emotional well-being and general competence indicates that public policy ought to move in the direction of increasing the range of settings available to a full continuum of care sites (Lawton, 1981).

Potential pitfalls in the focus on informal services lie in the possibility that this emphasis may serve to reinforce the pessimism that views direct formal services, exemplified in our large-scale social programs, as having failed (Binstock & Levin, 1976). In an era of diminishing funds, such pessimism, frequently accompanied by the idea that formal services act to erode informal help giving (see Lasch, 1978), threatens the development of a full range of services directed at numerous intervention targets. Policy emphasis on informal support systems requires long-term responsiveness to the broad demographic and economic changes that threaten to reduce the availability of informal support to older people. Increasing divorce rates are producing larger numbers of "reconstituted" families whose sense of obligation to aged "ex-in-laws" and stepparents cannot be taken for granted (Tobin & Kulys, 1981); support for aged family members may also be reduced as employment rates continue to rise for women, particularly for the middle-aged women who traditionally have been and who remain the primary informal caretakers of the aged.

The growing proliferation of specialized expertise in diverse disciplines and settings and the increasing emphasis on community support systems inevitably create problems of "fragmentation." Local agencies operate with overlapping mandates; the proliferation of services in health and social service settings increases the tendency to treat older people as a series of fragmented problems rather than as whole people (Gatz et al., 1980). Coordination and planning efforts and linkage mechanisms designed to overcome these problems run the risks of introducing more red tape into service delivery, and of diverting funds from direct service delivery efforts.

Potential threats to direct delivery of basic services are also seen by Gatz et al. (1980) in the continued proliferation of the rhetoric of prevention. The goal of optimizing human development over the life span is easily compatible with the delivery of basic direct services to impaired older people (Danish, Smyer, & Nowack, 1980)). However, Gatz et al. (1980) warn that the introduction of preventive programs may be viewed by many as an alternative to basic, direct, life-supportive services to these more impaired elderly and thus may divert funds from needed direct services. Preventive services have tremendous potential for overcoming the unfortunate tendency of ameliorative services to induce dependency and passivity in clients; and the tremendous cost-benefit potential of preventive services (Price, Ketterer, Bader, & Monahan, 1980) alone requires that their use be accelerated. Gatz et al. (1980) recommend that preventive services be applied within an optimizing framework that ensures continued support of direct service delivery efforts.

Settings, Services, and Future Success

The success of future services will be influenced by the settings in which they are carried out and in which developing professionals are trained. Because organizations set norms and embody values that shape the attitudes and behaviors of their occupants (Wicker, 1974), the organizational auspices of services and the basis for their delivery will affect the range of solutions likely to emerge for the problems that have hampered our efforts to deliver mental health services to the elderly in the past.

One setting characteristic that has been seen as having potential for improving on past efforts is that of age segregation. Whether services are organized on an "age-specific" basis or on an "age-irrelevant" basis presumably affects the amount of bias and the extent of negative attitudes shown toward older people. Butler (1975) has proposed that, in view of the prevalence of agism among professionals, services to the aged must be age-specific, at least early on in our experience of treating older people and of training professionals.

Arguments against age-specific services and policies, however, are also grounded in concern about the effects of negative attitudes toward the aged. Estes (1979), in evaluating the impact of the Older Americans Act, has argued that using old age as the basis for according services institutes a powerful differential that devalues older people's own definitions of their problems and minimizes important differences among older people.

The issue is complex; one approach to its solution is to make decisions based on a cost-benefit analysis of the likely harms and benefits of the services offered and of the labeling that their offering imposes. Currently it seems that, although being old is still an occasion for "social distance" (Tringo, 1970), being old has less stigma attached to it than do some other characteristics. Thus we have been able to preserve for older people the "dignity" of being poor for reasons of forced retirement by instituting transfer payment programs that separate such people from those receiving funds on the basis of other, less "deserving," causes of poverty. Older adults with mental health problems may similarly benefit from "geron-tology" clinics or, for that matter, from nursing homes that effectively label their problems as due to having become old rather than due to things "mental." Social evaluations of varied statuses change over time (Bengs-ton, Kasschau, & Ragan, 1977), however, and developing a diversity of forms of service delivery may be the best route to maintaining the flexibility needed to maximize the benefits offered by different forms of service organization at different times.

The quality of knowledge available about older people and about the processes of aging and of social change will have an impact on the quality of mental health service offered to older people. An important set of organizational characteristics likely to affect the quality of our knowledge about late-life mental health consists of the organizational barriers to or incentives for interdisciplinary knowledge generation. Whether gathered and known as part of the "lore" of clinical treatment or gathered and known as part of the formalized research literature, information accumu-lated about mental health in the aged will be valuable, in part, according to its ability to encompass the complexities represented by different disci-plines. The interplay of biological, psychological, and social factors in the appearance of late-life mental health problems (Woodruff, 1975) requires concepts, methods, and treatment settings that can encompass events at several "levels." The field of gerontology, at this point, has the benefit of a multidisciplinary knowledge base, and some of its theoretical frameworks, such as those included under the "life-span developmental" rubric, describe ways of understanding the interface between levels of events in aging. It is important that the settings we develop in our efforts to meet the mental health needs of the aged preserve the benefits of this heritage.

To date, our efforts on behalf of the mental health of older people have been meager and, in some cases, destructive. Judging from our past efforts, successful future programs will require greater capacity to reverse, or at least avoid, negative attitudes toward the aged; the capacity to recognize mental health problems in late life and to understand the biological and sociological events that influence their emergence in psychological states; and the capacity to anticipate changes in the people who will become old and in the society that will form the context of their aging. Encouraging the development of the broadest range of settings for training, treatment, and "optimization" will promote the kind of flexibility that will be needed to meet the changing configurations of older people in their changing societal conditions.

References

Agate, J. D. *The practice of geriatrics.* Springfield, IL: Charles C Thomas, 1970.

Bengston, V. L., Kasschau, P. L., & Ragan, P. K. The impact of social structure on aging individuals. In J. E. Birren & K. W. Schaie (Eds.), *Handbook of the psychology of aging.* New York: Van Nostrand Reinhold, 1977.

Binstock, R. H., & Levin, M. The political dilemmas of intervention policies. In R. H. Binstock & E. Shanas (Eds.), *Handbook of aging and the social sciences.* New York: Van Nostrand Reinhold, 1976.

Busse, E. W., Dovenmuehle, R. H., & Brown, R. G. Psychoneurotic reactions of the aged. *Geriatrics,* 1960, 15, 97.

Busse, E. W., & Pfeiffer, E. (Eds.). *Mental illness in later life.* Washington, DC: American Psychiatric Association, 1973.

Butler, R. N. *Why survive? Being old in America.* New York: Harper & Row, 1975.

Butler, R. N., & Lewis, M. I. *Aging and mental health* (2nd ed.). Saint Louis: C. V. Mosby, 1977.

Campbell, A., Converse, P. E., & Rodgers, W. L. *The quality of American life.* New York: Russell Sage Foundation, 1976.

Caro, F. G. Professional roles in the maintenance of the disabled elderly in the community: A forecast. *Gerontologist,* 1974, 14(4), 286-289.

Carp, F. M., & Carp, A. It may not be the answer, it may be the question. *Research on Aging,* 1981, 3, 85-100.

Ciliberto, D. J., Levin, J., & Arluke, A. Nurses' diagnostic stereotyping of the elderly: The case of organic brain syndrome. *Research on Aging,* 1981, 3(3), 299-310.

Danish, S. J., Smyer, M. A., & Nowak, C. A. Developmental intervention: Enhancing life-event processes. In P. B. Baltes & D. G. Brim, Jr. (Eds.), *Life-span development and behavior* (Vol. 3). New York: Academic, 1980.

Dellario, D. J., & Anthony, W. A. On the relative effectiveness of institutional and alternative placement for the psychiatrically disabled. *Journal of Social Issues,* 1981, 37(3), 9-20.

Dohrenwend, B. P., & Dohrenwend, B. S. *Social status and psychological disorder: A causal inquiry.* New York: John Wiley, 1969.

Epstein, L. J. Depression in the elderly. *Journal of Gerontology,* 1976, 31(3), 278-282.

Estes, C. L. *The aging enterprise.* San Francisco: Jossey-Bass, 1979.

Fozard, J. L., & Popkin, S. J. Optimizing adult development: Ends and means of an applied psychology of aging. *American Psychologist,* 1978, 33(1), 975-989.

Gatz, M., Smyer, M. A., & Lawton, M. P. The mental health system and the older adult. In L. W. Poon (Ed.), *Aging in the 1980s.* Washington, DC: American Psychological Association, 1980.

Gurland, B. J. The comparative frequency of depression in various adult age groups. *Journal of Gerontology,* 1976, 31(3), 283-292.

Gurland, B. J., Bennett, R., & Wilder, D. Reevaluating the place of evaluation in planning for alternatives to institutional care for the elderly. *Journal of Social Issues,* 1981, 37(3), 51-70.

Haug, M. R. Age and medical care utilization patterns. *Journal of Gerontology,* 1981, 36(1), 103-111.

Jarvik, L. F. Aging and depression: Some unanswered questions. *Journal of Gerontology,* 1976, 31(3), 324-326.

Juel-Nielsen, N. Epidemiology. In J. G. Howells (Ed.), *Modern perspectives in the psychiatry of old age.* New York: Brunner/Mazel, 1975.

Kahn, R. L. The mental health system and the future aged. *Gerontologist,* 1975, 15(1), 24-31.

Kay, D.W.K. Epidemiological aspects of organic brain disease in the aged. In C. M. Gaitz (Ed.), *Aging in the brain.* New York: Plenum, 1972.

Kay, D.W.K., Beamish, P., & Roth, M. Old age mental disorders in Newcastle-Upon-Tyne, Part I. A study of prevalence. *British Journal of Psychiatry,* 1964, 110, 146-158.

Kidd, C. B. Misplacement of the elderly in the hospital: A study of patients admitted to a geriatric and mental hospital. *British Medical Journal,* 1962, 2, 1491-1495.

Klerman, G. L. Age and clinical depression: Today's youth in the twenty-first century. *Journal of Gerontology,* 1976, 31(3), 318-323.

Kramer, M., Taube, C. A., & Redick, R. W. Patterns of use of psychiatric facilities by the aged: Past, present, and future. In C. Eisdorfer & M. P. Lawton (Eds.), *The psychology of adult development and aging.* Washington, DC: American Psychological Association, 1973.

Kulka, R. A., & Tamir, L. *Patterns of help-seeking and formal support.* Paper presented at the meeting of the Gerontological Society, Dallas, November 1978.

Lasch, C. *The culture of narcissism.* New York: Norton, 1978.

Lawton, M. P. The impact of the environment on aging and behavior. In J. E. Birren & K. W. Schaie (Eds.), *Handbook of the psychology of aging.* New York: Van Nostrand Reinhold, 1977.

Lawton, M. P. Community supports for the aged. *Journal of Social Issues,* 1981, 37(3), 102-115.

Leighton, D., Harding, J. S., & Macklin, D. B. *The character of danger.* New York: Basic Books, 1963.

Lerman, P. *The origins of deinstitutionalization of the mentally ill.* Unpublished manuscript, 1980.

Maas, H. S., & Kuypers, J. A. *From thirty to seventy.* San Francisco: Jossey-Bass, 1975.

McDonald, C. An age-specific analysis of the neuroses. *British Journal of Psychiatry,* 1973, 122, 477-480.

Moroney, R. M., & Kurtz, N. R. The evolution of long-term care institutions. In S. Sherwood (Ed.), *Long-term care: A handbook for researchers, planners and providers.* New York: Spectrum, 1975.

Nowlin, J. B. Physical changes in later life and their relationships to mental functioning. In E. W. Busse & E. Pfeiffer (Eds.), *Mental illness in later life.* Washington, DC: American Psychiatric Association, 1973.

Nydeggar, C. N. (Eds.). *Measuring morale: A guide to effective assessment.* Washington, DC: Gerontological Society, 1977.

Palmore, E. B. Social factors in mental illness of the aged. In E. W. Busse & E. Pfeiffer (Eds.), *Mental illness in later life.* Washington, DC: American Psychiatric Association, 1973.

Pasamanick, B. A survey of mental disease in an urban population, VI: An approach to total prevalence by age. *Mental Hygiene,* 1962, 46, 567-572.

President's Commission on Mental Health. *Report to the president of the President's Commission on Mental Health.* Washington, DC: Government Printing Office, 1978.

Price, R. H., Ketterer, R. F., Bader, B. C., & Monahan, J. (Eds.). *Prevention in mental health: Research, policy, and practice.* Beverly Hills: Sage, 1980.

Redick, R. W., Kramer, M., & Taube, C. A. Epidemiology of mental illness and utilization of psychiatric facilities among older persons. In E. W. Busse & E. Pfeiffer (Eds.), *Mental illness in later life.* Washington, DC: American Psychiatric Association, 1973.

Riley, M. & Foner, A. *Aging in society* (Vol. 1): *An inventory of research findings.* New York: Russell Sage Foundation, 1968.

Schaie, K. W. A reinterpretation of age-related changes in cognitive structure and functioning. In L. R. Goulet & P. B. Baltes (Eds.), *Life-span developmental psychology: Research and theory.* New York: Academic, 1970.

Shanas, E., & Maddox, G. L. Aging, health and the organization of health resources. In R. H. Binstock & E. Shanas (Eds.), *Handbook of aging and the social sciences.* New York: Van Nostrand Reinhold, 1976.

Sherwood, S. (Ed.). *Long-term care: A handbook for researchers, planners and providers.* New York: Spectrum, 1975.

Shinn, M., & Felton, B. J. Institutions and alternatives. *Journal of Social Issues,* 1981, 37(3), 1-5.

Smyer, M. A. Guest editor's comments. *American Psychological Association Division of Community Psychology Newsletter,* 1981, 14(3), 1.

Srole, L., Langner, T. S., Michael, S. T., Kirkpatrick, P., Opler, M. K., & Rennie, T.A.C. *Mental health in the metropolis: The midtown Manhattan study* (Rev. ed.). New York: Harper & Row, 1975.

Sue, S. Clients' demographic characteristics and therapeutic treatment. *Journal of Consulting and Clinical Psychology,* 1976, 44, 864.

Test, M. A. Effective community treatment of the chronically mentally ill: What is necessary? *Journal of Social Issues,* 1981, 37(3), 55-62.

Test, M. A., & Stein, L. I. Community treatment of the chronic patient: Research overview. *Schizophrenia Bulletin,* 1978, 4, 260-264.

Tobin, S. S., & Kulys, R. The family in the institutionalization of the elderly. *Journal of Social Issues,* 1981, 37(3), 145-157.

Tringo, J. L. The hierarchy of preference toward disability groups. *Journal of Special Education,* 1970, 4, 295-306.

Veroff, J., Kulka, R. A., & Douvan, E. *Mental health in America: Patterns of help-seeking from 1957 to 1976.* New York: Basic Books, 1981.

Vladeck, B. C. *Unloving care: The nursing home tragedy.* New York: Basic Books, 1980.

Wicker, A. W. Processes which mediate behavior-environment congruence. In R. H. Moos & P. M. Insel (Eds.), *Issues in social ecology.* Palo Alto, CA: National Press Books, 1974.

Woodruff, D. S. Introduction: Multidisciplinary perspectives on aging. In D. S. Woodruff & J. E. Birren (Eds.), *Aging: Scientific perspectives and social issues.* New York: Van Nostrand Reinhold, 1975.

Zarit, S. H. *Aging and mental disorders.* New York: Macmillan, 1980.

3

Children

Facilitating New Directions
Sheila Namir
Rhona S. Weinstein
University of California, Berkeley

Existing mental health services are failing to meet the needs of children. Despite the all-too-frequent proclamation that children are our nation's most vital natural resource, children remain greatly underserved in the area of mental health. Further, we have yet to implement a national strategy that will maximize the development of these precious human resources as well as provide a coordinated system of treatment for those children who suffer from serious emotional and behavioral difficulties.

Childhood has been a social issue for at least a century now. The roots of this concern lie in a fertile and imaginative period of reform from about 1880 to 1914, when many social movements for children emerged and most modern professional services for children were first established (Levine & Levine, 1970; Takanishi, 1978). As far back as the first White House Conference on Children in 1909, this country has emphasized its intent to develop a strong program to care for emotionally disturbed children. Since that time, however, the care of such children has not improved, but instead has worsened (Joint Commission on the Mental Health of Children, 1969).

Concern about the state of mental health services for children in this country has been mounting. When the Joint Commission on Mental Illness and Health (1961) failed to address children, much pressure was directed toward funding a national study of the mental health needs of children. A historical stimulant for the resulting Joint Commission on the Mental Health of Children study (1969) lay in the assassination of President Kennedy by an individual who as a diagnosed mentally ill child had never received treatment.

In their report, the Joint Commission on the Mental Health of Children (1969, p. 2) declared: "This nation, the richest of all world powers, has no unified national commitment to its children and youth. The claim that we are a child-centered society . . . is a myth." This commission concluded that services for children were "grossly inadequate, antiquated and poorly coordinated" (p. 56).

A decade later, the President's Commission on Mental Health (1978a, p. 6) identified children and adolescents as critically underserved populations, concluding that "as the Commission traveled through America, we saw and heard about too many children and adolescents who suffered from neglect, indifference, and abuse, and for whom appropriate mental health care was inadequate or nonexistent."

Dismal statistics continue to be gathered. Edelman (1981) began her recent address to the American Psychological Association with sobering facts about the number of children who are not receiving even the most basic health care, let alone services to prevent and treat mental health problems. Further, the Select Panel for the Promotion of Child Health (1981a, p. 38), in reviewing the improvement in health status and access to health services in the past two decades, found that

> an equally powerful set of facts can be marshaled to demonstrate that recent improvements have not benefitted all segments of the child population equally. Indeed for some groups of children and in some categories of problems, things have improved little or are actually getting worse.

In what follows, we try to clarify the ways in which children are underserved by existing mental health services, and the factors that have led to this condition as well as those that stand in the way of improvements. Beginning with a look at the historical context of children's mental health services, we proceed to examine the current picture of underserved needs and the existing recommendations for change in the nature of children's services. We also suggest some inadequately considered problems that must be addressed before such changes can be realized.

The Historical Context and Legacy

Much has been written recently documenting the history of children and youth in America (Bremner, 1970, 1972, 1974), analyzing the historical roots of childhood as a social and economic issue (Katz, 1980;

Takanishi, 1978) and charting the development of helping services (Levine & Levine, 1970). Extracting the history of children's mental health services from these sources suggests two important features that have characterized the development of children's services. First, growth has been slow in recognizing the needs of children as distinct from adults, and as thus requiring a unique set of services. Second, services for children have developed in a fragmented way, oriented to special groups of needy children and to parts of each child, instead of to the whole child and all children. There has been no consistent, well-developed attempt to identify a comprehensive set of needs of children, and to provide a central structure for ensuring that the needs of children are met.

The first attention to children was primarily directed toward those who were physically handicapped, "feeble-minded," poor, or delinquent. In the eighteenth century, the concepts of juvenile delinquency and child health hardly existed (Bremner, 1970). However, beginning in the early nineteenth century, institutions were organized for children who were orphans, poor (1802-1805), deaf and dumb (1817), juvenile delinquents (1825), and blind (1832). These institutions were primarily concerned with the education of children with special needs. In the middle of the nineteenth century (1853), the first hospital exclusively for children was established.

In the early years of the twentieth century, the social reform movement attended to the health and welfare of mothers and children with attempts to change child labor practices and to provide infant and maternal hygiene and welfare reforms. In 1912, the Children's Bureau was established in response to these efforts, and its primary concern was directed toward maternal and child health services, including services for physically handicapped children, aid to dependent children, and welfare services for children needing special care. Mental health, however, was still very separate from physical health.

Mental health services for children were first addressed by Dorothea Dix (in the 1840s) in her attempts to improve the care of the insane. Shore and Mannino (1976) observe that this reform still did not separate child services from adults services, since children and adults were placed together in wards of the newly developed state mental hospitals. Mental health services for children followed a similar pattern to that for children's services in general, by focusing first on educational needs, second on physical health and social welfare, and, finally, rather late in the history, on mental health and psychological development. For example, in 1896, the first child guidance clinic was founded to assist children with learning difficulties. In 1909, the study and treatment of juvenile delinquents began with the founding of the Juvenile Psychopathic Institute in Chicago, and in 1921, the Commonwealth Fund and the National Committee on Mental Hygiene established demonstration clinics to prevent juvenile delinquency and maladjustment in children. It was not until 1963 that a National Institute of Child Health and Human Development was formed to bridge the gaps among domains of biomedical, behavioral, and developmental functioning.

One tends to forget how recently mental health has been addressed at a national level in this country. The first national survey of mental illness was provided for in 1955, with the Mental Health Study Act. The report of the ensuing Joint Commission on Mental Illness and Health (1961) mentioned mental health services for children, but this area remained a low priority and was not recognized as a distinct area requiring specialized training of professionals and different funding than adult services (Shore & Mannino, 1976). In contrast to reforms in the areas of physical health, education, and welfare, the development of mental health services began with adults and then turned to children and youth (Witmer, 1940; Shore & Mannino, 1976).

In response to this omission of children's needs, under PL 89-97 of the Social Security Act funds were allocated in 1965 to conduct a three-year study into the resources, methods, and practices for diagnosing and preventing emotional illness in children and for treating and rehabilitating children with emotional illnesses. Despite the comprehensiveness of the report regarding the state of children's emotional and social health, basic issues were left unresolved by the Commission on the Mental Health of Children. Shore and Mannino (1976) point out the incredible fact that it was not until 1972, after the visibility given to the mental health needs of children by the Joint Commission, that federal funds were allocated specifically for children's mental health services. The community Mental Health Center Act (Part F) allocated $10 million for these services. Just as astounding, and reflective of the typical short-term solutions to problems and the fickleness of legislative response to problems, in 1977 this money was rescinded.

This brief history of services to children reveals most glaringly how recently attention has been turned toward the mental health needs of children. The history also highlights the separation of education from juvenile delinquency, and health and from mental health. This separation has led to fragmented and specialized services dealing with only one facet of a child's development, and has failed to stimulate coordinated and long-term efforts to enhance the development of children and to treat multiple problems.

The Current Picture:
How Children Are Underserved

There exist multiple difficulties in assessing the extent to which children are underserved. First, there are no national survey data on the incidence and prevalence of mental health problems of children (Select Panel for the Promotion of Child Health, 1981a). This deprives us of a unified body of direct evidence on underservice.

Second, the data that are available on the incidence and prevalence of emotional and psychiatric problems among children are often ambiguous. It is frequently not clear if figures relate to incidence or prevalence. Duplication of cases is overlooked both among agencies and within agencies over time in what are allegedly reports of incidence. Compilation of data in this way may overestimate the incidence of disturbance as well as the number of different children actually being served.

Third, diagnostic categories of mental health problems are defined inconsistently. Estimates often confound psychopathology in childhood and cognitive and/or social lags in development. Data on substance abuse, emotional disorders, juvenile delinquency, conduct disorders, impairments or delays in psychological development, learning disabilities, child abuse, and mental retardation may often overlap. Furthermore, the President's Commission on Mental Health found that at the federal level, at least eight separate authorities request information from states in different formats and for different time cycles within a year. As well, various federal, state and local agencies request and compile information that varies regarding clinical diagnoses, the types of services provided, and the expenditures for services.

Finally, data are also compiled without systematic attention to the definition of age groups. The President's Commission on Mental Health used the ages of 3 to 15 in its estimate of mental health problems in children. Another recent estimate (Kramer, 1976) used the category of children and adolescents under 18 years of age. Therefore, it is difficult to compare incidence and prevailing estimates accurately.

Given these difficulties, the available statistics afford only crude estimates of the extent to which children are underserved by mental health services. However, across several types of evidence, a pattern emerges that is undeniably clear. Several types of evidence that exhibit this pattern will be presented. These include: (1) the incidence and prevalence of mental health problems based on surveys; (2) estimates of children receiving mental health services; (3) the percentage of mental health funds allocated for children's services relative to the population of children; and (4) differential access to services related to age, ethnicity, and socioeconomic class.

Estimates of Incidence and Prevalence

The President's Commission on Mental Health (1978a) placed the "overall prevalence of persistent, handicapping mental health problems among children aged three to fifteen" in a range from 5 percent to 15 percent. A recent survey conducted by the National Institute of Mental Health estimated that 18 percent or 12 million children and adolescents under 18 years of age suffer mental health problems (Kramer, 1976). Earlier, the Joint Commission on the Mental Health of Children (1973) had estimated that the incidence of emotional problems among children ranged from 8 percent to 10 percent.

The Select Panel for the Promotion of Child Health (1981a) reported that a recent study of 7 pediatric care facilities found that from 5 percent to 15 percent of the children treated at those facilities had behavioral, educational, or social problems. They also estimated that 25 percent of physician referrals for children are related to psychosocial or behavioral problems. Supportive evidence for this estimate is found in a recent telephone survey conducted by the Task Force of Pediatric Education. This survey revealed that 14 percent of mothers with children under age 5 reported that their children had growth and development problems, and 10 percent reported behavior or discipline problems (Select Panel, 1981a).

The Select Panel also called attention to the number of children who are handicapped and have emotional disturbances as well. Of the 3.6 million handicapped children being served under PL 94-142 (the Education for All Handicapped Children Act), 8 percent have emotional problems. Others have provided estimates of the percentage of children with school maladjustment problems. Glidewell and Swallow (1968) place the incidence at 30 percent, with 14 percent to 23 percent showing severe emotional problems.

It is unclear whether any of these figures include problems not directly documented by the mental health system. The high proportion of adolescents who abuse alcohol and drugs, the 1 million children each year who are victims of child abuse and neglect (Select Panel, 1981a), the 8,000 to 10,000 juveniles held in adult jails on any given day and the thousands of other children who are incarcerated in institutions for juvenile offenders (Albee, 1980), or the approximately 4 percent of children who are mentally retarded may not be included in estimates of mental health problems (Select Panel, 1981a).

In summary, the estimates of incidence and prevalence of mental health problems among children range from 5 percent to 23 percent. Of approximately 70 million children under the age of 18, anywhere from 3.5 to 16 million children are in need of mental health services.

Estimates of Children Receiving Mental Health Services

One of the major problems with estimating the number of children who receive needed mental health services is that the National Institute of Mental Health (NIMH) does not keep records on separate individuals. Each time a child is admitted to a federally funded mental health program, the record indicates a new case. This can lead to overestimations of the number of children who are served.

One of the most likely places for children to receive mental health services is in one of the 752 community mental health centers (CMHCs) of the United States (Select Panel, 1981b). These federally funded centers are mandated by law (amendments of the 1975 CMHC Act) to provide mental health services for children. However, in 1977 the centers served only 396,000 children. Based on the lowest estimate of the prevalence of mental health problems in children (5 percent, or 3.5 million), these centers are serving approximately 11 percent of the children in need. The Select Panel (1981b, p. 90) concluded their analysis of the CMHC program by stating that the program "has been grossly deficient in meeting the mental health needs of children and youth." In a document prepared for the National Institute of Mental Health, Kramer (1976) also found that 90 percent of the children who need services do not receive them. Further, a recent survey by the American Psychological Association (Vandenbos, Stapp, & Kilburg, 1981) found that only 11.2 percent of the clinical services provided by members of APA are delivered to children 11 years and younger. These figures reflect a prevalence rate of 5 percent of the child population. Hobbs (1981) in his recent address to the American Psychological Association, estimated that even if one uses a more likely but still moderate figure of 10 percent of children as needing services, only 4 percent of these children receive services based on existing NIMH records.

Even for programs developed expressly to reach a large proportion of children and meet their needs, the statistics are equally distressing. The Early and Periodic Screening, Diagnosis and Treatment Program for children eligible for Medicaid actually screened less than 25 percent of those children eligible (Children's Defense Fund, 1977), and of those who were screened and found to be in need of treatment, only 50 percent were treated (Edelman, 1981).

Funding Allocations

Basing estimates of underserved needs on the funds allocated for services to children does not improve the picture of the number of children being served. The Select Panel (1981a) stated that of the $2.2 billion expended for the CMHC program over the past 14 years, 7.3 percent of this amount was spent on services for children. The total population of the United States includes 30 percent under the age of 18.

Within state mental health departments, there is frequently inadequate funding for those services available. California's population consists of 28 percent under age 18, with no overall plan for their service (California Office of Statewide Health Planning and Development, 1980). The average percentage of county budgets for children's service was 12.3 percent of available funds. In Massachusetts, although children are 40 percent of the state population, they receive less than 18 percent of funds from the Department of Mental Health (Task Force on Children Out of School, 1972). Given that children are the prime target for the prevention of emotional problems, the promotion of positive mental health, and the early treatment of psychological problems, one wonders what the statistics of those needing mental health services would be if Hobbs (1969, p. 37) had been heeded when he wrote:

> Seventy-five percent of our resources should be devoted to the mental health problems of children. This is the only way to make substantial changes in the mental health of our adult population a generation from now. . . . But, alas, children are unprofitable clients, and furthermore, they don't vote.

Differential Access to Services

There are very few studies available on access to care and quality of care for mental health services to children. However, the little data available do indicate that for the small percentage of children who actually receive mental health services when needed, the quality and type of services vary on the basis of age, ethnicity, and socioeconomic class.

Different patterns of service delivery have been documented when comparing children, adolescents, and adults who receive mental health care. Data for 1975 from the Civilian Health and Medical Program of the Uniformed Services (CHAMPUS; Dorken, 1980) indicated that age was inversely related to length of hospitalization. Children were hospitalized longer than adolescents (average days, 38.9) and adolescents longer than adults (average days, 18.4 versus 4.6). This, however, did not correlate with the quantity or the quality of attention. Children, in fact, received substantially fewer professional visits than other groups while hospitalized (1 visit for every 4.1 days of hospitalization). Adolescents received more attention than children (1 visit per 2.4 days of hospitalization), but still less than half of the visits given to hospitalized adults. Based on these data, children and adolescents received more hospitalization days with less active treatment than adults. Dorken (1980, p. 14) concludes that "the combination of extended hospital stays for children and adolescents with the minimal care they receive while hospitalized . . . causes concerns about warehousing."

The work of Sankar (1979) illustrates some of the factors related to hospitalization of children for emotional and psychiatric problems. Analysis by length of hospital stay showed that the child who stayed longer was younger at first admission, had a lower IQ, was more often male, and was more often from a disadvantaged social class and a larger family. Males and children from minority groups were overrepresented in the population of first and second admissions to the same psychiatric hospital. Part of the high rate of readmission was attributed to the lack of an adequate continuum of care for children upon immediate release or before hospitalization (Sankar, 1979).

Two age groups are also particularly neglected in the area of care for mental health needs. During the period from birth until entry into school, most children are invisible to society, and their whereabouts are unknown unless they come to the attention of professionals through gross deficiencies or as victims of child abuse (JCMHC, 1973; Ross, 1974). Yet this is also the period of rapid and crucial development of early competence acquisition, emotional and intellectual capacities, and a sense of identity, purpose, and direction (Bloom, 1964; Lee, 1973; Escalona, 1973; White, 1979). Preventive work can be most effective here, and the promotion of skill development can have far-reaching impact on the mental health and academic achievement of children. Systematic attention to parents of children who are in their early years also may yield large dividends, preventing the deleterious effects of insufficient or problematic relationships with their children.

Another large group of children not receiving adequate mental health care is adolescents. There are few facilities specifically developed to address the multiple mental health needs and problems of adolescents. Even fewer professionals have been trained adequately to deal with adolescent problems. Adolescents are caught between the child guidance or play therapy modalities, which are no longer appropriate for them, and adult psychotherapy (Cohen, Granger, Provence, & Solnit, 1975). The Joint Commission the on Mental Health of Children (1969, p. 276) concluded their analysis of services for adolescents by stating: "To put it briefly, insofar as mental health care is concerned, as a society we fail our teenagers at almost every level."

When teenagers are parents we often continue the cycle of inadequate prenatal and perinatal care to a new generation of children, resulting in continuing mental health problems. The high rate of teenage pregnancies, the low rate of prenatal care, and the disadvantaged position teenage mothers occupy in the labor market contribute to poor physical and mental health for millions of children (Moore, Hofferth, Caldwell, & Waite, 1970).

Perhaps the saddest indictment of not meeting the needs of children and teenagers is the adolescent suicide rate. Since 1955, the rate of teenage suicide has tripled (Giovacchini, 1981; Gordon & Scales, 1979; Keniston & the Carnegie Council on Children, 1977), and suicide is now the second leading cause of death for teenagers, following accidents. Self-destruction among youth is also reflected in the high and increasing rates of substance abuse and juvenile delinquency among adolescents. Although mortality rates for all other age groups have declined since 1960, death rates for adolescents and young adults (ages 15-24) have actually gone up since 1960 (Select Panel, 1981a).

Ethnic minorities and the rural and urban poor are especially neglected by existing mental health services (PCMH, 1978a). Programs for mental health care often neglect the culturally diverse, and children are no exception. The President's Commission (1978a) found that appropriate services are not available to many of the 22 million Black Americans, 12 million Hispanic Americans, 3 million Asian and Pacific Island Americans, and 1 million American Indians and Alaska Natives, and, of these, at least 30 percent are children. Programs and services are not developed with attention to the lifestyles, languages, and expectations of the ethnic groups in need of service. Furthermore, the types of services obtained by minorities are often discriminatory. For example, the Task Force on Mental Health and American Families (PCMH, 1978b) found that for nonminority children, behavioral problems were addressed by appropriate mental health services in voluntary clinical settings. However, for these same behavioral problems, minority children received the attention of police and juvenile courts. As a second example, the number of hospital days per child under 17 was almost 4 times as great for the lowest income group as for the highest income group, with an average length of stay more than twice as long (Select Panel, 1981a).

Finally, the Select Panel for the Promotion of Child Health (1981a) also found that there was a strong correlation between high family income and two desirable patterns of care—the appropriate use of preventive care and the timely use of routine acute care. In addition, the panel documented that the pattern of care for those who are Medicaid eligible is discontinuous, with 20 percent of those eligible moving in and out of eligibility each year, creating variable access to care. Furthermore, Medicaid-eligible poor and the affluent may have roughly comparable use rates; however, the poor and near poor who are not eligible for care have lower use rates. It should be remembered that comparable use rates of services do not necessarily mean that equal quality or equal access to different services is assured.

Upgrading Children's Mental Health Services

Existing Proposals for Improving Services

We have at hand now a variety of commission and panel reports, all of which have offered a series of recommendations for the improvement of children's services. Within the commissions, each task force has also developed recommendations relevant to children. It is impossible to do justice to these recommendations in the scope of this chapter. However, it is important to characterize the overall direction of these recommendations.

Beginning with the Joint Commission on the Mental Health of Children (1969), the thrust of proposals for change has been to support the development of a coordinated set of services that would (a) address the total needs of the child, (b) cover the entire life span of the child from conception to adulthood, (c) link up with the natural settings of family, school, peer group, and community in which the child is embedded, and (d) prevent mental health problems in addition to treating them. Interest in a greater role for prevention services is also reflected in the report of the President's Commission on Mental Health (1978a, 1978b). Further, in their report, children were targeted as an underserved population as well as the priority population for prevention activities. The Select Panel for the Promotion of Child Health (1981a, 1981b) concurred in their recommendations to routinely provide preventive services. Again, both the President's Commission and the Select Panel stressed considering health and mental health problems in concert, as well as working through families and schools.

These reports have also recognized the need for structural changes that would support the development of these types of services. In particular, the Joint Commission on the Mental Health of Children (1973) recommended the creation of a child advocacy system at the neighborhood, local, state, and national levels in which comprehensive plans for children and youth would be developed and coordinated on an ongoing basis. Each neighborhood would have local Child Development Councils, which would be served by the county-level Child Development Authority and the State Child Development Agency. At the federal level, an Advisory Council on Children would be appointed to the President's Office, which would advise the government on the effectiveness of programs, on the needs of children, and on recommendations for changes. Through these structural changes, this nation would develop a comprehensive strategy for children and youth.

Given that 98 percent of all children in the United States live with one or both of their parents, the Carnegie Council on Children report (Keniston & the Carnegie Council, 1977) recommended that the national policy be a family policy that would strengthen the ability of families to raise children effectively. Whether the policy is child or family focused, the fact remains that this country is without a national commitment to children as comprehensive as its defense policy (Keniston & the Carnegie Council, 1977). Further, the need for structural supports for prevention programs was also reflected in the recommendation of the President's Commission on Mental Health (1978b) to establish a Prevention Center within the National Institute of Mental Health. Clearly, the various commission reports underscore the need for structural changes to support the redirection of children's services.

Addressing children's mental health needs more effectively requires major changes in the structure of mental health services, not only conceptual, but also organization. Although it is true that we need more professional services, and an expansion of services and of research, the most promising changes must come in organization, financing, and structuring of services to children. Access barriers are often the result of provider and system features that determine patterns of utilization (Select Panel,

1981b). For example, Gottlieb and Hall (1980) analyzed the utilization of preventive mental health services and found that low utilization was often the result of a lack of social network analysis that could have informed the development of services. In some communities, informal referral agents are far more successful than organized referral services in disseminating information about services and thus in increasing utilization.

Major structural changes are far more difficult to engineer. It is easier to seek programs focused on special needs of target groups than to seek broader policy reforms (Select Panel, 1981a). The path from commission proposals to implementation is thorny indeed. Sometimes stumbling blocks lie in the proposals themselves. Shore and Mannino (1976) argue that the Joint Commission on the Mental Health of Children struggled but failed to resolve the underlying issues of the priorities and conceptualizations of child mental health services. They suggest that

> what was highlighted instead was the struggle between treatment and prevention, clinical and social approaches, motivational dynamic approaches and learning approaches and the medical model as contrasted with the education model or the public health model [Shore & Mannino, 1976, p. 23].

Also, predictable shrinkage occurs from the initial task panel's recommendations to their ultimate impact on services (Swift, 1980). In describing the events that followed the President's Commission on Mental Health (1978a, 1978b), Swift (1980) cites broad issues raised by the task panel on prevention that were not incorporated into the final commission report. Further, the recommendation to establish an NIMH Prevention Center was not reflected in the ensuing Mental Health Systems Act. Instead, a milder version (an office of prevention) with less power and a smaller budget was legislated (Swift, 1980). It is also apparent that from legislation to implementation, many more of these proposed changes fail to be actualized. The EPSDT program as well as Medicaid programs are excellent examples of changes that were legislated but that have inconsistent availability across states (Select Panel, 1981b).

Finally, stumbling blocks are inevitable when the proposed structural changes are not encompassing enough to counteract the press of existing practices or realities. There exist several factors that have stood in the way of the development of children's services and that will continue to block their further development unless addressed directly by the proposed changes. Any reformation of children's services must be introduced into the context of historical, social, and political conditions that have earlier resisted redirection.

Constraints upon the Redirection of Services

Political realities. There have been many attempts to improve the welfare of children with laws, institutions, and organizations developed to meet their needs. Yet there exist several political realities that have interfered with these developments. First, the style of American politics has been predominantly crisis oriented (Albee, 1980; Katz, 1980). The interest shown within this type of a political climate results in short-range goals and quick solutions to problems—solutions that can provide favorable results in the brief span of the four years of elected terms. The sustained effort, money, and continuing expertise needed to make deep structural changes are not considered.

Hyman (1976, p. 16) describes a familiar scenario throughout the history of child advocacy movements. Individuals or groups expose the plight of children. The public becomes incensed and politicians then pass legislation for reform. The reform is implemented and the "public is then diverted to other problems, funding slacks off, and the programs deteriorate from lack of support and entrenched forces that are insensitive to change."

Also illustrative of this crisis mentality are the White House Conferences on Children and Youth held each decade since 1909. Beck (1973) provides a historical perspective on these conferences, indicating that each one involved different leadership (for example, political and social leaders in 1909, physicians in 1919, family and child psychologists in 1930), as well as different issues, reflecting the currently perceived crises of the times. For example, the first conference was concerned with child labor, the second with standards of maternal and child health care, and the third with broader issues of education, labor, and vocational training. The 1940 conference was concerned with patriotism, democracy, and freedom, whereas the midcentury conference addressed the effects of both the uncertain world situation and the effects of prejudice in the United States on personality development. The 1960 conference was concerned with adolescents and the disintegration of the family, and the 1970 conference addressed the rights of children, with a call for action and advocacy.

Beck (1973) discusses certain ironies in this history. In particular, each conference "was called specifically to gather information, plan programs and set priorities for the next decade, . . . (but) turned out to be more a reflection of the preceding decade than a plan for the future" (Beck, 1973, p. 663).

A second political constraint on developing adequate services for children lies in the fact that many of the proposed solutions have required broad-sweeping sociopolitical changes in order to counteract the debilitating effects of inadequate nutrition and housing, lack of birth-control information, poverty, and discrimination. Katz (1980, p. 37) has pointed out that there is a "long standing American response to crises of youth" that involves locating the sources of the crises in the social and economic fabric of society, but then turning to education and reform of schools to solve the problems. He argues that education has been seen as an easy solution to the problems or a "smokescreen" for the need to make broad-sweeping structural changes in society that would increase social justice, assure equal distribution of resources, and provide a genuine resolution to continuing crises.

Finally, children lack a political voice in this society. As Edelman (1981, p. 111) wrote: "Children are the easiest people in America to ignore. They do not vote, lobby, or make campaign contributions." Furthermore, they do not even know that they are being treated unjustly, and remain powerless to obtain just treatment without the help of adults to speak for their concerns and assure them the necessary resources. Without the backing of strong political power, children's services have often in the final analysis become the lowest priority relative to other programs (Shore & Mannino, 1976).

Prevailing social climate. Many reviewers of the development of children's services have pointed to powerful attitudes in our society that have constrained the growth of services for children. Among these attitudes is a strong resistance in our society toward recognizing the existence of emotional problems in children (Shore & Mannino, 1976). This occurs in part because once a child is identified as mentally ill or emotionally disturbed, those responsible for the child are implicated and blamed. Thus to recognize emotional problems in children is to recognize problems in the people or institutions caring for children.

Further, progress in children's mental health services has been constrained by an underlying tradition in our society of self-reliance and individualism (Edelman, 1981; Shore & Mannino, 1976). Families are expected to care for their own children, and often the need for help is viewed as shameful.

Closely related to this attitude, and reinforcing it, is the fear or belief since the first White House Conference in 1909 that government will encroach on the family's autonomy, as well as that of state and local authorities. It is considered better that the private sector respond to the needs of people (Beck, 1973; Shore & Mannino, 1976). Certainly, this latter attitude has culminated in disparate care for those who can afford private services and those who cannot. Apparently, it is permissible for the government to "encroach" on the rights and individualism of lower-income families, but not on those of higher-income families. In recent times, the governmental role in human services for any group has also been called into question.

The organization of services. An examination of the 1981-1982 *National Directory of Children and Youth Services* (Directory Services Company, 1981) illustrates the current organizational fragmentation of services. For example, at the federal level, there is the office for Maternal and Child Health in the Public Health Service, the Office of Human Development Services with the Title XX Social Security programs, a National Center for Child Advocacy, and the Administration for Children, Youth and Families, responsible for the Children's Bureau and Head Start programs. Under the Department of Education, one finds programs for handicapped children; under the Justice Department are programs for juvenile delinquency; and under the Health Care Financing Administration there are the Early and Periodic Screening, Diagnosis and Treatment programs as well as the Medicaid programs. In short, there are separations of responsibility and program development for juvenile justice, drug and substance abuse, social services for adoption and foster homes, social security, rehabilitation, physical disability, recreation, developmental disabilities, education, day care, and maternal and child health. "Fragmentation occurs among programs within the health care system, and between the health care system and equally complex delivery systems in the related fields of social welfare, education, corrections, and rehabilitation" (Select Panel, 1981b, p. 5). Further, within states and counties there is an equal degree of fragmentation.

At an individual level, the most serious problem created by this fragmentation is that the child and his or her family have tremendous difficulties in locating and coordinating the necessary services. Also, a great deal of time and effort is spent in obtaining the necessary assessment and care. When care finally is provided, children are subject to different individual plans at the same time (Select Panel, 1981b), resulting in conflict and confusion for the family and child, and the waste of personnel and financial resources. The sense of a whole person who has a coherent set of needs is lost in a system that moves people among separate service units. As Lenrow and Cowden (1980, p. 475) point out: "Bureaucratically organized services promote a client's sense of being fragmented and helpless."

Fragmentation also reflects the separation of health from mental health in children, and encourages overlooking the fact that mental health in children is related to physical health and economic, social, and emotional climates of families (JCMHC, 1973). These are all considered and addressed separately in the organization of services to children. Further, there is no one agency at any level that has responsibility and authority for the development and delivery of health services, for continuity of care and uniform accounting procedures, and for quality of care and data collection.

Weaknesses in our knowledge base. In their recent *Annual Review of Psychology* article on child psychopathology, Ross and Pelham (1981) underscore the difficulties inherent in improving our understanding of the etiology and treatment of childhood psychological disorders. They cite two characteristics unique to childhood that make childhood psychopathology far more complex to study than that of adults. First, psychopathology in childhood is confounded with cognitive and social development. Children are continually changing, and what is considered pathological in one developmental period may no longer be considered pathological in another. Second, during the course of development children are embedded in environments, with little choice and minimal control over what happens to them. Thus the assessment of problems in children is heavily dependent on institutional norms and powerful others. The reactions of significant adults in a child's life influence the course of a problem as well as its recognition. Ross and Pelham (1981) conclude that these difficulties inherent in unconfounding pathological from developmental effects, and child-based from environment-based influences, have resulted in a weak system for classifying childhood disorders and in relatively limited research about psychopathology.

The advent of DSM-III is considered by some (see Garmezy, 1978) to increase the problems of defining childhood psychopathology. As Garmezy notes, children with deficits and disabilities that are not mental disorders may now be coded diagnostically as having psychiatric problems. Subsumed now under the rubric of mental disorders are such disparate problems as delays in development, learning disabilities, and personality or temperamental characteristics (such as shyness).

Another problem is the question of who defines childhood psychopathology. Parents may see their child's functioning as adaptive, while a teacher may consider the child's behavior maladaptive. Psychologists and psychiatrists are empowered by society to determine who is disturbed or deviant and in need of psychological services. Kaswan (1981, p. 292) notes that the "ostensible reason (for psychological treatment) may be to correct the unacceptable behavior, but a major sociopolitical requirement is that some socially legitimate institution, like a mental health agency, take charge." Reiff (1974) argues that the consequence of this role for psychologists is that the mental health profession exerts powerful social control. The way in which these professionals define a problem determines what will be done about the problem (Caplan & Nelson, 1973).

The complexities of distinguishing between normal and abnormal development in children urge careful attention and understanding of diagnosis and treatment in children. As Cowan (1978, p. 332) states, "It is essential to explore a continuum ranging from adaptive to dysfunctional patterns of individual differences." Furthermore, it is important to assess which "patterns of structural, functional, and behavioral variation *in combination with situational contexts,* . . . lead to further developmental change without special interventions" (pp. 332-333; emphasis added), and which patterns will inhibit developmental progress unless therapeutic intervention is provided. Somewhere in between these poles, a determination must be made of when interventions may not be necessary but can stimulate increased or optimal development.

Our understanding of the normal course of development has also been limited by our inattention to the environmental contexts that foster or interfere with psychological growth (Bronfenbrenner, 1979). Bronfenbrenner has argued for an ecologically valid psychology of development, which would examine the developmental consequences of different environmental conditions. To date, our narrow and "out of context" understanding of child development further reduces the knowledge base about normal and maladaptive growth needed to create effective and far-reaching services for children (Masterpasqua, 1981).

With all the problems in definition, diagnosis, and the understanding of childhood development and psychopathology, it is perhaps no wonder that adequate treatment and preventive services are seldom provided. Clearly, much research is necessary for the adequate, humane, and systematic provision of services to children. This research must also depend on interdisciplinary cooperation. Masterpasqua (1981) urges cooperation between community psychology and developmental psychology in understanding human development, and in the planning of environments responsive to developmental needs. The same cooperation is needed among clinical psychology, psychiatry, and other disciplines to conceptualize and learn about the development of problems in children and to promote effective therapeutic measures and delivery systems for ameliorating these problems.

Underemphasized Problems in Reforming Services

The institutional vehicle for service delivery. Resolving the problem of the current fragmentation of services requires more than a monitoring and referral network. The psychological distance of current services from the lives of children, the need to support preventive interventions for all children, the interest in bridging the gaps among health, mental health, welfare, and education—all necessitate a different conception of the children's service system.

Coordination of federal, state, and community systems in the provision, management, and quality of mental health programs is essential, but it is not enough. Yet considerably less attention has been paid to the institutional vehicle needed for delivering services to children. What should be its form and where should it be located?

How do we frame services around the child in the family, the school, and the community? How do we provide access to multiple services that meet the needs of the *whole* child, including prenatal care, social services, physical care, early diagnosis and treatment, prevention and competency building, day care services, and consultation with parents and other socializing agents. Of course, this demands collaboration among mental health agencies, health agencies, schools, and families, as has been proposed by various commissions and panels (see PCMH, 1978b; Select Panel, 1981a). Interdisciplinary cooperation is also essential in order to deal with the whole child (JCMHC, 1973). Furthermore, one cannot separate mental health from physical health in children, and increased collaboration between health and mental health services is urgently needed (Berlin, 1969; Broskowski, Marks, & Budman, 1981; Stone, Cohen, & Adler, 1980).

This concept of unity is not new; it was at the heart of the child guidance movement in the 1920s. Levine and Levine (1970, p. 242) state that the goals of the movement were to "put the professional mental health worker in ever closer touch with the community setting so he could influence it" and to promote close relationships among interdisciplinary professionals, the schools, families, and other agencies responsible for child welfare. Levine and Levine also analyze the demise of collaborative and cooperative services, particularly noting that specialized training and the independence of the various professionals contributed to the eventual lack of cooperation among services.

The development of separate bureaucracies concerned with types of children or parts of the child, and the concomitant hardening of professional boundaries, must be averted in current plans for the reform of children's services. Examples of local coordination among primary care providers are infrequent, but they demonstrate simplification of bureaucracy and cost-effectiveness. Cambridge, Massachusetts, established a single health, hospitals, and welfare agency under a commissioner in 1967 and provided school-based primary care units to provide both sick and well child services (Select Panel, 1981a). Denver has likewise created a system of neighborhood comprehensive care clinics. Recently, Los Angeles County has begun developing a network of children's services by integrating all child services (including juvenile justice) under the Los Angeles County Children and Youth Services Bureau. This central bureau is responsible for services to children and youth between the ages of 1 and 18 years in the provision of direct mental health services, education and training, and child advocacy.

These attempts conform to proposals that multiservice centers be developed in local communities (JCMHC, 1973; PCMH, 1978a, 1978b). The Select Panel (1981a) believes it possible to increase both state autonomy and federal accountability simultaneously in working toward national objectives for meeting the needs of children. Their plan involves structuring the health system with state authority over funding streams and a federal role in establishing objectives and standards for services. It is then appropriately left to local initiative to establish service centers and improve methods of case management and case advocacy to ensure meeting the health care needs of children.

How can one utilize local initiative to develop a service vehicle that would meet the needs of children for preventive and treatment interventions? Instead of building new institutions that would result in the development of yet another bureaucracy, an alternative model would locate services at critical points in the pathway of a child's normal development. Thus one stream of services might be based in local hospitals or clinics, which, in concert with the provision of obstetrical and pediatric care, would offer prenatal services, parental education and child development programs, diagnostic services, and consultation with day care and other preschool programs. These hospital-based programs would be linked intimately with a second major institutional base, namely, the schools.

School-based services would bring together teachers and school personnel, families, pediatricians, psychologists, psychiatric services, juvenile justice services, services for the handicapped, and family case work (including adoption and recreation) personnel, and would target specific services at various grade levels. Both preventive and treatment programs would be earmarked for the primary grades as well as the high school years. At a time when schools face shrinking enrollments and the closure of neighborhood schools, and when existing special services are confronted with severe cutbacks, a pooling of resources would appear to be sound financially as well as conceptually. Most importantly, local control through family involvement in PTA, school boards, and newly created advisory boards would ensure that children's services meet the needs of the community.

The time is ripe for new models of service delivery for children. In the final analysis, the community mental health center has been overwhelmed by treatment and has been unable to provide structural support for prevention (Snow & Newton, 1976). Typically, children have received little attention from such services and involvement in school and health care problems has been minimal. A new institutional host for integrating services for children is needed, but existing services need support rather than additions to the number of institutions concerned with children.

The structure of funding. Financial realities are partly responsible for the state of children's services as well as for differential access to existing services as discussed earlier. But the problems lie as much in the structure of funding as in the amount of funding available. Structural changes in funding patterns are necessary in order to support the proposed changes in services (Kiesler, 1980; Levine, 1981).

As examples of these structural constraints, children are not receiving their fair share of mental health monies relative to their numbers. Their weak political position in this country has maintained their low-priority position. These disproportionate allocations of funds must be addressed directly.

Further, Medicaid reimbursement is available for restrictive inpatient care at true cost of service, but funds for less restrictive forms of care, including outpatient counseling and day treatment, are not reimbursed at cost, despite the lower actual cost for these services. Hence the funding structure penalizes community treatment. In addition, other than specific grants, such as the categorical grant program under the Mental Health Systems Act, there is little funding for preventive services. Preventive care is rarely covered by either public or private insurance. While the CMHC has been resourceful in relabeling prevention activities in order to receive reimbursement, the relabeling has redefined problems in clinical rather than normative terms (Swift, 1980).

Categorical funding also contributes to duplication and further fragmentation of services. Categorical funding separates the needs of a child and/or family. Treatment for the whole child needs to involve a plan that often crosses the boundary between direct and indirect services. While treating a problem in a family, preventive interventions are often part of a comprehensive plan. Yet the existence of categorical funds often makes this impossible to accomplish. Additionally, children are often labeled with diagnoses that meet the funding criteria; witness the spate of learning disabled children once money became available for learning disabilities.

The Select Panel (1981b) had very specific recommendations regarding funding levels for the five major programs they reviewed, as well as comments on ten other federal programs affecting children. However, all of the general cries for more money, and the more specific ones, seem rather unlikely to be heeded in the current economic and social climate of the legislatures and the federal government.

The situation is particularly acute regarding Medicaid and the Mental Health Systems Act. Loss of eligibility for Medicaid by a large percentage of those previously eligible will create even less EPSDT screening and general health care than currently exists. The limited amount of money originally allocated to children's services under the Mental Health Systems Act ($10 million) will probably become even more ridiculously small with the final appropriations by Congress.

Despite poor prospects for increased funding for mental health services, the underlying structure of the funding needs to be reevaluated as well. In its existing form, it does not support the proposed reformation of children's services.

The training of child professionals. One of the most crucial constraints and limitations to the development of adequate and appropriate treatment and prevention services for children is the shortage of trained professionals to work with children. Tuma (1975) recently addressed the crisis in training psychologists to work with children and suggested that the severe shortage will continue to be so for many years. The picture is not much better for child psychiatrists. Albee (1979) found, twenty years after his report on mental health manpower trends, that the situation is even worse today. Both the Joint Commission (1969) and the President's Commission (1978a, 1978b) recommended increased training of specialists to work with children and families.

Not only is there a shortage of trained professionals to work with children, but these limited resources are further divided among a fragmented field with territorial limitations and commitments. For example, within psychology there are pediatric psychologists working with children in nonpsychiatric medical settings and clinical child psychologists who diagnose and treat children in mental health settings. There are school psychologists, who specialize in school-related problems; educational and developmental psychologists with applied interests; psychologists working as child advocates; and community psychologists with interests in prevention. Each of these subspecialists is interested in children, but each has become a specialist in a particular element of the total ecology. Rather than training specialists of the whole child as the child participates in family life, school, community, and health settings, we continue to generate knowledge of child development and to create services based on pieces of children's lives. Rather than view the child as embedded in multiple environments, we have opted for "setting" specialists, not child specialists. This training mode maintains professionals separateness as well as professional preciousness (Sarason, Levine, Goldenberg, Cherlin, & Bennett, 1966) in the delivery of services and limits the development of a coordinated set of services. Professionals are not trained to treat, and often have difficulty thinking about, the whole child, the whole family, and the nature of coordinating a network of services.

In the model proposed, the training of professionals would include working in multiple ecological contexts and would require that teachers, doctors, psychologists, and many others build a broad-based model for the understanding of children's needs over the life span of childhood. Clearly, interdisciplinary collaboration in learning, as well as in the delivery of services, is a critical factor in the training of specialists of the whole child. It is important to train more mrofessionals to work together in providing the range of services for children in nontraditional settings. The multi-service center concept demands a high level of respect and collaboration among all those who work with children, and a sensitivity and knowledge of community needs and demands for the provision of effective and usable services. In addition, increased training of ethnic minority personnel and multicultural sensitivity are required to meet the needs of ethnically mixed communities.

Toward a Unified Picture:
Rethinking Relationships Among Families,
Schools, and Mental Health Professionals

In its health plan, the State of California (California Office of Statewide Health Planning and Development, 1980) recognizes the need for services to respect the rights and responsibilities of families. Egeland, in her testimony to the subcommittee on the Master Plan for Children and Youth, expressed what critics of psychological services (see Keniston & the Carnegie Council, 1977; Gross, 1978; Lasch, 1979) have also noted:

> But government's responsibility has tended to expand under the "parens patriae" ideology—often "taking over" the responsibility of the parent—thereby weakening further the family structure. In other words, we may be actually perpetuating and intensifying the source of many of the problems we are attempting to solve when we intervene in such ways as to weaken the primary responsibility of the parents to protect the child's physical and mental health [California Office of Statewide Health Planning and Development, 1980, p. 95].

Similarly, the Task Panel on Mental Health and American Families of the President's Commission on Mental Health (1978b, p. Fam-Inf 4) stated:

> Mental health services for children must also be delivered within a system of care that insofar as possible promotes and maintains a continuing relationship between child and family.

As Conger (1981, p. 1481) states, the large bureaucratic mechanisms of mental health services have "tended to increase the relative isolation of the family from effective communication with, and influence over other social institution."

In a similar way, children's services should ultimately strengthen the capacity of the schools to guide children's development. Yet, often the delivery of mental health services serves to weaken the relationship between child and school. While children's problems manifest themselves in schools, treatments typically have involved teachers only on their periphery. Yet teachers have been left to cope with children on a continuing basis. The labels and the stigma of treatment have often resulted in the creation of greater distance in the relationship between child and school. One can view the passage of Public Law 94-142, which is concerned with the mainstreaming of handicapped children into regular classrooms, as a recognition of the weakened bond between children with special needs and the lifeblood of schools. In the implementation of mainstreaming, however, little attention has been paid to the strengthening of teachers' ability to handle individual differences in the classroom or to changes needed in the classroom value system so that it could become more tolerant of diversity (Sarason & Doris, 1979). Again, schools and families are not always strengthened by services.

Just as children's services have eagerly taken over responsibility for children, schools and families have just as eagerly expelled their troubling members outward to each other and to experts. Each of these resources has only focused on one aspect of the child, defining itself and excluding itself from participation with others in promoting healthy maturation in the child. Traditionally, each resource has either directly or inferentially placed blame for the etiology or maintenance of deviant behaviors. Consequently, each has become isolated with a tradition and culture that supports its value system and depreciates the approach or value system of other agencies.

In attempting to provide services that enhance the capacities of the family and the school to promote the development of children as well as to handle problems that disrupt the course of development, we must address the relationships among families, schools, and mental health professionals. It is a time of confrontation. Conflicts rage between children's rights and parents' rights, between parents' rights and schools' rights, and between school control and government control. Underlying these conflicts are struggles for the right to treatment, the right to be integrated in the community, the right to equal opportunities, and the right to be culturally different.

While there is considerable distance to bridge, one step toward that goal involves an examination of values. The mental health field has conceptualized families in far too narrow terms; the schools have defined achievement in exceedingly limited ways. Cultural variation in family life, newer family constellations, and dual-career fmaily structures must be addressed in the delivery of services and in the structure of schooling. We must develop programs to meet the needs and desires of those to whom services are directed, instead of demanding that children and parents conform to a single standard of the normative family.

Further, as Sarason and Doris (1979, p. 394) so forcefully argue in their examination of educational handicap, schools must reassess their reliance on "production-achievement as the major criterion for judging people." Not only is achievement a major criterion in sorting children in schools, but achievement has been conceptualized in very narrow ways. The focus has been on social comparison rather than on task mastery (Nicholls, 1979). This conceptualization of ability inevitably produces more misfits than winners. The White House Conference Committee (1974) emphasizes this concern by suggesting that instead of "knocking off the individual's sharp edges," we might move in the direction of making our schools fluid enough to accommodate individual differences of style, attitude, and readiness. Thomas and Chess (1977, p. 105), in their extensive study of temperament and development, state that "a child's deviation from a single stereotyped concept of normality may be the healthy expression of his temperamental individuality and should be recognized and respected as such." Thomas and Chess urge parents, teachers, and mental health professionals to understand temperamental traits and the optimal approach for each pattern, instead of relying on general characterizations and a single criterion for judgment regarding the functioning of children. Further, environments need to be moved toward greater toleration of individual differences.

This reexamination of underlying values concerning the nature of families and schooling in the context of planning for children's services requires ample structural supports. By locating services close to families via pediatric care linkages and schools, by requiring interdisciplinary cooperation on a daily basis, and by involving parents, teachers, and pediatricians in the conceptualization and implementation of programs for children, a structure for strengthening relationships rather than undermining them is put in place.

If the intent is to improve the capacity of the school and the family to handle the problems of children, very different components have to be built into the institutional base for delivering services. In one example of such a school-based intervention (the creation of school mental health teams composed of teachers, principals, nurses, special service personnel, and psychologists), the representative and interdisciplinary membership in an ongoing structure (a weekly group meeting) facilitated the working through of differing value orientations and the development of integrative program plans (Weinstein, 1979, in press).

Concluding Comments

The underdeveloped nature of services for children can be understood as a function of several interactive sets of influences. The historical context for the development of services left a legacy of fragmentation that ignored the whole child in its failure to provide a continuum of care. With professional specialization and large bureaucratic structures for service delivery, little improvement has been made in correcting this fragmenta tion. Instead, increasingly disparate care is being provided to children—care that depends on the age, gender, and socioeconomic status of the child and the severity of the problem.

Although many recommendations have been made to improve the provision of services to children, gaps in our knowledge base regarding childhood development and psychopathology, as well as political realities and the prevailing social climate, have constrained the prospects for change. Given these realities, we can suggest at least three areas in which psychologists might make contributions toward supporting new directions in the delivery of children's services. First, it is important to reexamine our existing models of training. We need to train child psychologists who can address the developmental regularities as well as the problems of children as they participate in a variety of (rather than in single) ecological settings. Such training, encompassing both research and practice, will benefit our currently weak knowledge base.

Second, new institutional bases for the delivery of children's mental health services must be identified. By identifying more natural points of entry and by supporting parents, schools, and health agencies in their care of children, advocacy on behalf of children might be strengthened and resistance to mental health interventions might be diminished. More than ever, cooperative efforts between social institutions and mental health agencies are needed. If such cooperative services are made available at a community level and are framed around family and child as consumers of health and educational resources, more effective utilization of mental health services is likely.

Finally, shrinking financial resources, as well as the continuing escalation of the need for children's mental health services, make it imperative that we reevaluate how these limited resources are used. The continued emphasis on expensive treatment services may be shortsighted if many of the problems could possibly have been prevented with adequate provision of preventive care for *all* children. It is also difficult to separate prevention from treatment in early childhood, particularly when one considers the whole life span of an individual. It is not our purpose to catalogue the many successful and creative prevention programs (see Murphy & Frank, 1979, for such a list). What is important to note, however, is Murphy and Frank's finding that successful programs involve *sustained long-term* work with children, from infancy into the school years. Additionally, these programs involve mothers in the activities and need to involve fathers.

Funding must be reorganized to reflect a recognition that treatment and prevention (or direct and indirect services) often converge in a plan for the treatment of a family or child. Comprehensive services should be available in local communities and should be responsive to the desires and needs of the community. Planning for services must involve interdisciplinary teams, interagency collaboration, and consumer representatives. Without meeting these basic criteria, services will continue to develop in fragmented ways, reflecting the lack of a sustained and comprehensive approach to the care and optimal development of all of our children.

References

Albee, G. W. Psychiatry's human resources: 20 years later. *Hospital and Community Psychiatry*, 1979, 30, 783-786.

Albee, G. W. Social science and social change: The primary prevention of disturbance in youth. In *The third annual Gisela Konpka lecture*. St. Paul, MN: Center for Youth Development and Research, 1980.

Beck, R. The White House Conferences on Children: An historical perspective. *Harvard Educational Review*, 1973, 43, 653-668.

Berlin, I. N. Mental health consultation for school social workers: A conceptual model. *Community Mental Health Journal*, 1969, 5, 280-289.

Bloom, G. *Stability and change in human characteristics*. New York: John Wiley, 1964.

Bremner, R. H. (Ed.). *Children and youth in America: A documentary history* (Vol. I): *1600-1865*. Cambridge, MA: Harvard University Press, 1970.

Bremner, R. H. (Ed.). *Children and youth in America: A documentary history* (Vol. II): *1865-1933*. Cambridge, MA: Harvard University Press, 1972.

Bremner, R. H. (Ed.). *Children and youth in America: A documentary history* (Vol. III): *1933-1972*. Cambridge, MA: Harvard University Press, 1974.

Bronfenbrenner, U. Contexts of child rearing: Problems and prospects. *American Psychologist*, 1979, 34, 844-850.

Broskowski, A., Marks, E., & Budman, S. H. (Eds.). *Linking health and mental health*. Beverly Hills, CA: Sage, 1981.

California Office of Statewide Health Planning and Development. *Issues in planning services for California's children and youth*. Sacramento: Author, 1980.

Caplan, N., & Nelson, S. D. On being useful: The nature of consequences of psychological research on social problems. *American Psychologist*, 1973, 3, 199-211.

Children's Defense Fund. *EPSDT: Does it spell health care for poor children?* Washington, DC: Author, 1977.

Cohen, D. J., Granger, R. H., Provence, S. A., & Solnit, A. J. Mental health services. In N. Hobbs (Ed.), *Issues in the classification of children* (Vol. II). San Francisco: Jossey-Bass, 1975.

Conger, J. J. Freedom and commitment: Families, youth and social change. *American Psychologist*, 1981, 36, 1475-1484.

Cowan, P. A. *Piaget with feeling: Cognitive, social and emotional dimensions*. New York: Holt, Rinehart & Winston, 1978.

Directory Services Company. *National directory of children and youth services, 1981-1982.* Washington, DC: Author, 1981.

Dorken, H. Mental health services to children and adolescents under CHAMPUS: Fiscal year 1975. *Professional Psychology,* 1980, 11, 12-14.

Edelman, M. W. Who is for children? *American Psychologist,* 1981, 36, 109-116.

Escalona, S. Overview of hypotheses and inferences. In L. J. Stone, H. T. Smith, & L. B. Murphy (Eds.), *The competent infant.* New York: Basic Books, 1973.

Garmezy, N. DSM-III: Never mind the psychologists, is it good for the children? In B. L. Baker & M. J. Goldstein (Eds.), *Readings in abnormal psychology.* Boston: Little, Brown, 1978.

Giovacchini, P. *The urge to die: Why young people commit suicide.* New York: Macmillan, 1981.

Glidewell, J., & Swallow, C. *The prevalence of maladjustment in elementary schools.* Chicago: University of Chicago Press, 1968.

Gordon, S., & Scales, P. Preparing today's youth for tomorrow's family. In M. W. Kent & J. E. Rolf (Eds.), *Social competence in children.* Hanover, NH: University Press of New England, 1979.

Gottlieb, B. H., & Hall, A. Social networks and the utilization of preventive mental health services. In R. H. Price, R. F. Ketterer, B. C. Bade, & J. Monahan (Eds.), *Prevention in mental health: Research, policy, and practice.* Beverly Hills, CA: Sage, 1980.

Gross, M. L. *The psychological society.* New York: Random House, 1978.

Hobbs, N. Mental health's third revolution. In A. J. Bindman & A. D. Spiegel (Eds.), *Perspectives in community mental health.* Chicago: Aldine, 1969.

Hobbs, N. *Mental health services for children: The revolution that never happened.* Paper presented at the annual meeting of the American Psychological Association, Los Angeles, August 1981.

Hyman, I. A. A bicentennial consideration of the advent of child advocacy. *Journal of Clinical Child Psychology,* 1976, 5, 15-20.

Joint Commission on the Mental Health of Children (JCMHC). *Crisis in child mental health: Challenge for the 1970's.* New York: Harper & Row, 1969.

Joint Commission on the Mental Health of Children (JCMHC). *From infancy through adolescence: Reports of Task Forces I, II, and III.* New York: Harper & Row, 1973.

Joint Commission on Mental Illness and Health. *Action for mental health.* New York: Basic Books, 1961.

Kaswan, J. Manifest and latent functions of psychological services. *American Psychologist,* 1981, 36, 290-299.

Katz, M. B. Missing the point: National service and the needs of youth. *Social Policy,* 1980, 10, 36-41.

Keniston, K., & the Carnegie Council on Children. *All our children: The American family under pressure.* New York: Harcourt Brace Jovanovich, 1977.

Kiesler, C. A. Mental health policy as a field of inquiry for psychology. *American Psychologist,* 1980, 35, 1066-1080.

Kramer, M. *Report to the President's Biomedical Research Panel.* Washington, DC: Government Printing Office, 1976.

Lasch, C. *The culture of narcissism.* New York: Norton, 1979.

Lee, D. L. *From plans to planets.* Chicago: Broadside Press, 1973.

Lenrow, P., & Cowden, P. Human services, professionals, and the paradox of institutional reform. *American Journal of Community Psychology,* 1980, 8, 463-484.

Levine, M. *The history and politics of community mental health.* New York: Oxford University Press, 1981.

Levine, M., & Levine, A. *A social history of helping services.* New York: Appleton-Century-Crofts, 1970.

Masterpasqua, F. Toward a synergism of developmental and community psychology. *American Psychologist,* 1981, 36, 782-286.

Moore, K., Hofferth, S. L., Caldwell, S. B., & Waite, L. J. *Teenage motherhood: Social and economic consequences.* Washington, DC: Urban Institute, 1970.

Murphy, L., & Frank, C. Prevention: The clinical psychologist. *Annual Review of Psychology,* 1979, 30, 173-207.

Nicholls, J. G. Quality and equality in intellectual development: The role of motivation in education. *American Psychologist,* 1979, 34, 1071-1084.

President's Commission in Mental Health (PCMH). *Report to the president of the President's Commission on Mental Health* (Vol. 1). Washington, DC: Government Printing Office, 1978. (a)

President's Commission on Mental Health (PCMH). *Report of the Task Panel on Mental Health and American Families.* Washington, DC: Government Printing Office, 1978. (b)

Reiff, R. The control of knowledge: The power of the helping professions. *Journal of Applied Behavioral Science,* 1974, 10, 451-461.

Ross, A. O. Part I: Forecasting the future–1986. In G. J. Williams & S. Gordon (Eds.), *Clinical child psychology: Current practices and future perspectives.* New York: Behavioral Publications, 1974.

Ross, A. O., & Pelham, W. E. Child psychopathology. *Annual Review of Psychology,* 1981, 32, 243-278.

Sankar, D.V.S. A child psychiatric hospital's first and second admissions. *Evaluation and the Health Professions,* 1979, 2, 32-41.

Sarason, S. B., & Doris, J. *Educational handicap, public policy and social history.* New York: Macmillan, 1979.

Sarason, S. B., Levine, M., Goldenberg, I. I., Cherlin, R. L., & Bennett, E. M. *Psychology in community settings.* New York: John Wiley, 1966.

Select Panel for the Promotion of Child Health. *Better health for our children: A national strategy* (Vol. 1): *Major findings and recommendations.* Washington, DC: Government Printing Office, 1981. (a)

Select Panel for the Promotion of Child Health. *Better health for our children: A national strategy* (Vol. 2): *Analysis and recommendations for selected federal programs.* Washington, DC: Government Printing Office, 1981. (b)

Shore, M. F., & Mannino, F. V. Mental health services for children and youth: 1776-1976. *Journal of Child Clinical Psychology,* 1976, 5, 21-25.

Snow, D. L., & Newton, P. M. Task, social structure, and social process in the community mental health center movement. *American Psychologist,* 1976, 31, 582-593.

Stone, G. C., Cohen, F., & Adler, N. E. *Health psychology: Theories, applications, and challenges of a psychological approach to the health care system.* San Francisco: Jossey-Bass, 1980.

Swift, C. F. Primary prevention: Policy and practice. In R. H. Price, R. F. Ketterer, B. C. Bader, & J. Monahan (Eds.), *Prevention in mental health: Research, policy, and practice.* Beverly Hills, CA: Sage, 1980.

Takanishi, R. Childhood as a social issue: Historical roots of contemporary child advocacy movements. *Journal of Social Issues,* 1978, 34, 8-28.

Task Force on Children Out of School. *Suffer the children: The politics of mental health in Massachusetts.* Boston: Beacon, 1972.

Task Panel on Prevention. Report of the Task Panel on Prevention. In D. G. Forgays (Ed.), *Primary prevention of psychopathology* (Vol. 2): *Environmental influences.* Hanover, NH: University Press of New England, 1978.

Thomas, A., & Chess, S. *Temperament and development.* New York: Brunner/Mazel, 1977.

Tuma, J. M. "Pediatric psychology" . . . Do you mean clinical psychology? *Journal of Clinical Child Psychology,* 1975, 4, 9-12.

Vandenbos, G. R., Stapp, J., & Kilburg, R. R. Health service providers in psychology: Results of the 1978 APA human resources survey. *American Psychologist.* 1981, 36, 1395-1418.

Weinstein, R. S. *Group consultation in school settings: Constraints against collaboration.* Paper presented at the annual meeting of the American Psychological Association, New York, September 1979.

Weinstein, R. S. Group consultation in a middle school: Toward staff collaboration in the treatment of student problems. In J. Alpert (Ed.), *Psychological consultation in schools.* San Francisco, in press.

White, R. S. Competence as an aspect of personal growth. In M. W. Kent & J. E. Rolf (Eds.), *Social competence in children.* Hanover, NH: University Press of New England, 1979.

White House Conference Committee. The 1970 White House Conference on Children and Youth. In G. J. Williams & S. Gordon (Eds.), *Clinical child psychology: Current practices and future perspectives.* New York: Behavioral Publications, 1974.

Witmer, H. L. *Psychiatric clinics for children.* New York: Commonwealth Fund, 1940.

4

Rural People
Richard G. Blouch
Millersville State College

This chapter addresses (a) the problem of inadequate mental health services to rural people, (b) factors that contribute to this inadequacy, and (c) current efforts to correct or alleviate this problem. The literature shows that, although room for disagreement remains, rural people are underserved in regard to mental health services. They display an incidence of mental health disorders similar to those of their urban counterparts, yet have access to a substantially smaller per capita supply of mental health professionals.

Attention to the provision of mental health services to rural people has resulted in new understanding of the factors that contribute to their underservice and in efforts by government agencies and mental health professionals to develop appropriate service delivery systems. Although encouraging, reports of these efforts are only preliminary because they lack evaluative data and, considering the heterogeneity of communities described as rural, are not likely to be generally applicable.

Definition of "Rural"

Defining the target population of this chapter is complicated by the diversity of rural America and the variety of ways in which the rural community has been defined. Flax, Wagenfeld, Ivens, and Weiss (1979) discuss the economic, ethnic, and regional differences existing among rural communities to support their description of rural America as heterogeneous. While recognizing this diversity, they utilize the Census Bureau's definition of "rural" as communities with less than 2,500 people. They also present a classification system used by the Bureau of the Budget,

AUTHOR'S NOTE: Thanks to Steven R. Heyman for his helpful comments on this chapter.

which utilizes the terminology of the standard metropolitan statistical area (SMSA). Under this system a county with a city of 50,000 or more people and counties that are economically or socially connected with the central city are considered to be a single SMSA, and therefore urban.

Another definition of people to be served by rural mental health workers is provided by Jones, Wagenfeld, and Robin (1976). They use the National Institute of Mental Health definition of "rural catchment area" as one serving an area outside an SMSA and consisting of counties in which more than 50 percent of the population reside in communities of 2,500 or fewer people. This variety of definitions and the heterogeneity of rural communities cause confusion in identifying the target population of rural mental health workers.

Factors Contributing to Underservice

A variety of factors, ranging from the geographic distances between the people to be served and the mental health facility to differences in values between rural people and mental health professionals, contribute to the underservice of rural people. This section will discuss: (a) the effects on service delivery of physical distance, (b) migration patterns and economic factors, (c) attitudes and values of rural people, (d) community structure, and (e) cultural differences between residents of rural communities and professional mental health workers who come to these communities.

Folk-Urban Differences

This section, and much of the research reviewed here, assumes a "folk-urban continuum" (Miner, 1964). This continuum, an attempt to capture a crucial urban-rural distinction and resolve problems in defining rurality, is based upon increasing heterogeneity, social complexity, and population density as one moves from folk to urban societies. Other characteristics of folk societies include preference for informal education, reliance upon tradition and traditional values, emphasis on family unity, and pride in self-help within the community while resisting outside intervention. While rural people represent the folk end of the continuum, mental health professionals are trained in and prefer to practice in urban settings (Keller, Zimbelman, Murray, & Feil, 1980; Munson, 1980; Richards & Gottfredson, 1978). It is generally true, although certainly with exceptions, that mental health professionals and rural people represent different positions on the folk-urban continuum. These differences and their effect upon the provision of services to rural people must be a focus of concern.

Population Dispersion and Geographic Distances

Geographic distances separating rural people from mental health services have been cited as a major problem in providing services to rural people. Cohen (1972) reports that in a catchment area of 20 counties and 20,000 square miles, utilization rates for outpatient services dropped steeply outside a 30-mile radius from the center. The Prairie View Mental Health Center, which serves a catchment area of 3 counties, also reports differential usage of its services based upon distance from the center (Segal, 1973). The President's Commission on Mental Health (1978) found transportation to be the major variable in providing services to people living in rural catchment areas. Some catchment areas in sparsely populated regions include up to 65,000 square miles.

Ozarin (in press) traced the history of rural mental health concerns at the federal level and claims that insensitivity to rural concerns was in part responsible for the Community Mental Health Centers Act of 1963 requirement that catchment areas have populations of between 75,000 and 200,000 people. These population parameters create no problems in densely populated areas, but effectively serve to deny comprehensive services to many people living in sparsely populated areas.

Personal Visibility in Small Communities

Social as well as physical characteristics of rural communities contribute to problems in providing mental health services. Jeffrey and Reeve (1978) express concern with the almost constant visibility of the mental health worker. This community visibility can have a demoralizing effect upon workers accustomed to the anonymity of urban living. Other factors contributing to confidentiality problems in small towns are the information networks typical of such environments and the likelihood that an employee of the mental health center may know a majority of the people who come seeking services.

Outmigration and the "Dependency Ratio"

Another problem affecting service delivery is the incapacity of many rural areas to provide financial support for mental health services. This incapacity is due in part to the outmigration of the young and better educated. Thus Flax et al. (1979) report a "dependency ratio" of 78 for the general population and 88 for the rural population. This ratio indicates the number of persons considered not to be gainfully employed (persons under 18 and persons 65 and over) per 100 persons considered to be gainfully employed (ages 18 to 65). The higher dependency ratio in rural communities means that these communities expend a greater portion of their resources than urban communities to support larger segments of their populations.

Hines, Brown, and Zimmer (1975) studied population change between 1960 and 1970, using counties as the basic unit. The population of nonmetropolitan counties decreased 5.6 percent while the population of metropolitan counties increased by 4.7 percent. In relating migration patterns to economic factors, they conclude that outmigration resulted in distorted age distribution, low levels of educational attainment, and low levels of labor force participation. They also found 8.5 percent of the families with an employed male head of household to have incomes below the poverty level, whereas 3.4 percent of similar families in metropolitan counties had incomes below poverty level. Another indication of the limited economic resources of rural communities is the finding by Jones et al. (1976) that only 13 percent of the income of rural mental health centers is derived from fees for service, while urban centers derive 25 percent of their income from this source.

In contrast to the historical pattern of outmigration from rural areas, the past decade has witnessed a reversal of the pattern in some rural areas (Ploch, 1978). Ploch studied the rural immigrants of one northeastern state and concluded that their high levels of education, their managerial and professional careers or experience, and their concern for the quality of life may help them to be a resource to the rural communities to which they move. Flax et al. (1979) also call attention to the recent change in demographic trends, but point out that rural communities in some regions experience immigration while rural communities of other regions continue the more typical pattern of emigration.

The Traditional Values of Rural People

Concern with the folk-urban continuum has prompted research that has attempted to identify differences in rural and urban values. Smith and Petersen (1980) assessed the tolerance for nonconformity of permanent residents of rural, other urban, and large-city settings and of residents who had migrated to these areas by analyzing data taken from the General

Social Survey of the National Opinion Research Center. Rural respondents consistently received the lowest tolerance scores among the three categories of residence; however, the group of people who had been raised and currently lived in rural areas had the lowest tolerance scores, while persons raised in large cities and currently residing in other urban settings had the highest tolerance scores. The differences observed in the tolerance levels of permanent residents and migrant residents lend support to Srole's (1972) recommendation that attention be given to the study of migrants and nonmigrants.

In another study of rural and urban values, Glenn and Alston (1967) studied the responses of farmers to national opinion polls. They conclude that, in comparison to urban workers, farmers are more traditional in religious beliefs, more work oriented, less tolerant of divorce and ethnic groups, less informed, and more favorable toward marriage and child-bearing. Willits, Bealer, and Crider (1974) surveyed students in small-town and rural high schools and found strong support for traditional religious, family, and personal behavior values. Distance from the high schools to urban and metropolitan areas was significantly related to the degree of support for traditional values, with students in the most remote schools showing the greatest support.

In yet another study of the relationship between rurality and values, England, Gibbons, and Johnson (1979) found rurality to be the fourth best predictor of eleven selected value orientations. The best predictor was class position of the respondent, followed by maturity of the respondent and stratification of the respondent's community. This study confirms the relationship of rurality and traditionalism of values, but presents other factors to be considered equally in supporting traditional valuing. Its findings are similar to those of van Es and Brown (1974), who found sociocultural differences between rural and urban residents but were able to account for more of these differences in the social classes and incomes of the subjects than in the community in which they resided. The conclusion is that mental health workers moving from urban work or training locations may expect to find more traditional values as they move into small communities and open country; however, the degree of traditionalism will vary with individuals and communities in relation to income, occupation, and social stratification.

Attitudes Toward Mental Health

Of particular concern to mental health service providers and researchers have been the attitudes of rural people toward the mental health of individuals and also toward provision of mental health services. The mental health education efforts of Cumming and Cumming (1957) in a rural Canadian community were met with denial, anger, and communitywide resistance.

Similar attitudes of superstition and prejudice in regard to mental health and the stigmatizing of persons experiencing emotional problems were reported in a survey of rural mental health centers (Gertz, Meider, & Pluckman, 1975). This study found that public attitude was a major impediment to the entry of mental health systems into the community. A survey of mental health personnel employed by schools found a preference for traditional mental health services (Jason & Glenwick, 1979). This preference was expressed by both urban and rural personnel, but urban personnel were more receptive to community mental health services.

Mental health problems were seen in a pejorative light by the poor, rural people surveyed by Lee, Gianturco, and Eisdorfer (1974), who recommend a long-term community education program as a way of overcoming these negative attitudes. However, D'Augelli (in press) warns that mental health education programs focusing on mental illness can be expected to elicit results similar to those experienced in the work of Cumming and Cumming (1957). Bentz, Edgerton, and Hollister (1971) found more positive attitudes toward the mentally ill than those previously reported here in their study of residents in two rural North Carolina counties. Within the population of their study they found more stigmatizing of mental illness by people living in the countryside compared to people living in rural towns. They also found greater stigmatizing by people with less education, lower social status occupations, and lower incomes. Although rurality appears to be related to negative attitudes toward mental illness, the attitudes of rural people regarding mental illness are not uniform.

Urban-to-Rural Transition
of Mental Health Professionals

The transition of urban-trained mental health workers (Munson, 1980 Richards & Gottfredson, 1978) to rural settings poses a difficult adaption process (Riggs & Kugel, 1976). The difficulty of this transition both discourages prospective workers from entering rural settings and results in early termination for some mental health workers who move to rural communities. Riggs and Kugel claim that the transition is made difficult by the loss of attachment to city resources, scrutiny of the newcomer by the community, the rural community practice of personal evaluation rather than associating the newcomer with the clinic or professional status, and a sense of continuous exposure to the community.

Mental health professionals also experience conflict because they have been trained to relate to clients formally, within the client-therapist role. However, in the rural community, the therapist is likely to interact with the client in roles and settings outside the consultation room. Privacy versus personal sharing is another area of disagreement between mental health professionals and rural people. While mental health professionals value sharing their experiences, rural people have been found to prefer privacy.

Hollingsworth and Hendrix (1977, p. 237), after surveying rural community mental health centers, conclude that there is a "lack of fit between our urban-trained psychologists and the rural setting." Their observations are similar to those of Riggs and Kugel (1976). They appear to support the idea that the urban-oriented mental health worker, trained in traditional therapeutic methods but working in a rural community, may be a deterrent to providing mental health services in rural settings.

The Social Environment of the Rural Community

Dillon (1974) and Jeffrey and Reeve (1978) suggest that an understanding of the rural community social system is basic to the success of rural mental health programs. Blouch and Snowden (1980) agree on the need for understanding the social systems of traditional rural communities. They cite Kelly's (1969) study of social environments in two high schools as a model for gaining this understanding. Kelly classifies social environments as fluid or constant and provides a model that is useful for classifying rural communities, predicting community reaction to specific interventions, and designing mental health interventions.

Kelly based the constant versus fluid distinction on low and high rates, respectively, of population exchange in the schools. His study of the constant social environment describes the social relationships in that school as having minimal interchange between social groups; subdued affect and low voice levels; unresponsiveness to new students; intolerance of exploratory behavior; and high structure, with a clearly defined hierarchy of leadership positions. Kelly's description of the constant social environment parallels Robert Redfield's description of folk society as quoted by Miner (1964) in his aforementioned discussion of the folk-urban continuum.

The applicability of Kelly's (1969) constant social environment model to the description of many rural communities is supported in several ways. Both rural communities and constant social environments have a low level of population exchange. This characteristic of rural communities is seen in the previously cited study by Hines et al. (1975), in which they found the lowest level of population mobility to be in rural communities. Also, Kelly's description of constant environments as intolerant of exploratory behavior and placing high value on conformity parallels a description by several researchers of rural attitudes and values (Glenn & Alston, 1967; Smith & Petersen, 1980). Thus the concept of a constant social environment characterizes what has been called the conservative rural ethic, reported to be a barrier to adaptation among urban-trained psychologists (Gertz et al., 1975).

Viewing rural communities as constant environments leads to several useful predictions. Like the constant environment, many rural communities will resist the work of change agents such as mental health interveners. This resistance gives the intervener the responsibility to understand the properties of the system and to take these properties into account when formulating community interventions. Kelly (1969) states two conditions for acceptance into a constant environment: contributing one's skills and allowing oneself to be absorbed by the social system. It follows that resistance to mental health interventions is reduced if the interventions are designed to meet existing needs and to utilize community resources and subsystems. To meet these conditions, the intervener must be informed about the community's needs, subsystems, and resources; therefore, other conditions of acceptance are assessing community needs and attitudes, bearing in mind rural diversity, and focusing on conditions of the particular rural community. Improvement of mental health services to rural people requires that mental health professionals understand the social environment of the rural community and work within the structure of that environment.

Underservice of Rural People:
Real or Imagined

Distribution of Mental Health Professionals

The answer to real or imagined mental health underservice for rural people can best be found by comparing the adequacy of services to rural people with those of persons living in urban, suburban, and other local-ities. Although, as Richards and Gottfredson (1978, p. 7) note, "there is no optimal ratio of providers to population," the practitioner-to-population ratio remains a good measure of comparison.

Richards and Gottfredson (1978) studied the distribution of psychologists throughout the 50 states and the District of Columbia and found them concentrated in affluent, urban states. Similarly, the distribution of psychiatrists, school guidance counselors, and clinical social workers was not found to provide "special advantages for serving poor people, black people, rural people, or other groups" (Richards & Gottfredson, 1978, p. 5).

Keller et al. (1980), in their study of 19 northeastern states and the District of Columbia, also found a concentration of psychologists in densely populated counties and an absence of psychologists in sparsely populated counties. Although factors other than population density contributed to the distribution of the psychologists, and only those listed in the *National Register of Health Service Providers in Psychology* were included in the study, the tendency of psychologists to locate in densely populated areas is evident.

Studies of the distribution of psychologists and other mental health professionals are complicated by the difficulty of identifying the areas in which professionals actually offer their services and the classification of these areas as rural or urban. Although methodological questions open these studies to debate regarding the exact interpretation of the data, the trends expressed support the claim made by the National Institute of Mental Health (1978) that it is difficult to induce mental health personnel to serve in rural areas. This publication, which focused on hours of service rather than on numbers of providers, reported that community mental health centers (CMHC) located in inner-city poverty catchment areas had average total facility staff hours of 8,566.2 per 100,000 population. The CMHCs located in rural poverty catchment areas had average total facility staff hours of 2,687.1 per 100,000 population. Despite the limited knowledge of the quantity and quality of services provided during these staff hours, these data support the claim of underservice to rural communities.

Incidence of Psychological Disorders

Justification for the provision of similar per capita mental health services in rural and urban areas must be based upon evidence of similar needs for such services. Dohrenwend and Dohrenwend (1972) conclude that rates of psychiatric disorder are higher in urban than in rural popula-tions. They base their conclusion on nine studies employing both urban and rural subjects. Challenging this view, Srole (1972) points to the remote geographical and economically marginal character of several of the cities and the questionable research methodology used in some of the studies. He also questions the applicability of data gathered in undeveloped coun-tries or developing countries to the industrialized nations. Srole further contends that folk knowledge, including Old Testament descriptions of the evils of the city and Thomas Jefferson's perception of the city as "the cancer of the body politic," has contributed to an antiurban bias in theory, research, national attitudes, and social policy. This bias tends to describe the city as plagued with problems, while freedom from these problems is to be found in the country.

Another source of evidence for higher rates of mental morbidity in rural settings is found in a comparison, adjusted for differences in methodology, of the Midtown and Stirling County studies. In still another reexamination of previously gathered data, Srole found *lower* rates of psychological distress among urban populations surveyed by the National Center for Health Statistics. He recommends that research turn from studying the effects of community differences to comparing the character-istics of people who stay in a community with those of people who move to other kinds of communities.

Still other studies find no significant difference in psychiatric disorder or emotional well-being between rural and urban populations. Webb and Collette (1979) used the prescription of stress-alleviating drugs in rural and urban areas as a measure of stress and found very little variation across the rural-urban continuum. Lee and Lassey (1980) reviewed the literature comparing rural and urban elderly people, and found that urban people had advantages in objective measures, such as transportation and housing, but they found no advantage in subjective measures, such as emotional well-being.

Link and Dohrenwend (1980) studied true and treated rates of psycho-logical disorder in rural and urban populations by examining data obtained by Warheit in a study of emotional distress in a developing county in Florida and data from a national study conducted by the National Opinion Research Center. The Warheit study found 33.3 percent of the rural population and 25.9 percent of the urban population reporting distress. The National Opinion Research Center reported 32.1 percent, 27.5 per-cent, and 32.9 percent, respectively, of rural, suburban, and urban people reporting emotional distress. The percentage of true cases treated showed a much wider difference, with 5.3 percent of the rural true cases to 9.3 percent of the urban true cases treated in Warheit's study and 18.9 percent of the rural, 26.2 percent of the suburban, and 23.1 percent of the urban true cases treated in the survey of the National Opinion Research Center. From these data Link and Dohrenwend (1980, p. 147) conclude that "people living in urban areas are more likely to receive treatment than people in rural areas." They do not provide a comparison between rural and urban people for prevalence of emotional distress, but examination of the reported ratios reveals only a small difference that, if anything, would suggest greater distress among rural people.

Additional evidence for higher levels of emotional distress in the rural population is found in a report by Flax et al. (1979) of a study by J. M. Derr. The study found higher Selective Service rejection rates for psychosis and neurosis among rural recruits than among urban recruits. Even this study with a large population distributed across the nation cannot be said to be a representative sample because of the single sex and narrow age range of the population.

On the other hand, a recent study lends some support to the notion of higher emotional distress levels among urban populations. Husani and Neff (in press) used the Health Opinion Survey, the General Well-Being Schedule, and the Center for Epidemiologic Studies-Depression Scale (CES-D) to determine the prevalence of psychopathology in predominantly rural counties in Tennessee and Oklahoma. Comparison between residents of these rural counties and residents of Kansas City, Missouri, on the CES-D showed higher levels of depression in the urban population; however, income was the best predictor of impairment without regard to place of residence.

Conclusion: Underservice to Rural People

These epidemiologic studies are plagued by methodological errors, variations in assessment techniques, and lack of uniformity in definition of psychiatric impairment. Nevertheless, Flax et al. (1979, p. 26) are led to conclude: "Although the accumulating evidence seems to support the notion that the mental health of rural areas is worse than that of urban, the conclusions are far from unambiguous." Considering the variety of conclusions reached in the previously cited research and the difficulties inherent in making comparisons, it is probably more accurate to say that true prevalence rates continue to be an unknown factor requiring more study. However, the assumption of healthier rural communities is unwarranted.

Clearly, mental health workers are concentrated in the more densely populated and more affluent areas. This pronounced geographic imbalance of service providers, coupled with the absence of an advantage in mental health for rural populations, makes it reasonable to conclude that rural people are, in fact, underserved.

Developments in the
Improvement of Services

Federal Government Legislation and Programs

Decisions made by the federal government have had pronounced effects upon the quality of mental health services provided to rural people. Ozarin (in press) reviews these developments in providing a historical perspective on the concern of federal agencies for mental health services to rural people.

The Community Mental Health Centers Act of 1963 was to have been a vehicle for providing services to rural people. However, the system it envisioned was based on urban standards of population density and resource availability. This urban orientation has resulted in rural catchment areas of large geographic size. Also, the available financial and manpower resources of these rural areas are strained by standards that assume a concentrated, mobile population, low communication and travel costs, a strong tax base, and an availability of physicians and mental health specialists (Clayton, 1977).

Ozarin (in press) says that the first assignment of an NIMH staff member to work specifically on rural mental health occurred in 1967, when Dorothea Dolan became Special Assistant for Rural Mental Health. In 1975, Ozarin was designated Coordinator of Rural Mental Health and shortly thereafter established the Rural Mental Health Work Group. This group sponsored a conference in 1977, which led to the formulation of research questions regarding rural mental health and rural mental health services.

However, recent work to assess rural community health needs and to recommend legislaton to meet these needs has not succeeded in bringing about legislative action. This failure was documented by the Task Panel on

Rural Mental Health of the President's Commission on Mental Health (1978), which found rural people to have disproportionately fewer mental health professionals and facilities than urban residents. Furthermore, this panel found the research on mental health needs of rural people to be "sporadic and fragmented" and concluded that this research inadequacy symbolizes "the mental health resource imbalance in rural America" (Vol. III, p. 1160). Despite recognition of these problems, the Report of the President's Commission on Mental Health made no recommendations for correcting them (Ozarin, in press). Also, the 1980 Mental Health Systems Act does not make any specific provision for correcting this underservice (Congressional Research Service, 1980). Activity at the federal level in support of mental health services for rural people has resulted in advocacy by NIMH and the President's Commission on Mental Health but not in legislation specifically designed to correct the underservice of rural people.

Rural Mental Health Research and Literature

The purposeful development of mental health services for rural people requires the guidance of research that evaluates methods of service delivery and literature that reports the research to the practitioner. Flax, Ivens, Wagenfeld, and Weiss (1978) note the rich diversity contained in descriptions of rural mental health services; however, they also report a lack of properly designed, evaluative studies of these services. The President's Commission on Mental Health (1978) was more critical in its assessment of research relevant to rural mental health.

Recent concern for mental health services to rural people has resulted in an increased volume of literature that may be useful in developing staff and programs effective in meeting the needs of the rural underserved. Segal's (1973) publication provides case histories of five rural mental health centers and reports on research and demonstration projects designed to identify both the needs of rural people and methods to meet these needs. Flax et al. (1979), in another NIMH-sponsored publication, provide an overview and annotated bibliography of literature relevant to rural mental health.

Other sources of information about rural mental health services include an annotated bibliography on the topic "Rural Mental Health"[1] and two recent publications addressing themselves specifically to rural mental health. These publications are a handbook by Keller and Murray (in press) and the *Journal of Rural Community Psychology,* first published in

1980.[2] However, the reports and articles contained in these publications can be criticized for being descriptive rather than evaluative.

Training Programs for Rural
Mental Health Workers

The provision of adequate mental health services to rural people requires the training or retraining of mental health professionals for the rural setting. Because the rural general practitioner is the person most likely to work with the emotionally distressed person in the rural community, most continuing education programs have been designed to improve the psychiatric skills of the general practitioner. Segal (1973) mentions a variety of continuing education programs in which general practitioners may attend training programs at a university or be visited in their offices by an itinerant psychiatrist. Another summary of continuing education programs for physicians and nurses is provided by Flax et al. (1979).

Although retraining of persons through continuing education programs provides mental health workers for rural communities, the shortage of rural mental health workers requires that persons be trained specifically for placement in rural settings. Segal (1973) cites several training programs supported by NIMH; however, most of these programs were limited to field experiences or specialties within a program rather than giving primary focus to practice in rural settings.

A more recent study of the availability of rural mental health training programs is not optimistic about the growth and development of these programs. Munson (1980) found social work training programs to be concentrated in urban states, and Keller and Prutsman (in press) conclude that only a handful of training programs for psychologists prepare their graduates for work in rural communities. Also, Flax et al. (1979) report only two programs designed to train psychiatrists for practice in rural settings and find few publications regarding the training of nonpsychiatrist rural mental health professionals. In summary, the training of rural mental health professionals has had a tentative start and is only beginning to develop an identity of its own.

Paraprofessional Caregivers
and Natural Helpers

The shortage of mental health professionals in rural settings has been a stimulus to the training and utilization of paraprofessional caregivers.

Accounts of training programs and uses of paraprofessional caregivers are provided in several articles (Hollister, Bentz, Miller, Edgerton, & Aponte, 1973; Kelley, Kelley, Gauron, & Rawlings, 1977; Naftulin, Donnelly, & O'Halloran, 1974; Segal, 1973). These caregivers represent a wide variety of helpers, including apprentice Navajo medicine men, homemakers, school personnel, and the clergy. However, this literature is lacking in evaluative studies that assess the effectiveness of the paraprofessional caregivers.

On the other hand, mental health workers have been cautioned against intrusion into delicate natural helping networks. D'Augelli (in press) urges professional mental health workers to resist the temptation to mold indigenous helpers into urban-type psychotherapists, and Libertoff (1980) warns against interventions that upset the balance of these systems. Hanton (1980) is also concerned with the appropriate use of natural helpers and urges mental health workers to become familiar with community patterns for utilizing formal, informal, and natural helpers. The recommended relationship of the mental health worker to the natural helper is one of observation and support. This relationship is appropriate for gaining entry to a constant social system but presents a difficult task for the professional who expects to lead and direct.

Utilizing Community Resources

Faced with limited financial resources and a lack of trained personnel, the rural mental health worker must rely upon agencies and helpers already in the community. The general practitioner is one such community resource. Cooperative relationships between a mental health center and community physicians, reported by McConnell (1980), were shown to improve the services of the center to the community. Also, Clayton (1977) believes that the 1975 enactment of the Rural Health Initiatives (RHI) and Health Underserved Rural Areas (HURA) programs presents even greater possibilities for cooperation between mental health centers and medical services projects in rural areas.

The community school system provides another resource for extending the services of the mental health center. In a primary prevention program reported by Noonan and Thibault (1974), mental health workers recognized a relationship between school absenteeism and later emotional distress and worked with the school to improve school attendance. In another rural community psychologists went into the school to provide direct services to students (Solomon & Hiesberger, 1980).

Faced with financial and human resource limitations and folk culture preference for self-help, rural mental health workers have learned to utilize the resources of the community. The Prairie View Mental Health Center provides an example of community involvement through cooperation with community theater, services to schools, developing community leaders, and the training of ministers and personnel directors (Segal, 1973). Although few rural mental health centers are afforded the opportunities that Prairie View enjoys, utilization of community resources has become a way of life for most rural programs.

Summary

Flax et al. (1978, p. 7) asked, "How does one systematically and objectively *generalize* from this wealth of experience?" Generalization about the delivery of mental health services to rural people is also made difficult by variations in the ethnic and racial composition, the economic base, and the degree of isolation of rural communities. However, one factor shared by many rural communities is underservice by mental health workers. This is shown by studies of both the geographic distribution of mental health workers and the prevalence of emotional distress in rural and urban communities.

The correction of this underservice is progressing at a slow pace. Federal agencies have called attention to this problem but have not been able to secure legislation that will correct it. Also, mental health professionals at training facilities and in the field have moved slowly in establishing training programs for rural mental health workers and in designing and evaluating delivery systems that are sensitive to the rural community.

Notes

1. National Clearinghouse for Mental Health Information, Alcohol, Drug Abuse, and Mental Health Administration, National Institute of Mental Health, Rockville, Maryland 20857.

2. *Journal of Rural Community Psychology,* Fresno Campus of the California School of Professional Psychology, 1350 M Street, Fresno, California 93721.

References

Bentz, W. K., Edgerton, J. W., & Hollister, W. G. Rural leaders' perceptions of mental illness. *Hospital and Community Psychiatry,* 1971, 22, 143-145.

Blouch, R. G., & Snowden, L. R. *Toward the assimilation of mental health interventions by constant environment communities.* Manuscript submitted for publication, 1980.

Clayton, T. Conference report: Issues in the delivery of rural mental health services. *Hospital and Community Psychiatry,* 1977, 28, 673-676.

Cohen, J. Effects of distance on use of outpatient services in a rural mental health center. *Hospital and Community Psychiatry,* 1972, 23, 27-28.

Congressional Research Service. *Major legislation of Congress* (MCL-072). Washington, DC: Library of Congress, 1980.

Cumming, E., & Cumming, J. *Closed ranks—An experiment in mental health education.* Cambridge, MA: Harvard University Press, 1957.

D'Augelli, A. R. Future directions for paraprofessionals in rural mental health, or how to avoid giving indigenous helpers Civil Service ratings. In P. A. Keller & J. D. Murray (Eds.), *Handbook of rural community mental health.* New York: Human Sciences Press, in press.

Dillon, J. Community mental health in a rural community. In G. Caplan (Ed.), *American handbook of psychiatry* (Vol. II, 2nd ed.). New York: Basic Books, 1974.

Dohrenwend, B., & Dohrenwend, B. Psychiatric disorders in urban settings. In S. Arieti et al. (Eds.), *American handbook of psychiatry.* New York: Basic Books, 1972.

England, J. L., Gibbons, W. E., & Johnson, B. L. The impact of a rural environment on values. *Rural Sociology,* 1979, 44, 119-136.

Flax, J. W., Ivens, R. E., Wagenfeld, M. O., & Weiss, R. J. Mental health and rural America: An overview. *Community Mental Health Review,* 1978, 3(5/6), 1, 3-15.

Flax, J. W., Wagenfeld, M. O., Ivens, R. E., & Weiss, R. J. *Mental health and rural America: An overview and annotated bibliography* (NIMH Monograph, U.S. Department of Health, Education and Welfare Publication No. [ADM] 78-753). Washington, DC: Government Printing Office, 1979.

Gertz, B., Meider, J., & Pluckman, M. L. A survey of rural community mental health needs and resources. *Hospital and Community Psychiatry,* 1975, 26, 816-819.

Glenn, N. D., & Alston, J. P. Rural-urban differences in reported attitudes and behaviors. *Southwestern Social Science Quarterly,* 1967, 47, 381-400.

Hanton, S. Rural helping systems and family typology. *Child Welfare,* 1980, 59, 419-426.

Hines, F. K., Brown, D. L., & Zimmer, J. H. *Social and economic characteristics of the population in metro and non-metro counties, 1970* (Economic Research Service, U.S. Department of Agriculture, Agriculture Economic Report No. 272). Washington, DC: Government Printing Office, 1975.

Hollingsworth, R., & Hendrix, E. M. Community mental health in rural settings. *Professional Psychology,* 1977, 8, 232-238.

Hollister, W. G., Bentz, W. D., Miller, F. T., Edgerton, J. W., & Aponte, J. F. *Experiences in rural mental health IV: Strengthening existing resources—Helping the helpers.* Unpublished manuscript, 1973. (Available from W. G. Hollister, M.D., Division of Community Psychiatry, University of North Carolina, Chapel Hill, North Carolina 27514.)

Husani, B. A., & Neff, J. A. The prevalence of psychopathology in rural Tennessee and Oklahoma. In P. A. Keller & J. D. Murray (Eds.), *Handbook of rural community mental health.* New York: Human Sciences Press, in press.

Jason, L. A., & Glenwick, D. S. Urban and rural perspectives towards traditional and community-oriented mental health services in the schools: An initial investigation. *Journal of Community Psychology*, 1979, 7, 50-52.

Jeffrey, M. J., & Reeve, R. E. Community mental health services in rural areas: Some practical issues. *Community Mental Health Journal*, 1978, 14, 54-62.

Jones, J. D., Wagenfeld, M. O., & Robin, S. S. A profile of the rural community mental health center. *Community Mental Health Journal*, 1976, 12, 176-181.

Keller, P. A., & Murray, J. D. (Eds.). *Handbook of rural community mental health*. New York: Human Sciences Press, in press.

Keller, P. A., & Prutsman, T. D. Training for professional psychology in the rural community. In P. A. Keller & J. D. Murray (Eds.), *Handbook of rural community mental health*. New York: Human Sciences Press, in press.

Keller, P. A., Zimbelman, K. K., Murray, J. D., & Feil, R. N. Geographic distribution of psychologists in the northeastern United States. *Journal of Rural Community Psychology*, 1980, 1, 18-24.

Kelley, V. R., Kelley, P. L., Gauron, E. F., & Rawlings, E. I. Training helpers in rural mental health. *Social Work*, 1977, 22, 229-232.

Kelly, J. G. Naturalistic observations in contrasting social environments. In E. P. Willems & H. L. Raush (Eds.), *Naturalistic viewpoints in psychological research*. New York: Holt, Rinehart & Winston, 1969.

Lee, G. R., & Lassey, M. L. Rural-urban differences among the elderly: Economic, social, and subjective factors. *Journal of Social Issues*, 1980, 36, 62-73.

Lee, S. H., Gianturco, D. T., & Eisdorfer, C. Community mental health center accessibility: A survey of the rural poor. *Archives of General Psychiatry*, 1974, 31, 335-339.

Libertoff, K. Natural helping networks in rural youth and family services. *Journal of Rural Community Psychology*, 1980, 1, 4-27.

Link, B., & Dohrenwend, B. P. Formulation of hypotheses about the ratio of untreated to treated cases in the true prevalence studies of functional psychiatric disorders in adults in the United States. In B. P. Dohrenwend, B. S. Dohrenwend, M. S. Gould, B. Link, R. Neugebauer, & R. Wunseh-Hitzig (Eds.), *Mental illness in the United States*. New York: Praeger, 1980.

McConnell, S. C. A highlander hookup between psychologists and physicians. *Professional Psychology*, 1980, 11, 170-171.

Miner, H. The folk-urban continuum. In A. Etzioni & E. Etzioni (Eds.), *Social change—Sources, patterns and consequences*. New York: Basic Books, 1964.

Munson, C. E. Urban-rural differences: Implications for education and training. *Journal of Education for Social Work*, 1980, 16, 95-103.

Naftulin, D. N., Donnelly, F. A., & O'Halloran, P. B. Mental health courses as a facilitator for change in a rural community. *Community Mental Health Journal*, 1974, 10, 359-365.

National Institute of Mental Health. *New dimensions in mental health: A new day in rural mental health services* (NIMH Monograph, U.S. Department of Health, Education and Welfare Publication No. [ADM] 78-690). Washington, DC: Government Printing Office, 1978.

Noonan, J. R., & Thibault, R. Primary prevention in Appalachia, Kentucky: Peer reinforcement of classroom attendance. *Journal of Community Psychology*, 1974, 2, 260-264.

Ozarin, L. D. Federal perspectives: The activities of the National Institute of Mental Health in relation to rural mental health services. In P. A. Keller & J. D. Murray (Eds.), *Handbook of rural community mental health.* New York: Human Sciences Press, in press.

Ploch, L. A. The reversal in migration patterns Some rural development consequences. *Rural Sociology,* 1978, 43, 293-303.

President's Commission on Mental Health. *Report to the president of the President's Commission on Mental Health.* Washington, DC: Government Printing Office, 1978.

Richards, J. M., & Gottfredson, G. D. Georgraphic distribution of U.S. psychologists. *American Psychologist,* 1978, 33, 1-9.

Riggs, R. T., & Kugel, L. F. Transition from urban to rural mental health practice. *Social Casework,* 1976, 57, 562-567.

Segal, J. (Eds.). *The mental health of rural America: The rural programs of the National Institute of Mental Health* (NIMH Monograph, U.S. Department of Health, Education and Welfare Publication No. [HSM] 73-9035). Washington, DC: Government Printing Office, 1973.

Smith, L. W., & Petersen, K. K. Rural-urban differences in tolerance: Stouffer's "cultural schock" hypothesis revisited. *Rural Sociology,* 1980, 45, 256,-271.

Solomon, G., & Hiesberger, J. Community mental health in rural schools: A demonstration project. *Journal of Community Psychology,* 1980, 8, 353-356.

Srole, L. Urbanization and mental health: Some reformulations. *American Scientist,* 1972, 60, 576-583.

van Es, J. C., & Brown, J. R., Jr. The rural-urban variable once more: Some individual level observations. *Rural Sociology,* 1974, 39, 373-391.

Webb, S. D., & Collette, J. Rural-urban stress: New data and new conclusions. *American Journal of Sociology,* 1979, 84, 1446-1452.

Willits, F. K., Bealer, R. C., & Crider, D. M. The ecology of social traditionalism in a rural hinterland. *Rural Sociology,* 1974, 39, 334-342.

5

The New Chronic Patient

The Creation of an Underserved Population

Steven P. Segal
Jim Baumohl
University of California, Berkeley

Since 1955 the population of mental hospitals has been reduced from 560,000 to 148,000. However, 25 years into this noble experiment we have recognized a terrible problem. As elderly patients have been removed to nursing homes and similar institutions, state and county hospitals have been besieged with a growing population of younger patients, many of whom have become familiar, periodic guests. In this era of community care, these "new chronic patients" receive only "revolving door" treatment: They are hospitalized briefly, treated with major tranquilizers, and discharged. Their chronicity is defined not only by recurring episodes of disorder, but by long-term erratic use of community-based mental health services and inpatient facilities.

As the title of this chapter implies, we believe that changes in the care of the chronically mentally ill have created this new chronic population. This is not to say that deinstitutionalization has created mental disorder, but that reliance upon community care has changed the social circumstances and status of chronic patients. The decline of the hospital has recast the nature of chronicity, for, unlike chronic patients of 25 years ago, today's chronic patients must struggle to survive as free agents in local areas. They have no choice in this matter.

To be sure, there have always been chronically disordered individuals who have lived somewhat independently. Even in its heyday, the grasp of the asylum was not sure and some proportion of the chronically mentally ill lived with family or friends or drifted in the eddies of the homeless poor (Segal & Baumohl, in press). However, prior to 1963, when the community mental health movement gained enormous ground via the passage of the Community Mental Health Center and Facilities Construction Act

(P.L. 88-164), autonomous adaptation to chronic mental disorder was atypical. Now, the autonomy of the chronically disordered is an established fact of life to which the mentally ill and their potential benefactors must adjust. For better or for worse, the mental hospital no longer provides long-term life-sustaining services for the chronically disordered, nor does it offer easily accessible respite from the rigors of independent living, nor does it provide much treatment. These and other functions of the mental hospital have been left to community care.

The New Chronic Population

In some ways there is nothing new about today's chronic population. Like the chronic patients of 25 years ago, half are male and half are female, and their diagnoses span the full range of diagnostic categories (Miller, 1965; Pepper, Kirshner, & Ryglewicz, 1981). On the other hand, the characteristics of today's population reflect significant demographic changes in the American populace as a whole.

First of all, the new chronic population consists of people who are relatively young (average age about 35). This is due in part to the segregation of elderly patients in skilled nursing facilities, but it is also the result of the enormous "baby boom" birth cohort that is now passing through adulthood. Whereas the rate of mental hospital admission has remained constant among young adults, the size of this age group has grown tremendously, thus yielding a proportionately greater number of patients (Kramer, 1977).

Second, the number of nonwhites in the chronic population, especially among younger chronics, has increased for similar reasons. As the birthrate among nonwhites has been substantially higher than among whites, their representation as a percentage of the mentally ill population has increased along with their percentage of the total population (see Kramer, 1977).

Today's chronic patients also represent a generation of mental health clients whose relationships to the mental health system have been formed in an era of civil rights and consumerism. Few have experienced long-term hospitalization, and few exhibit the apathy, lack of initiative, or the resignation that numerous studies have found to characterize the long-term mental hospital resident. New chronic patients have not been socialized to docility, to the role of acquiescent mental patient, and they do not use mental health services in the docile fashion of their predecessors, but rather as wary consumers demanding response to their broad needs for social and economic support. Their demands for such services are quite appropriate, reflecting a perfectly normal response to their predicaments as chronically poor people and as people suffering from chronic emotional distress and disorder.

Numerous clinicians and researchers have also observed that today's chronic patients, especially in the younger age range (18-35), tend to resist the contention that they are mentally ill (see, for example, Pepper et al., 1981; Schwartz & Goldfinger, 1981; Segal, Baumohl, & Johnson, 1977). They often define their discomforture as derivative from their poverty or their isolation, or, in some cases, their denial is elaborately incorporated into a system of delusions. Thus they approach mental health services with mistrust and fear of confrontation about their psychiatric status.

Finally, the younger members of this new chronic population have the vices of their agemates, in particular their use of illegal drugs. Their sometimes prodigious consumption of street drugs complicates their psychiatric status, affects their social functioning, and makes them difficult and rebellious consumers of all mental health services (Pepper et al., 1981; Schwartz & Goldfinger, 1981; Segal & Baumohl, 1981).

In sum, today's chronic patients are younger, more contentious, and more diverse than their counterparts of 20 years ago, but most importantly they face a different set of social contingencies that have less to do with their different characteristics than with the fundamental reorientation of mental health services to the provision of community-based care. In the course of this reorientation the social and material support of chronic patients, previously provided by the mental hospital, have been neglected. Indeed, in some cases, the term "community care" has become a chilling euphemism for decentralized neglect. Let us now turn to an examination of the useful functions of the mental hospital and see how they have or have not been translated into community care for the benefit of today's chronic population.

Caring for the Individual

Inpatient Treatment

The first function of the mental hospital has been the provision of treatment that cannot be provided on an outpatient basis. However, during the past 25 years professional beliefs about the types of treatment that cannot be given on an outpatient basis have changed dramatically. There has also been growing awareness of the iatrogenic effects of long-term inpatient care.

The parameters of "institutionalization" have been outlined in the works of Barten (1966), Goffman (1961), Gruenberg (1967), and Hansell and Benson (1971). These writers have described the apathy, lack of initiative, inability to plan for the future, and sense of powerlessness—the resigned "settling in" (Segal & Moyles, 1979)—that have come to characterize the long-term mental hospital patient. Various studies have shown that the longer individuals stay in a hospital the less likely it is that they will *want* to leave (Wing, 1962) and the less likely it is that they *will* leave (Paul, 1969). Efforts to improve the hospital environment so as to ameliorate these effects have emphasized milieu treatment. Such intensive treatment programs have been shown to be effective in improving within-hospital adjustment and release rates, yet they have had little effect on posthospitalization outcomes (Fairweather, 1964; Sanders, Smith, & Weinman, 1967).

These findings strongly suggested that there was no carry-over of the effects of intensive, carefully designed hospital-based treatment programs. Exemplary inpatients failed in the community, thus raising serious questions about the location of social, psychological, and domiciliary care in hospital settings.

However, the efficacy of home care as an alternative is not universal. Three well-controlled landmark studies compared home and hospital treatment (Pasamanick, Scarpitti, & Dinitz, 1967; Langsley & Kaplan, 1968; Langsley, Machotka, & Flomemhaft, 1969, 1971; Rittenhouse, 1970). These studies concluded that home treatment was a viable alternative to hospital care *for a select group of patients* in that no obvious and negative differences could be discerned. Unfortunately, the characteristics of this select group of patients remained largely undefined.

The results of these and similar studies showing few differences between short- and long-term hospital treatment (Caffey, Jones, Diamond, Burton, & Bowen, 1968; Gove & Lubach, 1969; Weisman, Feinstein, & Thomas, 1969; Glick, Hargreaves, Drues, & Schourstack, 1976a, 1976b; Herz, Endicott, & Spitzer, 1977) have led to the conclusion that inpatient treatment should be limited in scope and differentially applied to the patient population. The use of high levels of antipsychotic medication during emergency admissions and the use of newer drugs requiring continuous observation for safe administration has become a primary rationale for the continued treatment function of the hospital. However, these medications may be unnecessary (Mosher & Menn, 1978) and even contraindicated (Crane, 1973; Goldstein, 1970; Rappaport, Hopkins, Hall, Belleya, & Silverman, 1974) for some portion of those admitted to the hospital.

In sum, various studies demonstrate the feasibility of nonhospital care, but emphasize that the necessity for treatment has not been eliminated. Although advances have been made in specifying the type of patient who can receive treatment outside the hospital—usually the young and less seriously disordered—even these people must receive continuous long-term support in the community if they are not to suffer severe setbacks resulting in a generally bleak downward spiral (see Segal & Baumohl, 1980). This point is underscored by the results of the five-year follow-up of the Pasamanick study group, in which it was found that differences between home treatment and hospital treatment disappeared over time, with many patients from both groups requiring repeated hospitalization (Davis, Dinitz, & Pasamanick, 1974).

As we move toward community care in the 1980s, deinstitutionalization cannot proceed effectively without the development of appropriate local treatment alternatives to address the deficiencies that disrupt effective behavior and that are associated with the progression of mental illness: lack of material resources, lack of appropriate skills, inadequate defenses, inadequate social supports, and lack of sustained motivation (Mechanic, 1978).

These five deficiencies are to some extent addressed by efforts at "training in community living" (Test & Stein, 1978) that have become the community care treatment focus of the 1980s. Stein, Test, and Marx (1975) and Test and Stein (1978) report findings on 130 admittable psychiatric patients. In a randomized trial 65 were assigned to the experimental program of training in community living (TCL) that used specially trained staff to promote daily activities in the community. A control group of 65 patients received short-term psychiatric hospital therapy in a unit with a high staff-to-patient ratio that offered partial hospitalization and aftercare. Patients were primarily young adults who had experienced a previous psychiatric hospitalization (mean duration, 14.6 months). Patients with severe organic brain syndrome or primary alcoholism were excluded. Global symptomatology ratings and 6 of 12 components of clinical assessment showed greater improvement in the TCL group. Further, the TCL group spent significantly more time than the control group living in independent settings, in sheltered employment, and in full-time competitive employment. The TCL group also had higher scores on a scale measuring satisfaction with their personal circumstances. No significant differences were found in time spent in medical penal, or supervised settings such as halfway houses, family care homes, and boarding homes.

Sheltered-living arrangements, day hospital treatment programs, halfway houses, psycho/social rehabilitation programs, and programs emphasizing community support and training in community living have been developed to prevent the deterioration of patients that occurs even in the absence of any negative influence of the mental hospital. Experimental programs have demonstrated either no difference or differences favoring the new experimental programs over traditional inpatient care. Still, while progress seems to have been made, conclusions must remain tentative for two reasons. First, the nature of the inpatient care provided in these experiments has been largely unspecified. This undermines any detailed comparison between inpatient and alternative treatment modes. Outcome, therefore, is not attributable to any specific treatment practices. Second, the blush of creativity present in alternative modes, as compared to the routinized practices of most inpatient care, may create a Hawthorne effect that accounts at least in part for observed outcomes.

Yet even if we assume the effectiveness of community programs, their success has been confined to select, apparently healthier, and younger population groups. Unfortunately, people admitted to the mental hospital today are more clearly dangerous to themselves or others, more gravely disabled, and more drug-involved, and they lack the social and material resources to gain admission to current "enriched" community treatment programs or to make it on their own. We have a long way to go before the availability of community-based services even begins to match the need for services traditionally offered in inpatient settings.

Protecting the Individual

The second function of the mental hospital has been to protect the individual from his or her own uncontrolled, self-endangering impulses or the consequences of his or her self-neglect. This justification for involuntary commitment has been challenged by U.S. civil rights activists who argue in favor of the individual's right to fail and the right to be different (Kittrie, 1971). With respect to self-neglect, formally construed as "grave disability," mental health professionals have been criticized for their arbitrary use of this commitment criterion (Warren, 1977, 1979). Definitions of who is gravely disabled and what constitutes grave disability appear to vary from hospital to hospital. Similarly, the prediction of self-endangerment is fraught with considerable error, thus allowing the retention of many people who are, in fact, not dangerous to themselves (Monahan, 1976). Consequently, some states have legislated stringent regulations concerning conditions under which an individual may be detained involuntarily due to mental disorder. These regulations limit the amount of time that individuals may be held involuntarily for treatment and/or protection against their own dangerous impulses or grave disability.

Further, federal courts have established minimum evidentiary requirements for involuntary commitment. In Addington v. Texas (1979) the chief justice of the Supreme Court of the United States ruled that evidence must be at minimum "clear and convincing" before an involuntary admission may be used in the case of an individual dangerous to her- or himself or gravely disabled. A recent federal district court ruling (Doe v. Gallinot, 1979) declared that any individual held by reason of grave disability due to mental disorder must receive a judicial hearing in order to be held beyond 72 hours. Thus the courts have expressed great skepticism about the clarity of admission criteria and continue to tighten procedural requirements for involuntary detainment. As these procedural requirements become more severe, the number of such admissions is reduced.

Judicial decisions and legislation have an immediate impact on community care. Aviram and Syme (1974) have shown that such decisions have been the most influential factors in the reduction of mental hospital populations and the restricted use of mental hospital beds. The medical director of psychiatric emergency at San Francisco General Hospital recently said: "When a patient came into the hospital after having slit his wrists in an obvious suicide attempt, I was unable to simply admit him I first had to find out if there was anyone he could stay with who could take care of him." Thus the hospital has become a "residual resource" of use only when the individual's problem cannot be resolved by other preferred means (Bittner, 1967).

The mental hospital's function as a residual resource is distinctly different from its previous function as a bed of last resort. In days past, the hospital functioned as a poorhouse, sheltering on thin pretext many of society's dispossessed. Today's hospital errs in the direction of underadmission, taking only those among a strictly limited, psychiatrically eligible population who have nowhere else to go and who, if found to be competent, cooperate with the hospital's effort to maintain them as inpatients. Competent and uncooperative or ambivalent patients now possess easily exercised rights to release, and these freedoms coincide exactly with administrative pressure to minimize the utilization of inpatient beds. There is, then, a happy coincidence between fiscal efficiency and the desires of the uncooperative patient, which, in the short run, suits the needs of the mental health system and the desires of the patient.

To the extent that other resources exist for the homeless poor and the mentally ill among them who resist patienthood, this is a humane development. However, in the absence of such resources this represents the abandonment of the social support and protection of extremely vulnerable individuals. In short, it is indicative of the mental health system's failure to reorient itself to the needs of its clientele prior to their complete deterioration.

The tragedy of hospitalization as a residual resource is not only that hospitalization is difficult under these circumstances, but that other preferred means are largely unavailable. A vacuum in community resources often leaves the individual in crisis utterly adrift and lends an aura of draconian indifference to the actions of the courts and legislatures. Crisis houses and community-based nonhospital facilities have been developed and funded in very few areas. Thus it is the family that is implicitly required to take responsibility for its disabled member. But are families ready to accept such responsibility?

Although only a few first admissions to mental hospitals are totally isolated or have little family support available to them, each progressive cohort of returns has a larger proportion of people with no family support or limited interaction with family members (Miller, 1965; Pasamanick et al., 1967; Davis et al., 1974). In a study of former mental patients, aged 18-65, living in community-based sheltered-care facilities in California, Segal and Aviram (1978) found that 52 percent of the residents rarely, if ever, had access to family members. In addition, 60 percent had never been married, and 35 percent had dissolved their relationships. When examined by sex, these figures revealed that 73 percent of the men, as opposed to 44 percent of the women, had never been married, 22 percent of the men and 50 percent of the women were either separated or divorced, and only 4 percent of the men and 5 percent of the women were currently married.

An important by-product of chronic mental disorder is attenuated family support. It seems extraordinarily naive to expect that family members can or will respond to the intermittant crises of *chronic* patients. In the absence of crisis houses the hospital has a key role to play in community care by managing the psychiatric emergencies created by self-endangerment and grave disability. In this capacity the local psychiatric hospital makes community care possible. However, it appears that in the immediate future the mental health professions must work with the courts to provide better and more consistent definitions of civil commitment criteria if this important function of the hospital is to be preserved. Further, inpatient care must be readily available on a basis that is both voluntary and acceptable to consumers who find the trade of freedom for treatment to be a frightening and onerous quid pro quo. Community care has absorbed a specific piece of the hospital's role in providing the bed of last resort. A whole system of community-based sheltered-care facilities, including halfway houses, board and care homes, and family care homes, has developed throughout the United States to support the adult mentally ill who do not have shelter. With the availability of funds from Titles 18 and 19 of the Social Security Act, the nursing home has taken responsibility for the care of the aged mentally ill, along with sheltered-care homes licensed specifically for the elderly and providing lower levels of nursing supervision.

However, sheltered care, while more diverse and flexible than hospital care, and while more workable for many of the chronically mentally ill, has inherent limitations common to all institutional care. No matter how "patient centered" and benign, sheltered care demands conformity to the basic requirements of group living and to law and propriety. Those of today's new chronics who are sexually active, drug-involved, or simply very private have difficulty adjusting to such demands. We have yet to devise much that is both useful and appealing to them.

In part as response to this problem there have been several joint housing and social services initiatives, such as that under a demonstration program for deinstitutionalization of the chronically mentally ill sponsored by the U.S. Department of Health and Human Services (DHHS) and the Department of Housing and Urban Development (HUD). These departments have funded almost 2000 housing units in the past 3 years. Community-based organizations are receiving nearly $20 million to sponsor housing for chronically mentally ill individuals. HUD direct-loan funds to nonprofit sponsors will pay for construction or rehabilitation of 621 housing units. These residential units will be either group homes serving up to 12 persons or small apartment complexes of up to 10 units (Social Legislation Information Services, 1980).

However, despite the 1975 amendments to the Community Mental Health Centers Act, which, among other things, called for more services to the poor and chronically mentally ill, and despite the 1978 recommendations of the President's Commission on Mental Health, which focused attention on housing problems, little has changed for the better. Indeed, in many cities the problem of homelessness has grown progressively worse as gentrification, nonresidential conversion, condominium conversion, and tourist hotel conversion have eroded the supply of units in rooming houses and single-room occupancy hotels (Silvern & Schmunk, 1981; Kowal, 1981; San Francisco Department of City Planning, 1980). The San Francisco Department of City Planning (1980, p. i) concludes: "If conversion continues at the same rate as the past five years, vacancies in hotels will disappear within one or two years." The department further notes:

> Given the limitation of social and economic resources, residential hotel tenants will be severely affected if their current homes are converted. . . . The proximity of the hotels to the downtown area, and the accessibility to a host of service agencies which are situated close to the hotels all provide an opportunity for the tenants, particularly the elderly and the handicapped, to live a relatively independent life [San Francisco Department of City Planning, 1980, p. 18].

It is imperative that immediate efforts be made to preserve existing low-income housing stock; however, the prospects are not good. Federal subsidies to individual renters and low-interest loans for rehabilitation to owners or community groups with master leases have been suspended or proposed for drastic reduction or elimination by the Reagan administration (State of California, Department of Housing and Community Development, 1981). The funds of local governments are for the most part extremely limited, and the prospect of private financing has been virtually eliminated by the high cost of debt service (Kowal, 1981). Thus the only road currently available appears to be that taken in San Francisco, where only litigation, civil disobedience, and prolonged and acrimonious debate produced a political compromise resulting in the contribution of preservation funds by several major hotel firms involved in conversion and demolition, their private developer, local banks, and the city and county governments.

In the absence of community housing, older institutions have filled the gap left by the demise of the state hospital. Most notably, and perhaps most problematically, jails house increasing numbers of the mentally ill. Jail administrators now frequently ask for funds to finance mental health services. These requests pose a dilemma, for to satisfy the jailers would be to encourage the development of services which, though needed, might lead to the development of total institutions for the mentally ill within the correctional system. This, of course, would be contrary to the philosophy of community care.

Forensic or "criminal justice mental health" units, whether in local hospitals or jails, are still rare, as are community-based sheltered-care facilities that will accept serious ex-offenders. The fate of mentally ill ex-offenders will not be determined only by the availability of resources, however, but by the interaction among the general public, the courts, and the mental health professions on the matters of dangerousness and culpability for wrongdoing. We will discuss these issues presently.

Sanctuary

The third function of the hospital has been to provide the individual with brief sanctuary from environmental stress. While this function of the hospital is still significant, pressures to reduce the use of inpatient care are eroding it. During the late 1950s and early 1960s, innovative state hospital programs such as that implemented by the Dutchess County Unit of Hudson River State Hospital in Poughkeepsie, New York, maintained as many as two-thirds of their inpatients in the community. This unit promoted an "easy-in and easy-out" policy through which the hospital supported its patients but did not necessarily house them. The program's major goal was to help patients maintain their role in the family and to provide them with a temporary respite from environmental stress. As a statistical reflection of this easy-in and easy-out policy on a nationwide basis, the number of hospital residents declined while the number of admissions increased (Kramer, 1977).

While the "revolving door" policy has been criticized severely, it did serve some patients very well. Now, with fewer patients admitted to the hospital, local areas must develop alternative settings to fulfill the hospital's previous function of sanctuary. Examples of such facilities are those provided by the organization called Families of Adult Schizophrenics. Their facilities cater particularly to the short-term needs of schizophrenic patients living at home.

Mental Illness and the Justification of Humane Care

The fourth function of the mental hospital has been as the seat of practice and research that has defined and promoted the ideology of mental illness and the attendant model of scientifically based medical care. The scientific vagaries of theories of mental disorder have been oft analyzed (see Szasz, 1961; Scheff, 1966) and the medical model of diagnosis and treatment has been thoroughly worked over by numerous critics (see Rosenhan, 1973). Nonetheless, the ideology of mental illness, for better or worse, couches its explanations in the neutral language of disease and lifts an oppressive burden of culpability from the afflicted individual. Further, even in its purely custodial capacity, the mental hospital, in the tradition of medical care, has provided a more humane form of quarantine than existed in poorhouses, jails, and other repositories for the deviant and the outcast.

The decline of the mental hospital has been accompanied by an erosion of belief in the reality of nonorganically diagnosed mental disease. How widespread this belief ever became in the United States is a matter of conjecture, but its political potency appears to be ebbing (Benson, 1980), especially as more sensational crimes are attributed to those claimed to be disturbed and thus unfit for retribution (Sosowsky, 1978, 1980), and as more expert psychiatric witnesses contradict each other in the public theater of the courtroom. Thus the ideology of mental illness is in vulnerable disarray. Its epistemology is in question; its methods are of variable effectiveness. In short, there is no elegant cloak of comforting theory and practice to shield the mentally ill from accusations of premeditated evil and full human responsibility.

This development does not indicate that Americans have returned to a view of the mentally ill as incarnations of evil. It does, however, presage a more legalistic view of the mentally ill that presumes reason over delusion unless proven otherwise. As a result, the courts and the legislatures have become the principal arbiters of the madman's identity. As noted above, the courts have limited available involuntary treatment, and legislatures, by limiting all inpatient bed utilization, have indirectly handicapped the provision of voluntary care. Combined with the inadequate development of community-based alternatives, the result has been the accumulation of the mentally ill in settings such as jails and transient shelters where humane care is either a contradiction in terms or a financial impossibility.

The principle of humane care is founded upon the belief that all people ought to have the opportunity to experience life in all its richness, including its joys and, to some extent, its pains. But most importantly, humane care is founded upon a belief in self-direction. This includes the right to make decisions about use of time, privacy, and personal possessions, the right to fail in ways that are not severely self-destructive, and the chance to attribute success or failure to one's own efforts. While grounded in the ethic of self-sufficiency, the principle of humane care provides for the exception of certain people from the expectation of self-support and offers, instead, a regimen of kindness intended to allow them to function with whatever independence they can achieve.

The medical conceptualization of mental illness provided a scientific rationale for the exceptional status of the mentally ill and, as a consequence, an elaborate scientific approximation of humane care largely focused on the provision of treatment, sanctuary, and protection within a hospital setting. Moreover, the notion of mental disorder as a potentially chronic disease provided a basis for long-term substitutive care, or the consistent provision of the rudiments of survival over the course of a patient's life.

In theory, the community mental health movement is based on the principle of humane care. It is designed to promote this principle with an array of services that might be classified as supportive and substitutive. The supportive services are designed to maintain people in their social roles in their own homes. They include outpatient services (such as counseling, psychotherapy, and social casework in the form of evaluation), case management, crisis intervention, medication prescription and supervision, and vocational and rehabilitation services. Substitutive services involve the provision of community-based sheltered care in the least restrictive environment. This involves the provision of an alternative supervised home environment with limitations, in theory, designed to allow individuals to maintain the maximum degree of independence of which they are capable. These facilities include—in order of their legal abilities to impose physical restrictions on their residents—the mental hospital (full-time inpatient care or partial hospitalization, involving weekend, evening, or daytime stays), the locked crisis and long-term care facilities, the treatment-oriented halfway house, and the board and care, or unlocked, nursing home.

Unfortunately, the decline of the ideology of mental illness and its implicit recognition of chronicity has undermined provisions for long-term substitutive care. There was promise offered by provisions in the 1975 amendments to the Community Mental Health Centers legislation, the recommendations of the President's Commission on Mental Health (1978), and the Mental Health Systems Act signed into law October 7, 1980. The thrust of these measures would have been to develop the community-based alternatives that would adequately transfer the important substitutive care functions of the mental hospital to local facilities. That such humane care functions for long-term patients may be adequately fulfilled outside the hospital is indicated by the results of studies by Brown, Bone, Dalison, and Wing (1966), Marx, Test, and Stein (1973) and Linn, Caffey, and Klett (1977). However, programs proposed under the Systems Act exist largely on paper due to lack of funds, although there have been encouraging program reorientations by some community mental health centers with sufficient financial flexibility. However, the Reagan administration's block grant proposals, which in effect would constitute a repeal of the Mental Health Systems Act, may lead to the elimination of efforts to provide for more diverse and effective forms of substitutive care.

Serving the Community

Protection Against Danger

An important service performed by the hospital for the community has been to protect it from individuals thought to be dangerous. In this respect the mental hospital and the jailhouse have been perennial competitors for the custody of a sizable group of individuals who, in addition to whatever mental disorders they may suffer, commit belligerent or antisocial acts that warrant confinement.

There is extreme difficulty in defining jurisdictions in this area. As we have noted, the ideology of mental illness and its derivative methods of practice have provided neither a consistent explanation of nor a satisfactory solution to disruptive or threatening behavior, especially insofar as drug dependency, alcoholism, and personality or character disorders are concerned. Indeed, as Rabkin (1979) observes, it appears that "antisocial behavior and mentally ill behavior apparently coexist, particularly among young, unmarried, unskilled, poor males, especially those belonging to ethnic minorities." Thus agents of the mental health and criminal justice systems wrangle among themselves to determine which members of this unpopular group belong in which custodial facility. As a practical matter, decisions are made on a case-by-case basis and are influenced by available bed space in hospitals and jails, the procedural dilemmas of backlogged courts, and the sensibilities of particular judges, police officers, and psychiatric emergency room personnel. It is a sorting process that, if not purely random, lacks procedural coherence.

It has been this lack of procedural consistency in the protection of individual civil rights that has prompted the courts to limit the involuntary hospitalization of the gravely disabled. In combination with legislatively ordained limits on hospital utilization, this has narrowed the field of eligible hospital residents, often to those in a "present state of dangerousness" whose recent threat or attack upon another individual is thought to be due to mental disorder. These are often the individuals described by Rabkin (1979), who have past histories of arrest and who personify the prevailing jurisdictional dilemma in that they are veterans of both systems of control. When their viciousness is attributable to mental disorder they are hositalized; when it is attributable to a nonpathological orneriness, they are jailed. It is not surprising, then, that the criminal justice system is concerned with "mental cases" in its midst and the mental health system is distraught over the growing proportion of inpatients with records of arrest for serious crimes.

The large proportion of inpatients with previous arrest records has also created a serious political problem for proponents of community care. In addition to the widely publicized, hideous crimes committed by a few expatients, there have been several studies that demonstrate that ex-patients are more likely, as a group, to be a threat to the community than other residents (for a review, see Rabkin, 1979). However, the composition of the inpatient group has been changed drastically by different patterns of hospital utilization. A greater proportion of current patients are young, male, and members of ethnic minorities (Kramer, 1977). Thus this discernible greater threat issues from a more concentrated group of individuals whose lives have been spent in the badlands between poverty and the mental health and criminal justice systems.

The problem for proponents of community care concerns whether or not to abandon this group of people to a custodial institution under one or another auspice. Clearly, this tortuous interplay between the criminal justice and mental health systems affects that group of people who, as we have seen, are least likely to be acceptable to or successful in community-based alternative treatment. Their presence in the community under current circumstances seems to pose a real threat and comes at the expense of the social group. On the other hand, most of these individuals are not dangerous and those who may be are not predictable as such (Monahan, 1976). It is a case in which the continued confinement of many is necessary to prevent the damage caused by a few. Livermore, Malmquist, and Jeehl (1968) put it well:

Assume that one person out of a thousand will kill. Assume, also, an exceptionally accurate criterion is created which differentiates with 95% effectiveness those who will kill from those who will not. If 100,000 people were tested, out of the hundred who would kill, 95 would be isolated. Unfortunately, out of the 99,900 who would not kill, 4995 people would also be isolated as potential killers.

In short, community care has not and probably cannot replace the hospital's function of quarantining dangerous individuals. However, the interplay between the mental health and criminal justice systems may be the single most important issue in community care today, for public perceptions of dangerousness attributable to former patients at large can be mobilized politically to affect the character of specific treatment modes (Robles, 1981) and to restrict the liberty of former patients in general. Whereas the courts have recently issued many libertarian decisions, the populace has not changed its mind much about the threat associated with mental illness, and does not make the distinction between association and causation in implicating mental disorder in the increased actuarial risk of dangerous behavior observed in the group of individuals released from today's mental hospitals. This group is not representative of the mentally ill in general, but, given current restrictions on hospital admissions, represents a small, exceedingly troubled and troublesome subgroup that bears only a demographic resemblance to the total population of the mentally ill.

Protection of the Family

The second major function of the hospital in service to the community has been the protection of the family. Now, for the first time in 150 years, the burden of care has been transferred back to the family. The United States has for all intents and purposes abandoned the Mann-Dix doctrine of *parens patriae* in the care of the mentally ill. Is the family ready to accept such responsibility? What will be the impact of this responsibility on the family system and on the long-term adjustment of the patient to the community?

These issues have been discussed in some detail elsewhere (see Segal, 1979). It has also been noted that, especially for chronic mental patients, only a limited amount of support from family members can be expected. Yet research does indicate that when the family is available the attitudes of its members toward released patients are significantly better than those found among the general population (Phillips, 1963; Schwartz, Myers, & Astrachan, 1974; Swanson & Spitzer, 1970); that family members are often willing to take the former patient back into their home, though their enthusiasm is dampened considerably when the ill family member is severely symptomatic (Freeman & Simmons, 1963; Doll, 1976); and that family members tend to underestimate the actual costs to the family of having their relative at home (Hoenig & Hamilton, 1969).

From the perspective of the patient, research shows that the family home is not always the best place to be. For many, a destructive interaction pattern has developed within the family, and the critical goals of preventing the patient's chronic social disability and institutionalism are not attainable within the family context (Brown, Birley, & Wing, 1972).

Thus community care faces, once again, the problem of tailoring the most appropriate response for different types of patients. For many, community care must provide support within the family context through the outreach efforts of community mental health centers. For others, placement outside the family in a sheltered-care facility seems most appropriate. In the interim, several voluntary organizations of family members of ex-patients have been formed to fill service gaps that they now experience, for current services do not provide the discriminating responses that research has indicated are so necessary to an effective system of community care.

Conclusion

The mental hospital has been a great procrustean bed that many patients could neither like nor leave. Community care, on the other hand, holds enormous potential for diversity, for tailoring services to the needs and tastes of an ex-patient population as various as the American people. So it seems in the mind's eye. At this writing, however, community care has been slow to unfold its dazzling, multicolored wings. Paradoxically, a concoction of people of vision and people of parsimony, it has coughed and sputtered from the outset, an expensive creation of a frugal era. Like our War on Poverty, it has been programmed for failure by a government enamored of an idea but unprepared to pay for its realization.

However, a lack of money is not the only substantial impediment to community care. There has been a major flaw in its implementation: the failure to reorient the mental health system to the social and economic needs of its consumers.

Since the codification of the Mann/Dix doctrine in the New York State Care Act of 1890, which guaranteed complete state care for the seriously mentally ill, the state has been in the business of providing a home for chronic mental patients. From the outset the terms of this obligation have focused upon the rudiments for survival: food, shelter, clothing, and, of course, "humane care" or simple human kindness. In the mental hospital, in the bosom of *parens patriae*, the children of chaos were to find an orderly parental household where the bills were paid and brows were cooled with kind attention. Such a relationship between the state and the mentally ill has, until very recently, assumed a degree of ready dependence on the part of the patient, who, by forfeiting his or her autonomy, could be assured of stability and security through the medium of a ready-made home.

The hospital was a monolithic institution that covered all needs from birth to burial. The community mental health system that has replaced it is a threadbare and patchwork system of supportive and substitutive services. Unfortunately, this system of community-based mental health services was developed on the assumption that it could rely on competent and cooperative patients whose primary needs would be supportive in nature. It has invested most of its efforts in supportive services, focusing progressively fewer of its new resources on substitutive services. It has, until recently, denied the need for long-term substitutive care, and now finds itself confronted with a population of militant consumers whose needs are exactly the opposite of its investment, whose demands for services are not always put cooperatively, and whose needs, because of the reversed priorities in the system, cannot be fulfilled given the resources available to mental health practitioners.

To remedy these problems we must emphasize services that begin with the dilemmas of clients, thereby placing their lack of material resources and social skills and supports in the forefront of mental health service priorities. Specifically, we must (1) treat clients while training them for community living; (2) protect them by making the process of emergency hospitalization less threatening and by making crisis facilities more available to provide voluntary treatment or respite care that would prevent the erosion of resources; (3) provide sanctuary via brief and long-term sheltered-living situations; (4) maintain the system's emphasis on the protection of civil rights, thereby enabling clients to take full advantage of the community to meet their own particular needs; and (5) ensure the continued commitment of the family as a major source of social support by developing more adequate respite resources and independent living situations.

In a system of mental health care in which coerced compliance is impossible, it is essential to engage clients in a cooperative effort to cope with their disorders. This can be achieved only by aligning the priorities of mental health care with the most important needs of its consumers

Today's chronic patients are not only chronically disordered, but chronically poor. This is a direct result of changes in our system of mental health care, and we must accept this responsibility and remedy our neglect.

References

Addington v. State of Texas. 441 U.S. 418, 99 S. Ct. 1804, 1979.

Aviram, U., & Syme, L. *The effects of policy decisions and administrative programs on mental health hospitalization trends.* Paper presented at the Fifth International Congress of Social Psychiatry, Athens, Greece, September 1974.

Barton, R. *Institutional neurosis.* Bristol: John Wright & Sons, 1966.

Benson, P. Labeling theory and community care of the mentally ill in California. *Human Organization,* 1980, 39, 134-141.

Bittner, E. Police discretion in emergency apprehension of mentally ill persons. *Social Problems,* 1967, 14, 278-292.

Brown, G. W., Birley, J.L.T., & Wing, J. K. Influence of family life in the course of schizophrenic disorders: A replication. *British Journal of Psychiatry,* 1972, 121, 241-258.

Brown, G. W., Bone, M., Dalison, B., & Wing, J. K. *Schizophrenia and social care.* London: Oxford University Press, 1966.

Caffey, E. M., Jones, R. D., Diamond, L. S., Burton, E., & Bowen, W. T. Brief hospital treatment of schizophrenia—Early results of a multiple hospital study. *Hospital and Community Psychiatry,* 1968, 19, 282-287.

Crane, G. Clinical psychopharmacology in its 20th year. *Science,* 1973, 181, 124-128.

Davis, A. E., Dinitz, S., & Pasamanick, B. *Schizophrenics in the new custodial community.* Columbus: Ohio State University Press, 1974.

Doe v. Gallinot. 486 U.S. 983, 1979.

Doll, W. Family coping with the mentally ill: An unanticipated problem of deinstitutionalization. *Hospital and Community Psychiatry,* 1976, 27, 183-185.

Fairweather, G. W. (Ed.). *Social psychology in treating mental illness.* New York: John Wiley, 1964.

Freeman, H., & Simmons, O. *The mental patient comes home.* New York: John Wiley, 1963.

Glick, I. D., Hargreaves, W. A., Drues, J., & Schourstack, J. A. Short versus long hospitalization: A prospective controlled study. IV. One-year follow-up results for schizophrenic patients. *American Journal of Psychiatry,* 1976, 133, 509-514. (a)

Glick, I. D., Hargreaves, W. A., Drues, J., & Schourstack, J. A. Short versus long hospitalization: A prospective controlled study. V. One-year follow-up results for non-schizophrenic patients. *American Journal of Psychiatry,* 1976, 133, 515-517. (b)

Goffman, E. *Asylums.* Garden City, NY: Doubleday, 1961.

Goldstein, M. Premorbid adjustment, paranoid status, and patterns of response to phenothiazine in acute schizophrenia. *Schizophrenia Bulletin,* 1970, 3, 24-37.

Gove, W., & Lubach, J. E. An intensive treatment program for psychiatric inpatients: A description and evaluation. *Journal of Health and Social Behavior,* 1969, 10, 225-236.

Gruenberg, E. The social breakdown syndrome: Some origins. *American Journal of Psychiatry,* 1967, 123, 1481-1489.

Hansell, N., & Benson, M. L. Interrupting long-term patienthood: A cohort study. *Archives of General Psychiatry,* 1971, 24, 238-243.

Herz, M. T., Endicott, J., & Spitzer, R. L. Brief hospitalization: A two year follow up. *American Journal of Psychiatry,* 1977, 134, 502-507.

Hoenig, J., & Hamilton, M. *The desegregation of the mentally ill.* London: Routledge & Kegan Paul, 1969.

Kittrie, N. *The right to be different.* Baltimore: Johns Hopkins Press, 1971.

Kowal, C. *Financing residential hotel improvements: National case studies and approaches.* Paper presented at the conference on Residential Hotels: A Vanishing Housing Resource. San Francisco, June 11-12, 1981.

Kramer, M. *Psychiatric services and the changing institutional scene, 1950-1985.* Rockville, MD: U.S. Department of Health, Education and Welfare, 1977.

Langsley, D. G., & Kaplan, D. M. *The treatment of families in crisis.* New York: Grune & Stratton, 1968.

Langsley, D. G., Machotka, P., & Flomemhaft, K. Follow up evaluation of family crisis therapy. *American Journal of Orthopsychiatry,* 1969, 39, 753-759.

Langsley, D. G., Machotka, P., & Flomemhaft, K. Avoiding mental hospital admission: A follow up study. *American Journal of Psychiatry,* 1971, 127, 1391-1394.

Linn, M. W., Caffey, E. M., & Klett, C. J. Hospital vs. community (foster) care for psychiatric patients. *Archives of General Psychiatry,* 1977, 34, 78-83.

Livermore, J. M., Malmquist, C. P., & Jeehl, P. E. On the justifications for civil commitment. *University of Pennsylvania Law Review,* 1968, 117, 75-96.

Marx, A. J., Test, M. A., & Stein, L. I. Extra-hospital management of severe mental illness. *Archives of General Psychiatry,* 1973, 29, 505-511.

Mechanic, D. Alternatives to mental hospital treatment: A sociological perspective. In L. Stein & M. A. Test (Eds.), *Alternatives to mental hospital treatment.* New York: Plenum, 1978.

Miller, D. *Worlds that fail.* Sacramento: California State Department of Mental Hygiene, 1965.

Monahan, J. The prevention of violence. In J. Monahan (Ed.), *Community mental health and the criminal justice system.* New York: Pergamon, 1976.

Mosher, L., & Menn, A. Lowered barriers in the community: The Soteria model. In L. Stein & M. A. Test (Eds.), *Alternatives to mental hospital treatment.* New York: Plenum, 1978.

Pasamanick, B., Scarpitti, F., & Dinitz, S. *Schizophrenics in the community.* New York: Appleton-Century-Crofts, 1967.

Paul, G. L. Chronic mental patients: Current status—future directions. *Psychological Bulletin,* 1969, 71, 81-94.

Pepper, B., Kirshner, M. C., & Ryglewicz, H. The young adult chronic patient: Overview of a population. *Hospital and Community Psychiatry,* 1981, 32, 463-469.

Phillips, D. Rejection: A possible consequence of seeking help for mental disorders. *American Sociological Review,* 1963, 28, 962-963.

Rabkin, J. G. Criminal behavior of discharged mental patients: A critical appraisal of the research. *Psychological Bulletin,* 1979, 36, 1-27.

Rappaport, M., Hopkins, H., Hall, K., Belleya, T., & Silverman, J. *Selective drug utilization in the management of psychosis.* Progress report, National Institute of Mental Health Grant 16445.

Rittenhouse, J. D. *Without hospitalization: An experimental study of psychiatric care in the home.* Unpublished manuscript, 1970.

Robles, N. *From the therapeutic to custodialism.* Unpublished doctoral dissertation, University of California, Berkeley.

Rosenhan, D. L. On being sane in insane places. *Science,* 1973, 179, 250-258.

Sanders, R., Smith, R. S., & Weinman, B. S. *Chronic psychosis and recovery.* San Francisco: Jossey-Bass, 1967.

San Francisco Department of City Planning. *The conversion and demolition of residential hotel units.* San Francisco: Author, 1980.

Scheff, J. J. *Being mentally ill: A sociological theory.* Chicago: Aldine, 1966.

Schwartz, C., Myers, J., & Astrachan, B. Psychiatric labeling and the rehabilitation of the mental patient. *Archives of General Psychiatry,* 1974, 31, 329-334.

Schwartz, S. R., & Goldfinger, S. M. The new chronic patient: Clinical characteristics of an emerging sub-group. *Hospital and Community Psychiatry,* 1981, 32, 470-474.

Segal, S. P. Community care and deinstitutionalization: A review. *Social Work,* 1979, 24, 521-527.

Segal, S. P., & Aviram, U. *The mentally ill in community based sheltered care.* New York: John Wiley, 1978.

Segal, S. P., & Baumohl, J. Engaging the disengaged: Proposals on madness and vagrancy. *Social Work,* 1980, 25, 358-365.

Segal, S. P., & Baumohl, J. *No place like home: Sheltering a diverse population.* Keynote address, New York State Department of Mental Hygiene, Spring Conference, Wards Island, New York, June 4, 1981.

Segal, S. P., & Baumohl, J. *The mentally ill and the homeless poor.* In press.

Segal, S. P., Baumohl, J., & Johnson, E. Falling through the cracks: Mental disorder and social margin in a young vagrant population. *Social Problems,* 1977, 24, 387-400.

Segal, S. P., & Moyles, E. W. Management style and institutional dependency in sheltered care. *Social Psychiatry,* 1979, 14, 159-165.

Silvern, P. J., & Schmunk, R. *Residential hotels in Los Angeles: A case of benign neglect.* Paper presented at the conference on Residential Hotels: A Vanishing Housing Resource, San Francisco, June 11-12, 1981.

Social Legislation Information Services. Housing assistance program reauthorized and monitored new grants stress housing, social service coordination. *Washington Social Legislation Bulletin,* 1980, 26, 181-184.

Sosowsky, L. Crime and violence among mental patients reconsidered in view of the new legal relationship between the state and the mentally ill. *American Journal of Psychiatry,* 1978, 135, 33-42.

Sosowsky, L. Explaining the increased arrest rate among mental patients: A cautionary note. *American Journal of Psychiatry,* 1980, 137, 1602-1605.

State of California, Department of Housing and Community Development. *Residential hotel rehabilitation demonstration: A progress summary.* Sacramento: Author.

Stein, L. I., Test, M. A., & Marx, A. J. Alternative to the hospital: A controlled study. *American Journal of Psychiatry,* 1975, 132, 517-532.

Swanson, R., & Spitzer, S. Stigma and the psychiatric patient career. *Journal of Health and Social Behavior,* 1970, 11, 44-51.

Szasz, T. *The myth of mental illness.* New York: Harper & Row, 1961.

Test, M. A., & Stein, L. I. The clinical rationale for community treatment. In L. I. Stein & M. A. Test (Eds.), *Alternatives to mental hospital treatment.* New York: Plenum, 1978.

Warren, C. Involuntary commitment for mental disorder. *Law and Society,* 1977, 11, 629-649.

Warren, C. The social construction of dangerousness. *Urban Life,* 1979, 8, 359-384.

Weisman, G., Feinstein, A., & Thomas, C. Three day hospitalization: A model for intensive intervention. *Archives of General Psychiatry,* 1969, 21, 620-629.

Wing, J. K. Institutionalism in mental hospitals. *British Journal of Social and Clinical Psychology,* 1962, 1, 38-51.

PART II

UNDERSERVED ETHNIC GROUPS

6

Raza Populations

Manuel Barrera, Jr.
Arizona State University

When the Community Mental Health Centers Act was signed by President Kennedy in 1963, one of its effects was to establish mental health care as a civil right (Bloom, 1977). Not only were comprehensive mental health services to be provided independently of one's ability to pay, but centers were viewed as having a responsibility to act affirmatively in reaching out to those segments of the community who were in greatest need of mental health care. There was also a concomitant concern for equal opportunity hiring practices that would provide opportunities for ethnic minority professionals and paraprofessionals to serve as staff members of these centers. It was no accident of history that this act came in close temporal proximity to the Civil Rights and Economic Opportunities Acts of 1964. These three acts had common origins in the recognition that inequities existed in the distribution of goods, services, and opportunities across the diverse racial and socioeconomic strata of our country. Mental health took its place alongside education, employment, housing, and criminal justice as key targets for public scrutiny and change.

With this federal legislation serving as the backdrop, the stage was set for historical have-nots such as ethnic minorities to forcefully ask the question of the decade: "Are we getting our fair share of the action?" It was predictable that as Chicanos we would eventually come to examine mental health practices to determine the extent to which we received services and participated professionally in the delivery of these services.

AUTHOR'S NOTE: This chapter was completed while the author was partially supported by a Faculty Development Fellowship awarded by Arizona State University. Appreciation is extended to Martha Bernal and Amado Padilla for their permission to reprint Table 6.1, and to Ricardo F. Muñoz for his review of an earlier version of the manuscript.

Prior to 1970, the mental health of La Raza was rarely a topic of research or discussion in the behavioral science literature (Padilla, Olmedo, Lopez, & Perez, 1978). During the past decade this situation has improved substantially, to the point where mental health has emerged as one of the most popular topics of behavioral research on Raza populations. The purpose of the present review is to bring together recent studies that are related to the mental health of Mexican Americans and other Hispanic subgroups, to summarize what we know from this literature, and to highlight what I feel are the critical mental health issues currently confronting Raza communities. First the often-reviewed literature on Mexican American mental health service utilization will be examined. An analysis of previous reviews will serve as a departure point for considering more recent work on factors that are thought to influence Chicanos' use of these services. In contrast to these traditional mental health topics, the closing section of the chapter advocates a more fundamental and broad-based analysis of "mental health" issues that confront Mexican Americans. This approach would call for "mental health" professionals to work on problems related to education, labor, housing, political participation, and other nontraditional topics, rather than to continue to emphasize mental health services and their utilization.

A Review of Reviews

The interest in Mexican American mental health service utilization has resulted in at least seven distinct literature reviews in the past decade (Acosta, 1979a; Barrera, 1978; Griffith, 1981; Keefe & Casas, 1980; Lopez, 1981; Padilla, Ruiz, & Alvarez, 1975; Ramirez, 1980). For the most part these reviews have jointly examined the evidence regarding the relative use of services by Mexican Americans, as well as factors hypothesized to explain the resultant utilization patterns. Some of the reviews have had special emphases or limitations in their scope. For example, Lopez's (1981) analysis focuses almost exclusively on the underutilization question. In contrast, Keefe and Casas (1980) discuss assumptions regarding Mexican Americans' mental health without explicitly evaluating the plausibility of these assumptions for explaining utilization. In addition to examining utilization patterns and their possible causes, Padilla et al.'s (1975) paper includes sections that describe innovative treatment models for improving mental health services to Hispanics. There is a degree of cross-referencing among these reviews, yet several of them were apparently written independently of each other. Comparing these reviews reveals several points on which there is considerable agreement, as well as those issues that are more controversial.

Do Mexican Americans Underutilize Mental Health Services?

Reviews have consistently cited numerous studies that found underutilization of mental health services by Mexican Americans or Hispanics. In my earlier literature review (Barrera, 1978), I note that underutilization was reported in California state services (Karno & Edgerton, 1969), a San Jose mental health center (Torrey, 1973), Denver facilities (Kline, 1969), Colorado and New Mexico (Weaver, 1973), Texas state hospitals (Pokorney & Overall, 1970), and Seattle mental health agencies (Sue, Allen, & Conaway, 1978). Furthermore, a national survey of state and county inpatient services found that "Spanish Americans" had lower utilization rates than other whites or nonwhites (Bachrach, 1975). Despite agreement among these studies, the picture is not a simple one. Studies of the *incidence* of treated disorders in *public* facilities did not report lower utilization rates for Mexican Americans (Bloom, 1975; Jaco, 1960; Wignall & Koppin, 1967). In addition, some reviews describe innovative practices on the part of mental health facilities (for example, Karno & Morales, 1971; Phillipus, 1971) that appeared to result in increased utilization by Chicano consumers.

Lopez (1981) recently conducted a comprehensive review of mental health service use by Mexican Americans that includes studies that had not been reviewed previously. His analysis is noteworthy in that it spans three decades, draws distinctions between studies of single and multiple institutions, and deals strictly with Mexican-American consumers (as opposed to Hispanics more generally). Based on the findings of over 40 studies reported in 27 papers, it is clear that underutilization has not been reported consistently, particularly in the last decade of research. Of the reports that appeared between 1960 and 1970, 11 indicate underutilization by Mexican Americans, while 2 show proportional utilization or overutilization. In the period between 1970 and 1980, there are 15 studies that show underutilization, but 16 report representative utilization or overutilization.

From these analyses of the literature, there is no question that Mexican Americans have underutilized mental health facilities in a number of locales. It is also clear, however, that there have been a number of exceptions to this pattern. Ethnicity, in and of itself, was not a reliable predictor of utilization across the considerable diversity of treatment settings, consumers, and locations that were included in the studies reviewed.

Mediators of Service Use

There is considerable agreement on the factors that reviewers have selected to discuss as possible mediators of Mexican Americans' service use. Many of these factors, including those that were originally listed by Karno and Edgerton (1969), have been reorganized into major categories:

(1) lower "true incidence/prevalence" of mental disorder
    (a) preventive influence of natural support systems, particularly the family
    (b) preventive effects of community (barrio) integration
(2) Use of non-mental health services
    (a) physicians
    (b) natural support system members (such as family members, compadres, other friends)
    (c) curanderos
    (d) priests
    (e) prisons
    (f) drug-abuse treatment facilities
(3) person variables
    (a) tolerant criteria for perceiving and labeling disorder
    (b) negative attitudes toward mental health professionals and facilities
    (c) lack of knowledge about available services
(4) service variables
    (a) physically inaccessible facilities
    (b) language/culture of therapists and staff different
    (c) inadequate treatment modalities

The suggestion that Chicanos actually manifest lower "true" rates of mental disorder is not accepted by a single reviewer, although it is generally acknowledged that this question had not been studied adequately at the time of the reviews. Jaco's (1960) survey of mental disorder in Texas was typically cited as the original source of this suggestion, but it should be recalled that Jaco used treatment rates as the basis for his analysis and eventual conclusions. By the conclusion of this chapter, one point should become completely clear: Relying on treatment data to determine the incidence or prevalence of psychiatric disorder among Mexican Americans is questionable, since it is unlikely that existing ser vices are as available to and relevant to the needs of Mexican Americans as they are to other groups.

Person variables, particularly attitudes toward mental health, were not viewed by most reviewers as being important factors leading to the underuse of services by Mexican Americans. The few studies conducted on the topic fail to show that Chicanos held negative perceptions of mental health professionals or services. Following their survey of over 200 Euro-American and 400 Mexican American residents of Los Angeles, Karno and Edgerton (1969, p. 237) comment, "Our initial analyses indicated that there are remarkably few statistically significant differences between the interview responses of Mexican Americans and Anglos involving perceptions and definitions of mental illness." In an analogue study of college students' perceptions of therapists who differed in ethnicity (Mexican or Euro-American) and professional status (professional or nonprofessional), Mexican American subjects actually showed more favorable attitudes toward psychotherapy's efficacy relative to Euro-American subjects (Acosta & Sheehan, 1976). Finally, Keefe (1979) found that Chicano nonutilizers of mental health facilities had generally positive perceptions of mental health services, and those Mexican Americans who had direct or indirect contact with these services overwhelmingly found the staff easy to talk to (90 percent) and believed in the efficacy of the care (88 percent). The reviewers' lack of enthusiasm for the role of negative attitudes toward mental health care as a mediator of service use appears to have been justified.

Previous reviews have been most consistent in pointing to characteristics of mental health services and professionals as the most probable factors contributing to underutilization. However, this consensus is not based on data, since it emerges from a literature that lacks research to evaluate directly the influence of service variables on utilization. Reviewers appear to be influenced primarily by two factors: (a) the face-valid importance of bilingual/bicultural staff in initially attracting and maintaining Raza clients, and (b) the apparent increase in utilization that resulted when facilities introduced changes to make their services more congruent with the cultural and linguistic character of Chicano consumers. Articles by Karno and Morales (1971), Phillipus (1971), and Bloom (1975) are sometimes cited to illustrate the favorable impact of modifying service characteristics and introducing bilingual/bicultural staff.

The use of alternative services and natural support systems were also identified by some reviewers as a viable explanation for Mexican Americans' underuse of formal mental health services. There is less consensus on this point, perhaps because its plausibility requires that several conditions be met. First, one must assume that a hydraulic relationship exists between the use of formal mental health services and non-mental health services such that use of the latter decreases the former. This does not appear to be true in the case of *curanderismo* and perhaps not with the use of physicians (see Keefe, 1979). Those Mexican Americans who report consulting curanderos often acknowledge that they concurrently used formal mental health services; in fact, curanderos have been known to make referrals to community mental health centers (Weclew, 1975). Similarly, Keefe (1979) found that neither the use of curanderos nor the use of physicians as sources of emotional support appeared to be significantly related to Chicanos' decreased utilization of mental health clinics.

Second, it is not sufficient to show that Mexican Americans simply use alternative services; it must be demonstrated that they overuse these services relative to non-Mexican Americans. Furthermore, in order for alternative service use to be a truly compelling explanation for underutilization of mental health clinics, Mexican Americans must receive alternative services in numbers compensating for their underutilization of formal services.

Finally, studies typically have focused on those types of alternative services that are likely to be utilized primarily by Mexican Americans. If Mexican Americans' use of formal services is depressed by their use of curanderos, for example, couldn't Euro-Americans' formal service use also be depressed by their use of fraternal organizations or clubs (that are not likely to be joined by Mexican Americans)? A fair test of alternative services' impact on formal service use requires an inquiry into the full array of possible alternative services.

Summary

From this review of reviews, the following conclusions emerge:

(1) There have been numerous reports of underutilization by Mexican Americans, primarily from public facilities in the Southwest.
(2) However, several studies, particularly those conducted in the past decade, have reported equitable use or overuse of mental health services by Mexican Americans.
(3) There is little direct support for the contentions that Mexican Americans underutilize services because of a lower true prevalence of psychological disorder, negative attitudes toward mental health professionals or services, or the widespread use of curanderos.

(4) Service characteristics, such as the availability of bilingual/bicultural therapists, is the factor most consistently identified as a chief influence on the utilization rates of Mexican Americans. To a lesser extent, reviewers cite the role of gatekeepers (such as physicians and priests) and informal support systems as keys to understanding Raza utilization of formal services.

An Update of Some Old Issues

Since the publication of the major reviews discussed in the preceding section, a number of relevant articles have appeared that bear on these same issues. These more current reports have been organized around four areas: (a) epidemiological studies, (b) use of social support systems, (c) attitudes toward and efficacy of psychotherapy, and (d) service characteristics.

Epidemiological Studies

Epidemiological studies have special importance for the study of mental health service use by Raza groups. As previously mentioned, underutilization has been attributed to the lower "true" incidence of mental disorder that is enjoyed by Mexican Americans (Jaco, 1960). Even without accepting this broader claim, epidemiological studies are obviously principal methods of assessing need, and ultimately for evaluating the extent to which services are being obtained by those who "truly" manifest psychological distress.

Published epidemiological studies on Raza populations are rare and have not been cited frequently in previous reviews. Two separate reports grew out of a household survey of 1441 respondents in Houston, Texas (Antunes, Gordon, Gaitz, & Scott, 1974; Gaitz & Scott, 1974). Euro-American, Black, and Chicano men and women of diverse ages and socioeconomic levels completed a battery of measures that included the Langner 22-item symptom inventory and scales that were combined to form composite indices of "joy" and "angst." In the paper by Antunes et al. (1974), respondents were subdivided on the basis of both ethnicity and socioeconomic status. Results from the Langner scale showed that Euro-Americans reported more symptoms than Chicanos and Blacks for both high and low socioeconomic groups. Gaitz and Scott (1974) reported on the results of the "joy" and "angst" measures from this same survey. Scores on both "joy" and "angst" were highest for Anglo subjects, while

Mexican Americans scored in an intermediate position between them and Black subjects.

The Houston survey was presented as an implementation of the design described by Dohrenwend and Dohrenwend (1969) for testing the social selection/social stress hypothesis of psychopathology (Antunes et al., 1974). Antunes et al. interpret their findings as lending support to the social selection process while contradicting the social stress hypothesis. However, since Euro-Americans reported more symptoms than Blacks and Chicanos in both high and low socioeconomic groups, these results are also compatible with a response bias interpretation.

Quesada, Spears, and Ramos (1978) studied depression among 417 Mexican American and 97 Black women in a southwestern urban area. Blacks scored as more depressed on the Zung depression scale than did Mexican Americans. In addition, a composite socioeconomic index proved to be a significant predictor of depression for both ethnic groups.

Even more recently, Roberts (1980) reported the results of two large-scale surveys conducted in Alameda County (California). In comparison to Euro-Americans (and without adjusting for demographic variables), Chicanos and Blacks reported much greater dissatisfaction with leisure, marriage, and employment in the first study. In study 2, Chicanos again scored higher than Anglos on leisure and marital dissatisfaction, but not on job dissatisfaction.

Ethnic group differences for emotional or mental illness were not significant in either study. On chronic nervous trouble, Chicanos and Blacks appeared to be more distressed than Euro-Americans in the first study, but not in the second. In both studies Chicanos reported less positive affect than Anglos, but did not report greater negative affect. The overall pattern of results for these studies was not appreciably altered by adjusting for demographic variables. In summary, Roberts's (1980) study does not lend support to the hypothesis that Chicanos have a lower "true" prevalence of mental disorder.

The results of these three epidemiological surveys are not completely consistent. They report Chicanos to have both greater (Roberts, 1980) and less (Antunes et al., 1974) psychological distress than Anglos; and greater (Antunes et al., 1974) and less (Quesada et al., 1978; Roberts, 1980) distress than Blacks.

Rather than serving as a source of confusion, these inconsistent findings might serve as a further incentive for conducting epidemiological studies with Raza groups. Even without being concerned about broad generalizability, these studies have value as needs assessment tools within a particular locale.

Family and Social Support Networks

The social science literature typically portrays Raza groups as being embedded in supportive social networks composed of strong friendships and extended but cohesive family systems (see Casas & Keefe, 1978). The suggestion that the supportive milieu of the Mexican American family was responsible for their lower incidence of treated mental disorder was popularized by Jaco (1960), but this hypothesis was never formally evaluated in his research. Jaco's proposed explanation actually requires the confirmation of two assumptions: (a) Mexican Americans have more supportive families and friendships than Blacks and Euro-Americans and (b) the availability of natural social support systems decreases the likelihood of treated mental disorder.

In the intervening two decades since the publication of Jaco's (1960) study, there has been little research to directly address these two hypotheses. The most relevant research, which was conducted in three Southern California communities, has been described in an edited volume by Casas and Keefe (1978) and related articles (for example, Keefe, Padilla, & Carlos, 1979). In this project, Mexican American and Euro-American subjects were interviewed to ascertain information concerning family integration, mental health resources, and cultural characteristics. Results indicate that Mexican Americans were more highly integrated into kinship networks than Euro-Americans. Mexican Americans had more kin living nearby, and tended to visit them frequently and engaged them in mutual aid exchanges. In contrast, consistent ethnic group differences were not observed on items concerning provisions of emotional support. Chicanos, in contrast to Euro-Americans, were more likely to consult relatives, physicans, clergy, and community workers, whereas Euro-Americans were more likely to utilize friends for emotional support. This pattern was not replicated in interviews conducted a year later. Euro-Americans reported more consultation with friends, physicians, private therapists, group meetings, and neighbors in comparison to Mexican Americans. There was also a nonsignificant tendency for greater utilization of family members by Euro-Americans. The authors conclude that "natural helpers" are important social support resources for *both* Mexican Americans and Euro-Americans:

In sum, although our research shows that Mexican Americans rely greatly on familial support, there is no indication that this is a uniquely Mexican American trait. . . . Therefore, there is little reason to believe that the presence of the extended family can be the reason for an alleged lower incidence of mental illness among Mexican Americans [Keefe et al., 1979, p. 151].

In a related report from these same data, Keefe (1979) found no evidence that the availability of an extended family or use of relatives, friends, physicians, and curanderos influenced the use of mental health clinics. The only significant predictors of clinic use were being unmarried, a member of a female-headed household, and English speaking.

Mindel (1980) provides evidence to suggest that Mexican Americans, indeed, live within extended family systems and rely on them more for functional interactions (such as emergency help, advice, and financial aid) relative to Euro-Americans. Approximately equal groups of Euro-American, Black, and Mexican American adults with school-age children were drawn from neighborhoods in Kansas City. Results showed that relative to Blacks and Euro-Americans, Mexican Americans were most likely to have both nuclear and extended kin in the community and to interact with them frequently. Mexican Americans also were more likely to engage in supportive exchanges with their support systems compared to Euro-Americans, but slightly less than Blacks. In short, there were sizable differences between Chicanos and Euro-Americans in the availability and use of social support. Whether or not this support influenced use of formal mental health services was not addressed in this research.

In still another study, Blacks, Euro-Americans, and Mexican Americans were compared on their ratings of importance and satisfaction with family life (Raymond, Rhoads, & Raymond, 1980). The items from Flanagan's (1978) Quality of Life scale that constituted their measures are noteworthy in that they make reference to mutual assistance functions, that is, "things like communicating, visiting, understanding, doing things, and helping and being helped by them" (Raymond et al., 1980, p. 561). On a measure of family importance, Mexican Americans scored higher than Euro-Americans but not higher than Blacks. In contrast, Mexican Americans were not significantly different than Euro-Americans and were lower than Blacks on a measure of family satisfaction.

A fairly consistent picture emerges from recent studies on Mexican American support systems, which have largely consisted of research on the family. In brief, Mexican Americans appear to possess important, extensive, and readily accessible family ties relative to Euro-Americans and perhaps to Blacks. But this accessibility does not necessarily lead to comparatively greater actual support or satisfaction with these social ties. The supportiveness of kin and kith relationships is thought to be an integral, if not defining, characteristic of Raza culture. But, like so many topics in the social science literature concerning Raza groups, further research is needed to differentiate fact from fiction.

There are good indications that conceptual and empirical work on Hispanics will continue to grow in volume and sophistication. Valle and Vega (1980) have recently edited a book entitled *Hispanic Natural Support Systems: Mental Health Promotion Perspectives.* While the papers included in this publication provide no new data, they contain basic information on network concepts, numerous suggestions for utilizing networks in clinical practice, and some recommendations for future research. The recently completed National Survey of People of Mexican Descent in the United States, which was conducted by Carlos Arce and his colleagues at the University of Michigan, promises to increase substantially our understanding of Chicanos' use of natural support systems. Sizable portions of the survey instrument used in this nationwide study refer to family relationships and the role of informal helpers in coping with stressful events.

Finally, interest and research activities on social networks and social support processes is in vogue across a number of disciplines, such as anthropology, communications, psychology, sociology, and social work. The growing sophistication of paradigms and research methods should increase the likelihood that quality research will be conducted on the support systems of Chicanos and other Raza groups in the years to come.

Psychotherapy

Although comprehensive community mental health centers provide a diversity of services, psychotherapy still accounts for the bulk of the actual clinical contacts, and, no doubt, constitutes the prototypic mental health service in the minds of most potential consumers. In my earlier review I observed that studies have found Mexican Americans to have comparable (Karno & Edgerton, 1969) or even more favorable (Acosta & Sheehan, 1976) attitudes of psychotherapy's efficacy relative to Euro-Americans.

Despite these findings, interest in the area has persisted. Attitudes toward psychotherapy are still thought to influence the initial decision to utilize mental health services while actual reactions to psychotherapy (and therapists) could conceivably determine the duration of treatment.

In a study of outpatients in East Los Angeles, Mexican American and Euro-American subjects completed self-report measures of (a) expected therapist behaviors, (b) expected duration of therapy, and (c) definitions of various terms connoting mental illness (Acosta, 1979b). These scales were completed prior to their first therapy sessions. Results showed that almost identical percentages of Mexican and Euro-American subjects (49 percent and 4ε percent, respectively) expected their therapists to ask them questions and help them actively solve problems. Expected time duration of therapy showed some ethnic group differences, with Chicano clients expecting an average of 17 visits compared to 23 for Euro-Americans. Definitions for some of the mental illness concepts appeared to show ethnic group differences as well, but because tests of statistical significance were not reported, it is difficult to evaluate the reliability of these differences.

More recently, Keefe (1979) reported that 58 percent of a Mexican American subsample who had not used mental health services expressed a willingness to use one. Those who had direct or indirect contact with a mental health facility overwhelmingly found the staff easy to talk to (90 percent) and believed in the efficacy of the treatment (88 percent).

A few analogue studies have appeared that explored ethnicity effects in client-counselor contacts. In a study with Chicano community college students, both counselor ethnicity and attitudinal similarity were examined as possible influences on clients' perceptions of the counselor's credibility and attractiveness (Furlong, Atkinson, & Casas, 1979). The similarity of students' and counselors' attitudes toward cultural pluralism/assimilation proved to exert the only main effect on ratings of the counselors; counselor ethnicity did not appear to be a significant influence on these ratings. As predicted, analogue counselors whose expressed attitudes were similar to those of the subjects were rated more favorably than those with dissimilar attitudes.

The effects of information about the counselor, and client and counselor ethnicity were studied for their possible impact on client's willingness to see a counselor. There was some support for the hypothesis that greater information about the counselor increased the expressed willingness of the students to see that counselor. There was no support for the contention that these analogue clients would express a preference for a counselor of the same ethnicity and/or sex.

Cortese (1979) reviewed 15 experimental studies of psychotherapy or behavior modification that employed Hispanics as research subjects. After appropriately acknowledging the limited data base and the need for additional research, the author somewhat reluctantly concludes that: (a) there is some suggestion that treatment methods that deemphasize self-

MANUEL BARRERA, Jr. 131

disclosure (such as behavior therapy) are more effective than those methods that do, and (b) there is little evidence to suggest that it is preferable to match clients and therapists on ethnicity.

The tentativeness of these conclusions cannot be overemphasized. As Cortese points out, there are several limitations to the existing literature. In addition to its relative brevity, the list of studies in this area includes several analogue studies. An important question concerns the levels of acculturation represented in the samples of research participants. In some cases acculturation levels were unknown, while others used Raza college students who could be expected to differ in important ways from the general population of potential community mental health utilizers.

Service Characteristics

Many of the factors that have been studied as mediators of Mexican Americans' service use are person variables, that is, factors such as individuals' attitudes toward help seeking, their psychological adjustment, or their choice to utilize alternative forms of mental health care. An alternative approach, one that is less well represented in the literature, has as its emphasis the characteristics of the mental health services that are available to consumers. In this approach, features such as the ethnic composition of a center's staff, fee policies, the content of treatment modalities, and the physical environment of the clinic become principal targets for investigation, rather than intrapersonal variables.

Wu and Windle (1980) recently published a rare study of the relationship between minority staffing rates in community mental health centers and the center's relative use by minority clients. In total, 220 federally funded community mental health centers in a number of states were the subjects of this study. Results showed that for 72 centers that serviced sizable numbers of "Spanish Americans" there were reliable relationships between utilization by Spanish American clients and the presence of both Spanish American professional staff and other minority professional staff. While this study was not designed to determine a causal relationship between minority staffing and utilization, it is consistent with a policy of increasing the presence of Mexican American professionals as a method of facilitating utilization by Mexican American clients.

In another study the relationship between Mexican American's utilization of community mental health centers and the presence of Mexican American staff and administrators was investigated (Trevino, 1979). A total of 8 facilities in the state of Texas, all located in catchment areas with at least 20,000 Mexican American residents, were subjects of this research. Of these facilities, 4 had a low absolute proportion of Mexican American staff (less than 20 percent), while 4 had a high absolute proportion (greater than 46 percent). A central hypothesis of this study was that Mexican Americans would more heavily utilize the centers with a high proportion of Mexican American staff relative to those centers with a small proportion. The author concluded that the results did not support this hypothesis since Mexican Americans utilized the centers that had relatively few Mexican American staff members at a rate of 13.21 per 1,000 and at a rate of 12.02 per 1,000 in those centers with a high proportion of Mexican American staff. However, a reinterpretation of Trevino's findings would result in a different conclusion. Even though the absolute proportion of Mexican American staff members varied from a low of 5.8 percent to a high of 75.5 percent, in each case staffing proportions rather closely reflected the representation of Mexican Americans in that specific catchment area. In "low-proportion" centers Mexican Americans were a mean of 10.6 percent of the staff, 10.0 percent of the treatment population, and 9.9 percent of the general catchment population. For "high-proportion" centers, Mexican Americans were 55.8 percent of the overall staff, 58.2 percent of the clients seen in these centers, and 52.4 percent of the catchment area populations. Trevino's results are consistent with the assertion that when Mexican Americans' representation on the staffs of community mental health centers matches their representation in the catchment area, so too will their representation in the center's treatment population.

In an exploratory analysis of these data, Trevino (1979) also found a positive relationship between the presence of Mexican American administrators in the centers and subsequent utilization by Mexican American clientele. This finding is remarkable in light of the small sample size and the lack of glaring underutilization for any of the centers. Trevino suggests that administrators who are responsible for policy interpretation and program implementation can exert an important influence on the utilization of traditionally underserved populations.

Most of the evidence regarding the influence of agency characteristics (such as presence of bilingual/bicultural staff, fee schedules, accessibility and so on) has come from case studies of individual agencies. Several earlier reports of this type suggested that providing bilingual/bicultural staff, adapting the treatment environment to include artifacts of Mexican culture, and modifying fees and office procedures in order to accommodate Mexican American clientele can result in increased utilization by Chicano residents (Bloom, 1975; Karno & Morales, 1971; Phillipus, 1971)

An additional case report was provided for a community mental health center in the predominantly Mexican American city of Laredo, Texas (Trevino, Bruhn, & Bunce, 1979). This center adopted a sliding fee schedule and employed Mexican American bilingual staff members, including a physician and clerical personnel. Outpatient records for one year revealed that Mexican Americans represented 88.2 percent of the client population, which compared favorably to their representation of 86.3 percent in Laredo's general population. The authors note that if factors such as curanderismo, social supports, and proximity to Mexican culture operate to depress Mexican Americans' utilization of formal mental health services, then these factors should have surely been operative in Laredo. The fact that proportional service utilization was evidenced in this predominantly Mexican American border town is interpreted by the authors as support for the importance of community mental health center staffing patterns and procedures.

An update of Karno and Morales's (1971) initial description of a barrio mental health center showed that with the expansion of bilingual/ bicultural staff, the numbers of Mexican American clients also grew and continued to reflect the ethnic composition of the area surrounding the center (Flores, 1978). The author concludes that policies that led to the formation of a staff that was linguistically and culturally equipped to deal with Mexican American clients, the maintenance of a physical environment that reflected an appreciation for Mexican culture, and other policies that minimized financial and physical barriers to obtaining services all contributed to the ongoing success of the center.

Muñoz (in press) described some of his personal experiences as a Latino mental health professional working in a public facility that serves the ethnically diverse community in San Francisco. His observations capture what many people who deliver services to Raza communities believe to be 'truth,' but truth that suffers from too few empirical tests:

It has been my experience that when one makes it known that one is Spanish-speaking and that one is motivated to work with Latinos, the frequency of referrals increases rapidly. Sometimes the response is overwhelming, even in a setting where formerly Latinos came only rarely. Reasons for underutilization may thus be more a factor of availability and visibility of Spanish-speaking staff than a lack of need by the Spanish-speaking community [Muñoz, in press, p. 9].

Beyond the question of whether increased cultural relevance of services improves service utilization is the question of whether they lead to improved efficacy. In a pilot project at Colorado State Hospital, a Hispanic Treatment Unit was created to provide for the availability of bilingual staff, family involvement, cultural participation, and an emphasis on ethnic pride (Dolgin, Salazar, & Kort, 1980). In an initial evaluation of this project, 42 Hispanic patients were randomly assigned to either a traditional inpatient hospital unit or the Hispanic Treatment Unit. Upon termination, patients treated on the Hispanic Unit evidenced greater improvement on 8 of 9 outcome measures, including ratings of physical health, interpersonal relationships, substance abuse, and others. Although the development of culturally relevant treatment modalities has frequently been called for, this study represents one of the rare experimental tests of their efficacy.

In summarizing my earlier review I suggested that "variables associated with the responsiveness and quality of mental health services, particularly the availability of bilingual-bicultural staff, are advocated as the most relevant areas for future research" (Barrera, 1978, p. 35). The evidence that has appeared in the interim has been consistent with the importance that was placed on service characteristics in this earlier review. The certainty with which service variables are singled out as the principal factor in understanding Raza participation in community mental health services must be tempered by the relative shortage of empirical evidence. The work of Wu and Windle (1980), Trevino (1979), and Dolgin et al. (1980) exemplifies the brands of research that will contribute to our further understanding of the relationship between characteristics of community mental health centers (such as their staffing patterns, service policies, and treatment procedures) and subsequent utilization and efficacy of care.

Raza and Community Mental Health: A Reappraisal

The *Report to the President of the President's Commission on Mental Health* has been described as "a manifesto for a fourth mental health revolution" (Albee, 1978). Alternatively, the several volumes of findings and recommendations might be regarded as calling for an extension of the Third Revolution, a return to many of the principles that were articulated in the report by the Joint Commission on Mental Illness and Health (1961) that gave rise to the Community Mental Health Centers Act. While the President's Commission's call for a greater emphasis on prevention represented a relatively new focus, the central theme was clearly to provide services to the underserved. Hispanics proved to be but one of many subgroups that were identified as undeserved. Children, adolescents, the elderly, Blacks, American Indians, Asians and Pacific Islanders, women, inner-city residents, rural residents, seasonal farm workers, substance abusers, the physically handicapped, and still others were all viewed as underserved. Albee (1978, p. 550) observes that the only ones not identified as being underserved were "white educated males living in the affluent sections and suburbs of major American cities." I am not convinced that an argument could not be made to include even this subgroup.

The report of the Special Populations Subpanel on Mental Health of Hispanic Americans (1978) echoed the same concerns that were expressed twenty years ago at the birth of the community mental health movement. The call to "get our share of the action" that was sounded during the sixties was captured in the subpanel's (1978, p. 917) comments:

> Hispanic residents contribute to this country and are thus entitled to an equitable share of the Nation's mental health resources. They are not, however, receiving their fair share of health and mental health dollars as reflected by utilization statistics, the limited number of Hispanic professionals in the health fields, and the dearth of mental health organizations administered by Hispanics.

It is hard to argue with many of the subpanel's observations and recommendations that, for the most part, are anchored in the mainstream concerns of traditional community mental health. They express the need for more epidemiological research on Hispanics, particularly those studies that acknowledge the distinctness of Hispanic subgroups. The personpower shortage that they discuss is, in fact, significantly more acute than it is for Euro-Americans and certain other groups, and it is likely to become worse if affirmative action efforts are not expanded or at least continued. Their suggestions for prevention include strategies for preserving Raza culture and providing for mental health education. Yet, overall, mental health for Raza populations in the 1980s continues to be discussed in terms of clinics, psychotherapy, mental health professionals, utilization, and efficacy of services.

Not a Conclusion, but a Dangling Question

How should we go about serving Raza as an underserved population? I feel that I, like a number of others concerned with the mental health of Raza, have approached this question with the myopic view that services

TABLE 6.1 Hispanic Faculty and Graduate Students in Ph.D. Clinical Psychology Programs, 1970-1978

Faculty	1970[a]			1972[b]			1976[c]			1977-1978[d]	
	N	(N)	%	N	(N)[e]	%	N	(N)[e]	%	N	%
Chicano	2	(3)	.19	1	(1)	.08	7	(9)	.55	22	.64
Cuban	0			0			0				
Puerto Rican	2	(3)	.19	1	(1)	.08	3	(4)	.24		
Total Hispanic	4	(6)	.38	2	(2)	.16	10	(13)	.78	22	.64
Total faculty	1,041	(1,322)		1,251	(1,514)		1,275	(1,670)		3,458	

Graduate Students	1970a			1972b			1976c			1977-1978d Graduate School		Internship	
	N	(N)e	%	N	(N)e	%	N	(N)e	%	N	%	N	%
Chicano	6	(8)	.16	39	(47)	.82	74	(97)	1.24				
Cuban	0			0			11	(14)	.18				
Puerto Rican	19	(24)	.49	36	(44)	.76	45	(59)	.76				
Total Hispanic	25	(32)	.65	75	(91)	1.58	130	(170)	2.18	196	3.57	11	1.77
Total students	3,858	(4,900)		4,759	(5,758)		5,958	(7,805)		5,486		623	

SOURCE: Reprinted by permission from Bernal (1980, Table 1).

a. Boxley and Wagner (1971) mail survey of APA-accredited Ph.D. clinical programs. N = 103, response rate = 79%.

b. Padilla, Boxley, and Wagner (1973) mail survey of all Ph.D. clinical programs. N = 114, response rate = 82%.

c. Padilla (1977) mail survey of all Ph.D. clinical programs. N = 128, response rate = 77%. Includes part-time and graduate-student instructors.

d. Vidato (1979) survey. Includes only APA-accredited clinical programs and reports only on total SSSS faculty members and students. Data based on APA annual self-study reports. N = 100.

e. Due to differing response rates in the 1970, 1972, and 1976 surveys, the number of faculty members and students are adjusted by estimating what they would be if response rates were 100%. This estimate assumes that departments not participating in the surveys have similar minority group representations.

refer to those activities typically performed by mental health professionals within organizational structures and facilities we regard as community mental health centers. If the question is defined in this way I am fairly convinced that the answer rests with the kinds of specific changes that were discussed earlier in the context of service characteristics. However, since this proposed solution to the problem depends heavily on the supply of well-trained bilingual/bicultural mental health professionals, the likelihood of fully implementing these changes must be seriously questioned. Even strong advocates of accelerated training of Hispanic mental health professionals recognize the obstacles to supplying sufficient personpower to meet the mental health needs of Raza if traditional service mechanisms are to be used (see Table 6.1). After noting the gross underrepresentation of Raza faculty and graduate students in psychology, and the disproportionate growth of Raza populations, Bernal (1980, pp. 131-132) asserts:

> The implications of these data are straight-forward. The total number of current graduate students and the rate at which they are completing their training are so low that we cannot hope to meet the vast mental health personnel needs of the 10 to 17 million or more Hispanics in the United States at any time within the next 5 to 6 years that it takes to complete the doctoral degree.... As the demand for mental health services for these children and their families increases, Hispanic psychologists will be even less represented in psychology than they are now.

Bernal's observation represents a reverberation of Albee's (1959) analysis of personpower needs in mental health.

So how should we go about providing mental health services to Raza? Realistically we must recognize that the number of Raza service users is small. Only 2 percent of Keefe et al.'s (1979) Mexican American sample had used a mental health clinic in the preceding two years. Numbers are small even when Raza equitably utilizes community mental health services such as the 12 or 13 per 1000 reported in Trevino's (1979) paper. Our concern over the small segment of Raza who receives or should receive clinical services is perhaps another reflection of our reverence for the medical model. We value the principle that resources should be diverted to a small segment of those with truly severe problems—even when we realize the limitations that stem from shortages of appropriate personnel and the complexities of client-initiated help seeking.

An alternative approach would be to give greatest priority not to the problem of providing services to the few that could benefit from clini-

utilization, but to those problems that affect the greatest number of Raza people. This approach calls for a liberal definition of "mental health" in order to include problems that result in Hispanics failing to obtain basic resources such as education, housing, employment, and political power. If patterns that emerged from previous studies continue to characterize Hispanic groups, then some priority targets for intervention will become apparent. In 1977 over 20 percent of Hispanic families had incomes below the poverty level, compared to less than 10 percent for non-Hispanics (Brown, Rosen, Hill, & Olivas, 1980). This same report found that Hispanics had larger families, were twice as likely to live in central cities, and were less likely to complete high school than non-Hispanics. Of the population 25 years or older, 23 percent of Mexican Americans had completed less than 5 years of formal schooling, compared to 3 percent for non-Hispanics. Unemployment, a stressful event that has an impact on both the economic and psychological well-being of individuals (Gore, 1978), has been shown to effect a disproportionately high percentage of Raza workers (Kane, 1973; Newman, 1978). These problems exemplify just some of the "mental health" issues that should be addressed through service provision.

The suggestion to emphasize social-economic-political problems instead of problems related to clinical practices is certainly not a new one; it is largely embodied in what has been discussed as prevention. The special importance this approach has for Raza stems from the severity and prevalence of these problems that involve the basic resources necessary for meeting the daily demands of living. The problem of mental health clinic use seems pale in comparison.

In an ideal situation, personpower and economic resources could be devoted to a multifaceted plan to meet the mental health needs of Raza people—there would be an intense effort to provide culturally sensitive treatment in community mental health centers as well as broad-scale, imaginative interventions on pervasive problems in education, employment, and so on. Because this ideal situation does not exist, we must set priorities and, in a sense, choose between upgrading our services to the 2 percent of Raza who utilize community mental health facilities or administering to the needs of the 20 percent in poverty or the 20 percent who lack elementary school educations. If we, as mental health professionals, choose to concentrate our efforts in these latter areas, serving the underserved will take on an emphasis that differs from that described in the bulk of the studies reviewed in the present chapter. For some of us, this will require applying our skills and knowledge in unfamiliar areas, perhaps acquiring new skills, and enduring the threats to our self-identities that will come from relinquishing traditional roles.

References

Acosta, F. X. Barriers between mental health services and Mexican Americans: An examination of a paradox. *American Journal of Community Psychology*, 1979, 7(5), 503-520. (a)

Acosta, F. X. Pretherapy expectations and definitions of mental illness among minority and low-income patients. *Hispanic Journal of Behavioral Science*, 1979, 1(4): 403-410. (b)

Acosta, F. X., & Sheehan, J. G. Preferences toward Mexican American and Anglo American psychotherapists. *Journal of Consulting and Clinical Psychology*, 1976, 44, 272-279.

Albee, G. W. *Mental health manpower trends*. New York: Basic Books, 1959.

Albee, G. W. "A manifesto for a fourth mental health revolution?" (Review of *Report to the president of the President's Commission on Mental Health*, 1978, Vol. 1). *Contemporary Psychology*, 1978, 23(8), 549-551.

Antunes, G., Gordon, C., Gaitz, C. M., & Scott, J. Ethnicity, socioeconomic status, and the etiology of psychological distress. *Sociology and Social Research*, 1974, 58, 361-369.

Bachrach, L. L. *Utilization of state and county mental hospitals by Spanish-Americans in 1972*. (NIMH Division of Biometry Statistical Note 116, U.S. Department of Health, Education and Welfare Publication No. [ADM] 75-158.) Washington, DC: Government Printing Office, 1975.

Barrera, M., Jr. Mexican-American mental health service utilization: A critical examination of some proposed variables. *Community Mental Health Journal*, 1978, 14(1) 35-45.

Bernal, M. E. Hispanic issues in psychology: Curricula and training." *Hispanic Journal of Behavioral Sciences*, 1980, 2(2) 129-146.

Bloom, B. L. *Changing patterns of psychiatric care*. New York: Human Sciences Press, 1975.

Bloom, B. L. *Community mental health: A general introduction*. Monterey, CA: Brooks/Cole, 1977.

Boxley, R., & Wagner, N. Clinical psychology training programs and minority groups: A survey. *Professional Psychology*, 1971, 2, 75-81.

Brown, G. H., Rosen, N. L., Hill, S. T., & Olivas, M. A. *The condition of education for Hispanic Americans*. (National Center for Education Statistics.) Washington, DC: Government Printing Office, 1980.

Casas, J. M., & Keefe, S. E. (Eds.). *Family and mental health in the Mexican American community*. Los Angeles: Spanish Speaking Mental Health Research Center, 1978.

Cortese, M. Intervention research with Hispanic Americans: A review. *Hispanic Journal of Behavioral Sciences*, 1979, 1(1), 4-20.

Dohrenwend, B. P., & Dohrenwend, B. S. Social and cultural influences on psychopathology. *Annual Review of Psychology*, 1969, 25, 417-452.

Dolgin, D. L., Salazar, A. A., & Kort, G. A culturally-relevant treatment program for the Hispanic inpatient. *Borderlands*, 1980, 4(1), 131-142.

Flanagan, J. C. A research approach to improving our quality of life. *American Psychologist*, 1978, 33, 138-147.

Flores, J. L. The utilization of a community mental health service by Mexican Americans. *International Journal of Social Psychiatry*, 1978, 24, 271-275.

Franco, J. N., & LeVine, E. An analogue study of counselor ethnicity and client preference. *Hispanic Journal of Behavioral Science,* 1980, 2(2), 177-183.

Furlong, M. J., Atkinson, D. R., & Casas, J. M. Effects of counselor ethnicity and attitudinal similarity on Chicano students' perceptions of counselor credibility and attractiveness. *Hispanic Journal of Behavioral Sciences,* 1979, 1(1), 41-53.

Gaitz, C. M., & Scott, J. Mental health of Mexican-Americans: Do ethnic factors make a difference? *Geriatrics,* 1974, 29, 103-110.

Gore, S. The effect of social support in moderating the health consequences of unemployment. *Journal of Health and Social Behavior,* 1978, 19, 157-165.

Griffith, J. E. *Variables affecting Mexican American utilization of mental health services: Implications for strategies to improve service utilization.* Paper presented at the Third National Conference on Need Assessment in Health and Human Service Systems, Louisville, March 1981.

Jaco, E. G. *The social epidemiology of mental disorders.* New York: Russell Sage Foundation, 1960.

Joint Commission on Mental Illness and Health. *Action for mental health.* New York: Basic Books, 1961.

Kane, T. D. Structural change and Chicano employment in the Southwest, 1950-1970: Some preliminary observations. *Aztlan,* 1973, 4, 383-399.

Karno, M., & Edgerton, R. B. Perception of mental illness in a Mexican-American community. *Archives of General Psychiatry,* 1969, 20, 233-238.

Karno, M., & Morales, A. A community mental health service for Mexican-Americans in a metropolis. In N. N. Wagner & J. Haug (Eds.), *Chicanos: Social and psychological perspectives.* Saint Louis: C. V. Mosby, 1971.

Keefe, S. E. Mexican Americans' underutilization of mental health clinics: An evaluation of suggested explanations. *Hispanic Journal of Behavioral Sciences,* 1979, 1(2), 93-115.

Keefe, S. E., & Casas, J. M. Mexican Americans and mental health: A selected review and recommendations for mental health service delivery. *American Journal of Community Psychology,* 1980, 8(3), 303-326.

Keefe, S. E., Padilla, A. M., & Carlos, M. L. The Mexican-American extended family as an emotional support system. *Human Organization,* 1979, 38(2), 144-152.

Kline, L. Y. Some factors in the psychiatric treatment of Spanish-Americans. *American Journal of Psychiatry,* 1969, 125, 1674-1681.

Lopez, S. Mexican Americans' usage of mental health facilities: Underutilization reconsidered. In A. Baron, Jr. (Ed.), *Explorations in Chicano psychology.* New York: Praeger, 1981.

Mindel, C. H. Extended familialism among urban Mexican Americans, Anglos, and Blacks. *Hispanic Journal of Behavioral Sciences,* 1980, 2(1), 21-34.

Muñoz, R. F. The Spanish-speaking consumer and the community mental health center. In E. Jones & S. Korchin (Eds.), *Minority mental health.* New York: Holt, Rinehart & Winston, in press.

Newman, M. J. A profile of Hispanics in the U.S. workforce. *Monthly Labor Review,* 1978, December.

Padilla, A. M., Olmedo, E. L., Lopez, S., & Perez, R. *Hispanic mental health bibliography, II.* Los Angeles: Spanish Speaking Mental Health Research Center.

Padilla, A. M., Ruiz, R. A., & Alvarez, R. Community mental health services for the Spanish-speaking/surnamed population. *American Psychologist,* 1975, 30, 892-905.

Padilla, E. R. Hispanics in clinical psychology: 1970-1976. In E. L. Olmedo & S. Lopez (Eds.), *Hispanic mental health professionals*. Los Angeles: Spanish Speaking Mental Health Research Center, 1977.

Padilla, E. R., Boxley, R., & Wagner, N. The desegregation of clinical psychology training. *Professional Psychology*, 1973, 4, 259-264.

Phillipus, M. J. Successful and unsuccessful approaches to mental health services for an urban Hispano-American population. *Journal of Public Health*, 1971, 61, 820-830.

Pokorney, A. D., & Overall, J. E. Relationship of psychopathology to age, sex, ethnicity, education, and marital status in state hospital patients. *Journal of Psychiatric Research*, 1970, 7, 143-152.

Quesada, G. M., Spears, W., & Ramos, P. Inter-racial depressive epidemiology in the Southwest. *Journal of Health and Social Behavior*, 1978, 19, 77-85.

Ramirez, D. G. *A review of the literature on the underutilization of mental health services by Mexican Americans: Implications for future research and service delivery*. San Antonio: Intercultural Development Research Association, 1980.

Raymond, J. S., Rhoads, D. L., & Raymond, R. I. The relative impact of family and social involvement on Chicano mental health. *American Journal of Community Psychology*, 1980, 8(5), 557-569.

Roberts, R. E. Prevalence of psychological distress among Mexican Americans. *Journal of Health and Social Behavior*, 1980, 21, 134-145.

Special Populations Subpanel on Mental Health of Hispanics Americans. Report. In *Report to the president of the President's Commission on Mental Health*, Vol. 3: *Task Panel Reports*. Washington, DC: Government Printing Office, 1978.

Sue, S., Allen, D. B., & Conaway, L. The responsiveness and equality of mental health care to Chicanos and Native Americans. *American Journal of Community Psychology*, 1978, 6, 137-146.

Torrey, E. F. *The mind game: Witchdoctors and psychiatrists*. New York: Bantam Books, 1973.

Trevino, F. M. *Community mental health center staffing patterns and their impact on Hispanic use of services*. Paper presented at the Hispanic Health Services Research Conference, University of New Mexico, Albuquerque, September 6, 1979.

Trevino, F. M., Bruhn, J. G., & Bunce, H., III. Utilization of community mental health services in a Texas-Mexico border city. *Social Science and Medicine*, 1979, 13A, 331-334.

Valle, R., & Vega, W. (Eds.). *Hispanic natural support systems: Mental health promotion perspectives*. Sacramento: California State Department of Mental Health, 1980.

Vidato, D. *A data report on the 1977-78 academic year and trends of APA accredited programs: Student and faculty distributions*. Unpublished manuscript, 1979.

Weaver, J. L. Mexican-American health care behavior. A critical review of the literature. *Social Science Quarterly*, 1973, 54, 85-102.

Weclew, R. V. The nature, prevalence, and level of awareness of "curanderismo" and some of its implications for community mental health. *Community Mental Health Journal*, 1975, 11, 145-154.

Wignall, C. M., & Koppin, L. L. Mexican-American usage of state mental hospital facilities. *Community Mental Health Journal*, 1967, 3, 137-148.

Wu, I., & Windle, C. Ethnic specificity in the relationship of minority use and staffing of community mental health centers. *Community Mental Health Journal*, 1980, 16(2), 156-168.

7

American Indian and Alaska Native Communities

Past Efforts, Future Inquiries

Spero M. Manson

Oregon Health Sciences University

Joseph E. Trimble

Western Washington University

Over the last two decades, mental health services delivered to American Indians and Alaska Natives have grown dramatically in terms of general availability as well as in the range of care offered.[1] This growth can be attributed to a number of factors, notably changes in federal public health policies, increasing tribal resources and expertise, and community demands for more comprehensive and culturally relevant care. The rapid expansion of mental health services to Indians and Natives has, however, frequently preceded careful consideration of a variety of questions about several critical components of such care, specifically, the delivery structure itself, treatment processes, program evaluation, epidemiological data, and preventive strategies. Given the limitations and meager attempts at delivering formal services, it is not surprising that an immediate need led to explosive growth, which outstripped our knowledge for designing and implementing appropriate programs. The time has come to take stock of the current situation. Toward this end, in this chapter we selectively review the literature pertinent to each of the areas listed above. A series of questions

AUTHORS' NOTE: Inquiries about this chapter may be directed either to Spero M. Manson, Department of Psychiatry, Room 254 Gaines Hall, 3181 S.W. Sam Jackson Park Road, Oregon Health Sciences University, Portland, OR 97201, or to Joseph E. Trimble, Department of Psychology, Western Washington University, Bellingham, WA 98225. The first author wishes to acknowledge partial support from the Center for Epidemiologic Studies, NIMH, Grant 1-R01-MH33280-01.

are posed as points of departure for future inquiry, the answers to which will, in our opinion, form the basis for significant advances in the delivery of mental health services to Indian and Native people.

Before turning to a discussion of specific aspects of the delivery of mental health services to this special population, some mention of the broader context is in order, particularly for readers who may be unfamiliar with these communities. Preliminary estimates from the 1980 census indicate that the American Indian and Alaska Native population numbers approximately 1.5 million, nearly double the 1970 count (U.S. Department of Commerce, 1981). If past trends have continued, slightly more than half live in rural areas, on reservation or native lands. Indian and Native communities are culturally heterogenous, having been classified into distinct regions the number varies from 9 to 17 depending upon the criteria applied in terms of differences in language, social organization, religious practice, and ecological relationships. Of the over 200 major native American languages that existed immediately prior to European contact, 149 of them are still spoken, excluding hundreds of dialectal variations. At present, there are 253 federally recognized tribal entities, an additional 85 that have been afforded tribal status by the states in which they reside, and several dozen that are not formally recognized in any fashion. Here, too, many more distinctions are possible and are made by Indian and Native people.

Mental health services to Indians and Natives are delivered by a diverse array of providers, many acting through federal agencies, some through locally controlled organizations, and others as part of private as well as state-managed systems. Eligibility criteria are even more confusing and vary with the provider agency in question. Indeed, this confusion prompted a recent study sponsored by the U.S. Department of Education Office of Indian Education, to determine workable definitions of "Indian." Despite the "definition" of Indian study, bureaucratic ambiguity remains, employing tribally defined membership (criteria for which differ across tribes), blood quantum (frequently one-fourth, genealogically derived), personal identification/community consensus, and various permutations thereof. It is within this setting, then, that the following issues and concerns arise.

Delivery of Services

Mental health services to American Indians and Alaska Natives are provided through private agencies and practitioners, county and state agencies, community mental health centers, the Bureau of Indian Affairs the Indian Health Service, urban Indian health programs, and tribal health departments. The nature and extent of services delivered vary with each agency or community organization, as does our knowledge concerning their respective client populations, problems treated, and outcomes.

State and Local Services

Very little information exists on client profiles and diagnostic distribution for Indian people seeking services from private agencies. Given the availability of services provided by other institutions, it is likely that relatively few individuals seek private care.

Numerous Indians from both urban areas and reservations are served by county and state mental health facilities. However, the diverse points of entry into this system—such as state hospitals, day treatment centers, the Social Security Administration, CETA, and vocational rehabilitation sectors—yield a confusing and often unmanageable set of service use data. For example, in Oregon alone, there are over 30 service agencies that may see potentially disturbed individuals (Oregon State Commission on Indian Services, 1978). Yet, despite considerable overlap, record keeping is not coordinated. Nor do these records necessarily indicate patient ethnicity, further frustrating an account of service utilization patterns by minority groups.

Though established for the purpose of reaching high-risk minority populations, federal community mental health centers (CMHCs) tend to underserve them. This occurs in catchment areas that have significant numbers of non-White residents (over 2000; Wu & Windle, 1978). American Indians in particular appear to use these facilities far less than other segments of American society (Sue, 1977; Sue, Allen, & Conaway, 1978; Willie, Kramers, & Brown, 1973). Sue (1977), in a study that surveyed 17 Seattle, Washington, CMHCs over a 3-year period, reports the following distribution of diagnoses at intake of Indian patients: mental retardation, 2.7 percent; neurosis, 12.2 percent; personality disorder, 18.9 percent; behavior disorder, 4.1 percent; and other, 25.5 percent. Of these same Indian patients, 55 percent were highly unlikely to return to the centers after their initial contact; this is a more significant dropout rate than demonstrated by Black, Asian, Chicano, or White patients.

Bureau of Indian Affairs

The Bureau of Indian Affairs (BIA) maintains 123 offices across 12 geographic areas, serving 281 tribes with a total population of approximately 649,000. Its community service division houses educational and social service branches. The former is charged with consultant, advisory, and administrative responsibility for Indian youth and adult education. This responsibility is met through tribal and state contracts, federal boarding schools, and educational and vocational guidance programs. The latter branch encompasses child welfare (including care, supervision, and other services for delinquent, dependent, or neglected children) and family services (largely counselor intervention in problems that arise due to family breakdown and emotional instability). Mental health professionals and paraprofessionals are employed in both branches. However, their diagnostic observations are seldom a matter of formal record; at best they are expected to refer clients to mental health care providers, such as the Indian Health Service. Typically, there is little or no postreferral monitoring.

The Indian Health Service

The Indian Health Service (IHS) annually provides inpatient and outpatient care to more than .75 million American Indians, urban and rural, through direct or contract services. A relatively new but growing component administers social service and mental health programs in 8 regional areas through 72 units composed of hospitals, clinics, and satellite centers (Beiser & Attneave, 1978). Most patient contacts occur with paraprofessionals and social workers rather than with psychiatrists, psychologists, or psychiatric nurses. Record protocols enable staff to code a wide range of problem areas (67 categories), including, for example, alcohol misuse, anxiety, depression, cultural conflict, and suicide attempts. Individuals referred for psychiatric evaluation are diagnosed according to the International Classification of Diagnoses-Adapted (ICDA). Health service-wide ambulatory care data for the 1975 fiscal year—predicated on visits, not on individual patients—indicate the following distribution of treated disorders: neurosis (anxiety, depression, and the like), 38 percent; alcoholism, 31.5 percent; psychoses, 8 percent; drug abuse and dependence, 2.7 percent; personality disorder, 2.1 percent; organic brain syndrome, 1.1 percent; and "other," 16.6 percent (Rhoades, Marshal, Attneave, Echohawk, Bjork, & Beiser, 1980). A new patient information care system is being implemented throughout the IHS; ICDA codes for psychiatric diagnoses have been retained.

Urban Indian Health Care Programs

Beginning in the early 1970s, Indian and Native communities started to assume direct control of the management and provision of health services to their members. At present there are approximately 26 urban Indian health programs. These programs—authorized under Public Law 93-437, the Indian Health Care Improvement Act, and implemented on a contractual basis with the Indian Health Service—have only recently expanded to include mental health care, and then on a limited basis. Borunda and Shore (1978) characterize the general climate in which most operate and, in reporting the results of an attitudinal survey among Portland Indian residents, anticipate future service emphases. An unpublished summary of urban mental health problem areas compiled in 1978 by the American Indian Health Care Association indicate that: (a) Indian children, adults, and families have significant and multiple mental health needs, and (b) these needs lie especially in the areas of chemical dependency, vocational/employment/financial, family, learning, emotional and interpersonal, and cultural difficulties. The needs assessment that formed the basis for this summary included samples of patient caseloads over a period of 10 consecutive working days in 3 urban health clinics. During that time, 3 physicians saw 348 patients. Among the total population, the most frequent problem areas were determined to be: chemical dependency (32 percent), family strife (30 percent), learning disability or difficulty (10 percent), physical complaints (10 percent), and employment (3 percent). The sample of patient files closely coincided with the impressions of clinic staff and Indian and non-Indian mental health professionals in interfacing agencies. This pattern of diagnosis is thought to be representative of just a fraction of the Indian community, as some were no doubt referred to other helping agencies.

Tribal-Based Health Care Programs

A similar set of circumstances characterizes tribal health programs. Reservation communities are empowered to assume either partial or total responsibility for the delivery of a wide range of services, including mental health care, as part of Public Law 93-638, the Indian Self-Determination Act. To date, 61 different tribal health programs have been established under contract to the Indian Health Service. Less than half of these programs have a formal mental health component.

Service Delivery Considerations

The proliferation of services within the delivery structure outlined above raises a number of critical questions, the answers to which can guide future growth, even consolidation:

(1) Is there a relationship between the form of delivery structure and the degree of service utilization (frequency of return, as well as initial contact)?

(2) What are the channels by which information about service availability is communicated to and among Indians?

(3) What service programs have successfully engendered participation in planning and operation? How?

(4) Does participation relate to differential program effectiveness? How?

(5) What impact will pending federal policy changes (P.L. 437, Indian preference, and so on) in service delivery control and eligibility requirements have on delivery structure and subsequent organizational development?

(6) To what extent can service duplication be avoided through mutual referral?

(7) How can service delivery be restructured to render existing health resources more cost-effective?

(8) What is the rate of referral compliance by Indian patients?

(9) To what extent is it affected by different eligibility requirements across services?

(10) How can one increase such compliance?

Though this chapter focuses on the formal delivery structure, one should be aware of the important and extensive role that traditional healers play in mental health care among Indian people. Dinges, Trimble, Manson, and Pasquale (1981) discuss the social ecology of counseling and psychotherapy with Indians and Natives, providing a detailed overview of the function of traditional healers and their relationship to western health care professionals. Any effort to plan and deliver mental health services to this special population must take potential impact upon traditional mechanisms of care into account.

Treatment Approaches

Counseling and psychotherapy outcome research has emphasized the importance of client or patient variables, expectation, degree of distur bance, therapist characteristics, and the like. The development of a facilitative relationship or working alliance is also of considerable importance. This interpersonal climate is thought to result from the ability of the therapist to understand the client and to communicate this understanding adequately.

Therapy in cross-cultural settings—which characterizes the vast majority of Indian and Native mental health experiences—has its most serious problems in those very areas of interaction that have been demonstrated to effect psychotherapy outcome. Cross-cultural therapy implies a situation in which the participants are most likely to evidence discrepancies in their shared assumptions, experiences, beliefs, values, expectations, and goals. Several recent literature reviews (Rachman, 1973; Bergin, 1971; Pedersen, Draguns, Lonner, & Trimble, 1981) indicate that this situation, at its extreme, establishes conditions that are clearly unfavorable for successful therapy. This view is supported by the subjective reports of many clinicians involved in cross-cultural psychotherapy, as well as the limited cross-cultural research conducted in this domain.

Complexities in Counseling and Psychotherapy

Among the most notable difficulties is the client's inaccurate or inappropriate perception of the therapist's role (and the converse). Thus there is often a discrepancy between what the patient expects (for example, to take a passive-dependent role) and what the therapist interprets as the most beneficial role (for example, to facilitate self-exploration, problem or feeling clarification, insight, or the like). Montijo (1975), for example, discusses the problems of Puerto Rican clients and emphasizes that blocking occurs as a result of differing expectations on the part of the psychotherapy participants. Problems can result from feelings of powerlessness, fatalism, mistrust, superstition, externalization of control, and submission to authority figures.

This same theme is emphasized by Wax and Thomas (1965), Attneave (1974), and Trimble (1981) in their discussions of the difficulties often inherent in attempts by whites to work with American Indian clients. They suggest that, in general, traditional therapeutic forms of social or interactional control and influence are viewed by Indians as out of the realm of proper behavior of action and that Indian clients frequently react with disquiet, fear, or bewilderment. Higginbotham (1977) and Goldstein (1981) have reviewed the literature extensively with respect to culture and role expectancies in psychotherapy. Clear differences exist and do affect subsequent outcome.

In addition to expectation for role performance, the clients of cross-cultural therapy do not always find themselves motivated to change in ways that are congruent with the therapist's goals and value system. Although they may be motivated to seek treatment, they probably do not share as many valued directions of change as participants from the therapist's cultural background. Trimble (1981) makes exactly this point, citing major differences between White and Sioux (Bryde, 1970), Pueblo (Zintz, 1963), Hopi (Aberle, 1951), and Arapaho (Tefft, 1967) cultural values. Moreover, Indian clients may hold quite different beliefs about the etiology of their problems and the manner in which change can be accomplished (Trimble, Manson, Dinges, & Medicine, in press).

Characteristics of Service Providers

Certain therapist characteristics, qualities, and activities have been identified as contributing to positive and negative outcomes in psychotherapy in general. In fact, many clinicians believe these qualities to be the most important determinants of patient improvement. Therapist variables such as warmth, honesty, self-disclosure, empathic communication, specific personality characteristics, and personal adjustment are among those that have received the greatest attention in empirical studies. This research was initially summarized by Truax and Carkhuff (1967) and has been updated on several occasions (Truax & Mitchell, 1971; Mitchell, Bozarth, & Krauft, 1977; Lambert, De Julio, & Stein, 1978). The evidence indicates that the quality of the relationship correlates with positive outcomes. The absence of these qualities has been found to be associated with patient deterioration (Lambert, Bergin, & Collins, 1977). Cross-cultural research suggests that many of the same therapist characteristics are also related to positive outcome between participants from different cultures (Sue, 1981). Perceived expertness (Berman, 1979; Atkinson, Maruyama, & Matsui, 1978), trustworthiness (Vontress, 1971), positive regard and empathy (Calia, 1968; Jones & Seagull, 1977), comfort, and previous cross-cultural experience (Sue, 1981) have been shown to be related to different-culture patient improvement. Considerably more work needs to be done in this regard, especially with respect to the manner in which such variables are defined and operationalized. Little or no data are available on the therapist variables most closely linked to positive outcomes in psychotherapy among Indian patients. Speculation and anecdotal impressions abound, yet remain to be tested systematically (Dinges et al., 1981).

Treatment-Related Considerations

To this end, the following questions must be examined within American Indian and Alaska Native communities:

(1) What treatment modalities (indigenous and nontraditional) are available for various forms of psychopathology?

(2) What expectancy variables define the therapeutic relationships? From the Indian patient's viewpoint? From the therapist's viewpoint?

(3) What process variables occur between therapists and Indian patients?

(4) How does one appropriately measure outcome?

(5) What constitutes effective treatment?

(6) To what extent and under what conditions are treatment modalities differentially effective?

(7) Under what conditions and for what reasons are practices and techniques of traditional healers appropriate?

Program Evaluation

Program evaluation proceeds at a different level of analysis than does the measurement of treatment outcomes. It examines specified organizational and service delivery goals in the context of community needs and the subsequent impact of an intervention scheme. Planners and administrators of Indian programs advocate evaluation of this nature, but seldom practice it. In those few instances in which such efforts are carried out, program response (in the form of modification or redirection) rarely follows. This seems to be true of the delivery of mental health services in general as well as in the Indian case.

Utilization of Services

With one major exception, which is discussed at the end of this section, the evaluation of services delivered to Indian and Native communities has taken the form of studies of reasons for underutilization, or, more specifically, of barriers to service. Murdock and Schwartz (1978) surveyed 160 elderly Sioux residents of a South Dakota reservation and found the overall awareness of available services to be remarkably low. More than 40 percent of the respondents were unaware of 15 of the 21 service agencies on the reservation. Awareness of service availability closely paralleled previous differences in perceived need by household type. Elderly persons living alone were less aware of medical, home maintenance, and personal maintenance services than their counterparts residing as couples or with children. Moreover, the former were *more* aware of social and mental health services, for which they expressed considerable need, but that were sorely lacking.

Dukepoo (1980) interviewed 62 elderly Indians from the Southern California area. Of this group, 45 percent indicated that they actively sought some form of care from mental health services. However, 81 percent of those who did so on a regular basis spoke negatively about the quality of the services. Fear, mistrust, and insensitivity of agency personnel were cited as the predominant barriers to service use. In a study of institutionalized elderly Apache living in Phoenix, Cooley, Ostendorf, and Bickerton (1979) found service barriers similar to those discussed by Dukepoo.

A few articles describe service delivery problems among specific tribal groups. Hippler (1975) argues that Eskimos, for example, fail to respond to mental health care systems because of their intrinsic belief in magic. He further asserts that Eskimos will continue to be nonresponsive to such care as long as magic-thinking and beliefs in traditional healers persist.

Beliefs about the effectiveness of mental health care staff can affect use patterns. Reporting on their work among the Navajo, Schoenfeld, Lyerly, and Miller (1971) indicate that patient referrals are directly related to the attitudes that program staff hold toward the provider agencies. For example, few, if any, clients were referred to the BIA program since attitudes toward its staff were largely negative. Furthermore, whereas the mental health personnel were viewed positively, a great deal of mistrust existed between them and other agencies, hampering effective coordination of the delivery of services in this community.

Urban Indian leaders and community members share a mutual concern for mental health conditions and availability of services (Borunda & Shore, 1978). According to Barter and Barter (1974), urban Indians believe that their mental health needs are not being met adequately and that the federal government shares in the responsibility for providing care. Available services are viewed with suspicion and hence are underutilized—a recurrent finding among Indian populations and other ethnic minority populations (Sue, 1977; Sue & McKinney, 1975).

Nonurban and off-reservation Indians apparently experience problems similar to those of their urban counterparts. Bittker (1973), based upon a survey of Phoenix-area service delivery facilities, reports that off-reservation Indians have ambiguous status; state and federal governments typically consider them to be outside the realm of their responsibility. Nonetheless, their need for services is as great as those of Indians from other settings—perhaps greater, considering the few services available to them.

Evaluation-Related Considerations

This rather limited focus of past evaluation efforts suggests that we must begin to ask a series of broader, more comprehensive questions:

(1) What services currently maintain an active program evaluation component? What is this component's function? How are data collected and used to inform development?

(2) What evaluation models are available in general, especially those culturally appropriate for use in certain Indian areas? Are there program examples?

(3) Are certain types of evaluation more appropriate for one delivery structure than for another?

(4) What are the major barriers to program evaluation? How can these be overcome?

(5) How does one meaningfully apply evaluation data to program development?

(6) What efforts are being made to evaluate the effectiveness of traditional healers in providing services, or the effectiveness of collaborative efforts between professionals and healers?

(7) What are the competencies required for delivering effective mental health services in Indian areas? Must all programs fit the cultural needs of communities? Or must the orientation of the clientele be adjusted to accommodate the limitations of the programs? To what extent are these issues being researched and assessed?

Several large-scale evaluations by Beiser and Attneave of the mental health program within the Indian Health Service move us in this direction. Their first effort (Beiser and Attneave, 1975) covered the 1972-1973 fiscal year and employed a diverse set of methods, including participant observation at various service units, interviews with select staff, a review of archival data, and the examination of quantitative data describing case loads and patient characteristics. One year later, Beiser and Attneave (1977) conducted an extensive series of analyses of patient contact with the same program, using data generated by a computerized record-keeping system. The results of these linked studies are just becoming available and show great promise for future program design and modification (Rhoades et al., 1980; Beiser & Attneave, in press).

Epidemiology

Epidemiological data are requisite to the cost-effective deployment of mental health resources and are especially important when said resources are limited, as is the present case. Manson and Shore (1981) conducted an extensive review of the literature with respect to epidemiological studies of American Indian and Alaska Native communities and discovered three that were conducted on a communitywide basis. Shore, Kinzie, and Thompson (1973) interviewed one-half of the adult Indian population in a Pacific Northwest coastal village. Roy, Chaudhuri, and Irvine (1970) surveyed slightly more than one-quarter of the Indian population located on ten reservations under the jurisdiction of a Canadian administrative agency. Sampath (1974) interviewed virtually the entire adult population of a southern Baffin Island Eskimo settlement. All three of these studies report diagnostic distributions and prevalence rates, and explore the relationship between psychiatric morbidity and contemporary social pressures. Though open to various methodological criticisms, these kinds of data provide a broader and more divergent picture of the nature and pattern of disorder in Indian and Native communities than those that derive from service utilization studies, by far the more common approach to estimating such trends (Sue, 1977; Rhoades et al., 1980).

Epidemiological Considerations

Future epidemiological work among Indian and Native communities must address the following questions:

(1) To what extent are current diagnostic tools valid and reliable indicators of psychopathology as perceived and experienced by Indian people?

(2) What is the relationship between "treated" prevalence and incidence rates (derived from service records) and patterns of disorder as manifested in the community at large?

(3) Are the data that serve as the basis for "treated" prevalence and incidence rates collected in a reliable, systematic fashion?

(4) Can these data be organized, collated, and reported in a regular relatively current and accessible form?

(5) Can a mechanism be developed to translate such data into meaningful recommendations for the development of mental health services to Indian people?

Collecting and Measuring Mental Health Data

In response to the first question, two recent studies indicate the methodological and conceptual shortcomings of several diagnostic instruments when administered to members of this population. Pollack and Shore (1980) reviewed scores on the Minnesota Multiphasic Personality Inventory (MMPI) for 142 American Indian patients at Indian Health Service mental clinics in the Portland service area. Regardless of the scale of interest, the scores of nonpsychotic depressed Indian patients were indistinguishable from the scores of schizophrenic Indian patients. Nor were there any significant differences between antisocial-alcoholic patients and those with situational reactions. On the basis of these findings, Pollack and Shore conclude that the similarity of subgroup profiles demonstrates significant cultural influence on the response patterns, rendering the MMPI useless among American Indians. Manson and Shore (in press) describe an ongoing study of the relationships between ethnopsychiatric data and *Diagnostic and Statistical Manual III* (DSM-III) research diagnostic criteria for depression within the Hopi of northeastern Arizona. They offer a number of examples of the practical and conceptual difficulties in modifying select portions of the Diagnostic Interview Schedule (Robins, Holzer, Croughan, & Ratcliff, 1981) for administration to members of this tribe, echoing earlier warnings by Chance (1962). Clearly, answers to questions about reliability and validity of diagnostic tools among Indian communities await careful studies such as these.

There is little or no indication in the literature as to the relationship between "treated" prevalence and incidence rates and patterns of disorder at the community level in the Indian population. No service utilization records were available for comparison among the communities in which epidemiological studies have been conducted previously.

Mental health data are collected systematically by the Indian Health Service across its 72 service units. A new computerized patient care information system has been implemented in 2 service areas and, depending upon availability of funds, will be put into effect servicewide in the near future.[2] The protocols for collecting data of this nature have not been examined in terms of interrater reliability, which is further complicated by the disparate educational backgrounds and varied training of service providers. Manson and Shore (in press) demonstrate that diagnostic interviews can be conducted in a reliable manner by psychiatrists employing the Schedule for Affective Disorder and Schizophrenia—

Lifetime Version. However, until common diagnostic procedures are adopted and the reliability of the collection of patient information is established, this question will also plague future planning and delivery efforts.

Health care planning and policy are monitored by a diverse array of agencies and community organizations: the Indian Health Service and its advisory committees, tribal health departments, the National Indian Health Board and its constituent area offices, the Urban Indian Health Care Association, and the Bureau of Indian Affairs, to name a few. Some attention needs to be given to how the kinds of data described above can be introduced into such a network to ensure appropriate consideration in the design and modification of mental health services, both those currently delivered and those planned. Successful efforts in this regard will probably prove to have had multiple points of contact with unequivocal relevance and strong community support.

Prevention

Prevention concepts, especially those that involve mental health promotion and enhancement, have long held the interest of tribal planners and service providers, the Indian Health Service, local as well as national advisory boards, and American Indian and Alaska Native people in general. This interest stems from a community-derived sense of self and of others that lends itself to the public health model that underpins the western health care system introduced into Indian country through past treaty arrangements (Beiser & Attneave, 1978). Moreover, indigenous approaches to health and welfare—at the levels of the individual and of the tribe— provide fertile ground for the growth of such concepts. Traditional healers, their patients, significant others, social context, and common ethos are intimately linked in an attempt to realize many of the same goals as those expressed in the Alcohol, Drug Abuse, and Mental Health Administration (ADAMHA) prevention policy, namely:

> family cohesion and positive family relationships, positive self-esteem; a basic belief in one's self-worth and relative value to the world, however personally defined; respect for others; interpersonal and social skills necessary for effective functioning in society; positive coping capacities and generalized stress resistance, and availability of networks and positive community support systems [U.S. Department of Health and Human Services, 1981, p. 10].

However, despite this apparent receptivity, relatively little prevention research or service has been conducted in the area of Indian mental health, and much of what exists represents a very narrow focus (Manson, in press-a).

Prevention-Related Considerations

In light of the present state of the art, future research on and the delivery of prevention services to American Indian and Alaska Native communities must consider the following questions:

(1) What forms of psychopathology are thought to be preventable? By indigenous means? By nontraditional means?
(2) What are the available techniques?
(3) How does one appropriately measure outcome?
(4) What constitutes effective prevention?
(5) To what extent and under what conditions are these techniques differentially effective?
(6) How can "mental health" be sustained and promoted?

Primary Prevention Efforts

Primary prevention seeks to lower the prevalence of disease by reducing its incidence, which can be accomplished in three ways: health promotion and enhancement, disease/disorder prevention, and health protection.

Health promotion and enhancement involve building or augmenting adaptive strengths, coping resources, survival skills, and general health. In addition to focusing upon the capacity to resist stress, health promotion and enhancement require an understanding of the conditions that generate stress and that may affect psychosocial functioning negatively. There are very few efforts of this nature in the Indian mental health literature. Exceptions include work by Dinges, Yazzie, and Tollefson (1974) on developmental task accomplishment among Navajo parents and children; by Kleinfeld (1973b), in her study of the characteristics of successful boarding school parents for Alaska Native students; by Lefley (1974), in her research on the familial and social correlates of psychological health among Miccosukee children; by Goldstein (1974), in his evaluation of the Toyei Indian School model dormitory project; and by Manson (in press-b) and Manson, Murray, and Cain (in press) on the various features of support networks that facilitate situational problem solving among Indian elderly.

Disease/disorder prevention encompasses a much narrower spectrum of concerns. It targets a specific disorder and, based on an analysis of risk factors, attempts to manipulate one or more conditions to forestall the occurrence of the disease in question. The majority of primary prevention projects in Indian mental health are of this type, but they seldom move beyond the identification of risk factors to study the differential success of interventions according to the conditions manipulated. Hence the literature is replete with profiles of the "typical" Indian alcoholic, delinquent, addict, and suicide, and lacks data on the effectiveness of potential responses.

Health protection techniques employ regulatory and legislative action to reduce the probability that the disease agent and host will come into contact. Bonnie (1978, pp. 210-213) discusses health protection in terms of four legal strategies: establishing the conditions of content (availability), deterring undesired behavior through punishment, symbolizing an official posture toward the behavior, and influencing the contact of messages in the mass media. With respect to Indian communities, the classic "experiment" in health protection was the federally imposed (and in many places now tribal) prohibition of liquor sales and liquor consumption on reservation lands. Levy and Kunitz (1974) clearly demonstrate that the prevalence of "problem drinking" and of associated phenomena (accident, arrest, and homicide rates) is not necessarily lower and may be even higher on "dry" reservations than on "wet" reservations.

Secondary Prevention Efforts

Secondary prevention seeks to reduce the prevalence of disease or disorder through early case finding and treatment. A reduction in the duration of a case consequently decreases the total number of active cases at any given point in time. Efforts of this nature are extremely sparse in the Indian mental health literature. Manson and Shore (in press) have begun to identify the relationships among psychophysiological symptoms, indigenous categories of illness, and research diagnostic criteria for depression within a southwestern Indian tribe, permitting earlier intervention and more appropriate treatment. McShane and Plas's (1980) study of the psychoeducational impact of otitis media, specifically of parent reports of the number of a child's ear infections as a means of detecting psychoeducational problems earlier, is another example.

Tertiary Prevention Efforts

Tertiary prevention addresses the degree of disability that an individual suffers as the consequence of a disease/disorder. The most common approach is rehabilitation, complemented by community support programs to reduce the need for institutionalization. Despite a number of tertiary prevention programs in the area of Indian mental health, largely for chronic alcoholics and drug abusers, *virtually no research* has been conducted on the relative effectiveness of rehabilitation strategies, on the kind and nature of community support that best facilitates deinstitutionalization, or on *how* to engender and to maintain such support.

Summary and Conclusion

A special task panel report on the mental health of American Indians and Alaska Natives was submitted to the President's Commission on Mental Health (PCMH) in 1978. Many of the questions posed in this chapter echo the recommendations of that report. Those recommendations note that "at present services and service delivery systems to Indian people . . . are disjointed, disorganized, wasteful, fragmented, and counterproductive" (PCMH, 1978, p. 982) and call for an examination of ways in which to coordinate the delivery of mental health care more effectively. Concern is expressed over the lack of knowledge about the relative efficacy of nonindigenous forms of counseling and psychotherapy with American Indians and Alaska Natives and about mechanisms to enhance and support traditional practices. Thorough and ongoing program evaluation is set forth as the cornerstone for eliminating duplication of services, for achieving greater institutional accountability, and for increasing awareness of successful, appropriate methods of care. The lack of a solid epidemiological data base is recognized, as is the cultural bias of diagnostic instrumentation. Mental illness prevention is frequently cited in the context of the chronic physical ailments that plague Indian and Native people; mental health promotion is held out as a possible and desired function of boarding schools. Basic and applied research on the full range of phenomena associated with these aspects of service is a common theme across all the recommendations. In this chapter we have summarized that which is known with regard to the delivery structure, treatment processes, program evaluation, epidemiology, and prevention, and have offered a series of specific questions that can serve as guideposts to future inquiry.

Notes

1. Pursuant to a 1978 resolution by the National Congress of American Indians, people indigenous to North America are referred to as "American Indians" and "Alaska Natives," except when specific tribal designations are appropriate. For the sake of brevity, we employ the term "Indian" in referring to this special population.

2. Personal communication with William Douglas, Ph.D., Systems Analyst, Office of Mental Health Programs, Indian Health Service, 1980.

References

Aberle, D. F. The psychosocial analysis of a Hopi life-history. *Comparative Psychology Monographs,* 1951, 21(1), 80-138.

American Indian Health Care Association. *Six studies concerning assessing mental health needs in the Minneapolis-St. Paul area: A summary.* Minneapolis: Author, 1978.

Atkinson, D. R., Maruyama, M., & Matsui, S. Effects of counselor race and counseling approach on Asian Americans' perceptions of counselor credibility and utility. *Journal of Counseling Psychology,* 1978, 25, 76-83.

Attneave, C. L. Medicine men and psychiatrists in the Indian Health Service. *Psychiatric Annals,* 1974, 4(11), 49-55.

Barter, E. R., & Barter, J. R. Urban Indians and mental health problems. *Psychiatric Annals,* 1974, 4(9), 37-43.

Beiser, M., & Attneave, C. L. *Service networks and utilization patterns.* Mental Health Programs, Indian Health Service. Rockville, MD: Indian Health Service, 1975.

Beiser, M., & Attneave, C. L. *Analysis of patient and staff characteristics, presenting problems and attitudes towards mental illness* (Final report, U.S.P.H.S.) Rockville, MD: Indian Health Service, 1977.

Beiser, M., & Attneave, C. L. Mental health services for American Indians: Neither feast nor famine. *White Cloud Journal,* 1978, 1(2), 3-10.

Beiser, M., & Attneave, C. L. Mental disorders among Native American children Rates and risk periods for entering treatment. *American Journal of Psychiatry* 1982, 139, 193-198.

Bittker, T. E. Dilemmas of mental health delivery to off-reservation Indians *Anthropological Quarterly,* 1973, 46, 172-182.

Bergin, A. E. The evaluation of therapeutic outcomes. In A. E. Bergin & S. L Garfield (Eds.), *Handbook of psychotherapy and behavior change.* New York John Wiley, 1971.

Berman, J. Counseling skills used by black and white female counselors. *Journal of Counseling Psychology,* 1979, 26, 81-84.

Bonnie, R. J. Discouraging unhealthy personal choices: Reflections on new direction in substance abuse policy. *Journal of Drug Issues,* 1978, 8, 199-219.

Borunda, P., & Shore, J. H. Neglected minority: Urban Indians and mental health *International Journal of Social Psychiatry,* 1978, 24(3), 220-224.

Bryde, J. F. *The Indian student: A study of scholastic failure and personality conflict.* Vermillion: University of South Dakota Press, 1970.

Calia, C. F. The culturally deprived client: A reformulation of the counselor's role. In J. C. Bentley (Ed.), *The counselor's role: Commentary and readings.* Boston: Houghton Mifflin, 1968.

Chance, N. A. Conceptual and methodological problems in cross-cultural health research. *American Journal of Public Health,* 1962, 52(3), 410-417.

Cooley, R. C., Ostendorf, D., & Bickerton, D. Outreach services for elderly Native Americans. *Social Work,* 1979, 29, 151-153.

Dinges, N. G., Trimble, J., Manson, S., & Pasquale, F. The social ecology of counseling and psychotherapy with American Indians and Alaska Natives. In A. J. Marsella & P. Pedersen (Eds.), *Cross-cultural counseling and psychotherapy: Foundations, evaluation and cultural considerations.* Elmsford, NY: Pergamon, 1981.

Dinges, N. G., Yazzie, M. E., & Tollefson, G. D. Developmental intervention for Navajo family mental health. *Personnel and Guidance Journal,* 1974, 52(6), 390-395.

Dukepoo, P. C. *The elder American Indian.* San Diego: Campanile, 1980.

Goldstein, A. P. Evaluating expectancy effects in cross-cultural counseling and psychotherapy. In A. J. Marsella & P. Pedersen (Eds.), *Cross-cultural counseling and psychotherapy: Foundations, evaluation and cultural considerations.* Elmsford, NY: Pergamon, 1981.

Goldstein, G. S. The model dormitory. *Psychiatric Annals,* 1974, 4(11), 85-92.

Higginbotham, H. N. Culture and the role of client expectancy in psychotherapy. In R. W. Brislin & M. Hamnett (Eds.), *Topics in culture learning* (Vol. 5). Honolulu: East-West Center, 1977.

Hippler, A. E. Thawing out some magic. *Mental Hygiene,* 1975, 59, 20-24.

Jones, A., & Seagull, A. A. Dimensions of the relationship between the black client and the white therapist: A theoretical overview. *American Psychologist,* 1977, 32, 850-855.

Kleinfeld, J. *A long way from home.* Fairbanks, AK: Institute for Social, Economic and Government Research, 1973. (a)

Kleinfeld, J. Characteristics of successful boarding home parents of Eskimo and Athabascan Indian students. *Human Organization,* 1973, 32(2), 191-199. (b)

Lambert, M. J., Bergin, A. E., & Collins, J. L. Therapist-induced deterioration in psychotherapy. In A. S. Gurman & A. M. Razin (Eds.), *Effective psychotherapy: A handbook of research.* Elmsford, NY: Pergamon, 1977.

Lambert, M. J., De Julio, S. S., & Stein, D. M. Therapist interpersonal skills: Process, outcome, methodological considerations and recommendations for further research. *Psychological Bulletin,* 1978, 85, 467-489.

Lefley, H. P. Effects of a cultural heritage program on the self-concept of Miccosukee Indian Children. *Journal of Educational Research,* 1974, 67(10), 462-466.

Levy, J., & Kunitz, S. *Indian drinking.* New York: John Wiley, 1974.

McShane, D., & Plas, J. *Otitis media, psychoeducational difficulties, and Native Americans.* Manuscript submitted for publication, 1980.

Manson, S. M. (Ed.). *New directions in prevention among American Indian and Alaska Native communities.* Portland: Oregon Health Sciences University Press, in press. (a)

Manson, S. M. Daily problematic life situations among American Indian elderly: A comparison of urban and rural perceptions. *Gerontologist,* in press. (b)

Manson, S. M., Murray, C., & Cain, L. Ethnicity, aging, and support networks: An evolving methodological strategy. *Journal of Minority Aging,* in press.

Manson, S. M., & Shore, J. H. Psychiatric epidemiological research among American Indians and Alaska Natives: Methodological issues. *White Cloud Journal,* 1981, 2(2), 48-56.

Manson, S. M., & Shore, J. H. Relationship between ethnopsychiatric data and research diagnostic criteria in the identification of depression within a southwestern American Indian tribe. *Culture, Medicine and Psychiatry,* in press.

Mitchell, K. M., Bozarth, J. D., & Krauft, C. C. A reappraisal of the therapeutic effectiveness of accurate empathy, nonpossessive warmth, and genuineness. In A. S. Gurman & A. M. Razin (Eds.), *Effective psychotherapy: A handbook of research.* Elmsford, NY: Pergamon, 1977.

Montijo, J. The Puerto Rican client. *Professional Psychology,* 1975, 6, 475-477.

Murdock, S. H., & Schwartz, D. F. Family structure and the use of agency services: An examination of patterns among elderly Native Americans. *Gerontologist,* 1978, 18(5), 475-481.

Oregon State Commission on Indian Services. *First annual report.* Salem: Author, 1978.

Ostendorf, D., Hammerschlag, C. A. An Indian-controlled mental health program. *Hospital and Community Psychiatry,* 1977, 28(9), 682-685.

Pedersen, P., Draguns, J., Lonner, W., & Trimble, J. (Eds.). *Counseling across cultures.* Honolulu: University of Hawaii Press, 1981.

Pollack, D., & Shore, J. H. Validity of the MMPI with Native Americans. *American Journal of Psychiatry,* 1980, 137(8), 946-950.

President's Commission on Mental Health (PCMH). *Report to the president of the President's Commission on Mental Health,* Vol. 3: *Task Panel Reports.* Washington, DC: Government Printing Office, 1978.

Rachman, S. The effects of psychological treatment. In H. Eysenck (Ed.), *Handbook of abnormal psychology.* New York: Basic Books, 1973.

Rhoades, E. R., Marshal, M., Attneave, C., Echohawk, M., Bjork, J., & Beiser, M. Impact of mental disorders upon elderly American Indians as reflected in visits to ambulatory care facilities. *Journal of the American Geriatrics Society,* 1980, 28(1), 33-39.

Robins, L. N., Holzer, J. E., Croughan, J., & Ratcliff, K. S. National Institute of Mental Health Diagnostic Interview Schedule. *Archives of General Psychiatry,* 1981, 38, 381-389.

Roy, C., Chaudhuri, A., & Irvine, D. The prevalence of mental disorders among Saskatchewan Indians. *Journal of Cross-Cultural Psychology,* 1970, 1(4), 383-392.

Sampath, B. M. Prevalence of psychiatric disorders in a southern Baffin Island Eskimo settlement. *Canadian Psychiatric Association Journal,* 1974, 19, 363-367.

Schoenfeld, L. S., Lyerly, R. J., & Miller, S. I. We like us. *Mental Hygiene,* 1971, 55(2), 171-173.

Shore, J. H., Kinzie, J. D., and Thompson, J. L. Psychiatric epidemiology of an Indian Village. *Psychiatry,* 1973, 36, 70-81.

Shore, J. H., & Manson, S. M. Cross-cultural studies of depression among American Indians and Alaska Natives. *White Cloud Journal,* 1981, 2(2), 5-12.

Sue, D. W. Counseling the culturally different: A conceptual analysis. *Personnel and Guidance Journal,* 1977, 55, 422-425.

Sue, D. W. Evaluating process variables in cross-cultural counseling/therapy. In A. Marsella & P. Pedersen (Eds.), *Cross-cultural counseling and psychotherapy: Foundations, evaluation, and cultural considerations.* Elsmsford, NY: Pergamon, 1981.

Sue, S. Community mental health services to minority groups: Some optimism, some pessimism. *American Psychologist,* 1977, 32, 616-624.

Sue, S., Allen, D. G., & Conaway, L. The responsiveness and equality of mental health care to Chicanos and Native Americans. *American Journal of Community Psychology,* 1978, 6, 137-146.

Sue, S., & McKinney, H. Asian-Americans in the community mental health care system. *American Journal of Orthopsychiatry,* 1975, 45, 111-118.

Tefft, S. K. Anomy, values and culture change among teen-age Indians: An exploration. *Sociology of Education,* 1967, Spring 1967, 145-157.

Trimble, J. Value differentials and their importance in counseling American Indians. In P. Pedersen, W. Lonner, J. Draguns, & J. Trimble (Eds.), *Counseling across cultures.* Honolulu: University of Hawaii Press, 1981.

Trimble, J., Manson, S., Dinges, N., & Medicine, B. Towards an understanding of American Indian concepts of mental health: Some reflections and directions. In P. B. Pedersen & A. J. Marsella (Eds.), *Cross-cultural mental health services.* Beverly Hills, CA: Sage, in press.

Truax, C. B., & Carkhuff, R. R. *Toward effective counseling and psychotherapy: Training and practice.* Chicago: Aldine, 1967.

Truax, C. B., & Mitchell, K. M. Research on certain therapist interpersonal skills in relation to process and outcome. In A. E. Bergin & S. L. Garfield (Eds.), *Handbook of psychotherapy and behavior change.* New York: John Wiley, 1971.

U.S. Department of Health and Human Services. *ADAMHA prevention policy and programs, 1979-1982.* Washington, DC: Government Printing Office, 1981.

U.S. Department of Commerce, Bureau of the Census. *1980 census of population and housing: United States summary.* Washington, DC: Government Printing Office, 1981.

Vontress, C. E. Racial differences: Impediments to rapport. *Journal of Counseling Psychology,* 1971, 18, 7-13.

Wax, R. H., & Thomas, R. K. American Indians and white people. *Phylon,* 1965, 12, 1-8.

Willie, C. V., Kramers, B. M., & Brown, B. S. *Racism and mental health: Essays.* Pittsburgh: University of Pittsburgh Press, 1973.

Wu, I.-H., & Windle, E. *Ethnic and sex specificity in the relationship of minority staffing and in minority use of community mental health centers.* Rockville, MD: Center for Minority Group Mental Health Programs, National Institute of Mental Health, 1978.

Zintz, M. V. *Education across cultures.* Dubuque, IA: William C. Brown, 1963.

8

Blacks

Rethinking Service
Thom Moore
University of Illinois—Urbana-Champaign

From time to time a society must take a break from its everyday activity to step back and ask itself some questions: How are we doing? Are people happy? Are people realizing their dreams? Are people creative and productive? Do people think of their lives as meaningful and worthwhile? These are, of course, questions that have been put before the human race on many occasions and in numerous forms. The answers are often elusive and vague, but the questions are nonetheless worthy of contemplation if the society is to survive and grow. At one level Americans ask themselves these questions (more specifically, of course) every time a public election occurs, when the decision can be that we are doing just fine and should continue the present course or, for any number of reasons, we are not doing fine and we want things to be different.

If the above questions are asked in the right way, the answers can lend understanding to the concepts themselves. For instance, if we ask, "Are you happy?" and the reply is "Yes," a follow-up question might very well be "Why?" The answer to the "why" question will in turn identify the specific resources that indeed make people happy, such as family, children, employment, shelter, food, and any number of other things. These are the guidelines toward which society orients itself. By having such answers available, a society so inclined could decide to use its resources and energies to make opportunities available for its members to achieve the things they need and want in life. A growing society concerns itself not only with survival necessities, but with quality of life as well.

The purpose of this chapter is to consider these questions as they apply to mental health services to Black Americans. In essence, the chapter will ask, "How are Black Americans doing in general?" By comparing data on social indices over time and between Blacks and Whites, a clearer understanding of the answer will be developed. This method will allow for an evaluation of the absolute as well as the relative changes experienced by Blacks in the last two decades.

Primarily, the chapter is directed to the social level of analysis, where mental health problems are conceived in a broader context of social conditions and consequences. The decision to emphasize stressors attributable to the social system, instead of defective responses attributable to the person, is a conscious one. It does not originate in a desire to deny any role to the study and treatment of individual psychopathology. Rather, it springs from an intention to redress the imbalance against representation of social forces and to reaffirm their priority status.

In order to design treatments for mental health and illness, psychologists and other human service workers attempt first to establish the etiology of the disorder.

Beginning with the formal creation of clinical psychology, through the National Mental Health Act of 1945, person-oriented theories have guided research and treatment. Caplan and Nelson (1973) examined articles from the first six months' issues of the 1970 *Psychological Abstracts* that either mentioned Blacks specifically or were included under the index heading "Negro." In only 16 percent of the articles were problem characteristics identified as situationally or environmentally caused, and in 3 percent problem characteristics were viewed as causing situation of environmental characteristics. All remaining articles either explicitly or implicitly lead the reader to conclude that the person caused the particular problem. In addition, 48 percent of the remaining articles were of a comparison type that found Blacks lacking. Caplan and Nelson note that they do not condemn the person orientation; however, they say, it ignores other forces that operate on Black Americans. The significance of this article is that it points out the attitude with which psychological disorders are approached and it identifies the danger this presents for Black Americans.

Etiology

Twenty years after the inception of formal clinical psychology the social climate began to change. There was a clamoring for more new concepts, different treatments, a lessening of the doctor-client relationship, and a concern for the community at large. Dissatisfaction with psychiatric intervention experienced by researchers, practitioners, and society in general ushered in the community mental health movement, which supported a new search for understanding and treatment of mental

health and illness. Because much of the previous work had been conceptualized under the person perspective, there were few models relevant for
research or treatment. Faris and Dunham (1939) had pioneered a tradition
within sociology using surveys and epidemiological methodology to
describe existing mental disorder. Findings from that early study essentially indicated that high rates of schizophrenia were concentrated in the
center city and declined as one moved toward the surrounding areas. The
study has been reanalyzed and criticized for numerous reasons; however, it
gave legitimacy to an emerging thought that the sources of mental illness
existed outside of the person. Indeed, a few practitioners went so far as to
deny the existence of mental illness altogether.

Another study of great importance was that of Hollingshead and
Redlich (1958). They conclude that rate of disorder, types of disorders,
and treatment are related to social class. Hollingshead and Redlich found
that the lower class contributed both a higher proportion of patients than
they represented in the population and proportionally more than higher
classes. In terms of types of disorders, they conclude that "the sharp
increases in the rates for each type of psychotic disorder between classes IV
and V (lowest) indicate clearly that something is operating in the society
that gives rise to remarkable increases in the various kinds of rates at the
class IV and V levels." Among the many relationships they found between
treatment and social class was that lower-class patients invariably were in
treatment longer. Some of this was caused by the fact that they were
signed into state hospitals and virtually forgotten. Although the direct link
from situation (environmental, social system) to mental health and illness
was not found in this study, it again suggests that there is more to human
behavior than lies within the individual. The studies of Faris and Dunham
(1939) and Hollingshead and Redlich (1958) attracted others to frame
their mental health questions in terms of the aggregate rather than the
individual (Leighton, Harding, Macklin, Macmillan, & Leighton, 1959;
Jaco, 1960; Meyers & Bean, 1962; Srole, Langner, Michael, Opler, &
Rennie, 1962). According to Murphy (1969, p. 323):

> Such studies (Clark, 1948; Faris & Dunham, 1939; Jaco, 1959,
> 1960; and Malzberg, 1949) have demonstrated that stratification and
> rates of mental illness are correlated: in general, the higher the social
> economic position of the individual, the lower the rate of illness.
> Furthermore, among those receiving treatment for mental illness, the
> neuroses seem more characteristic among those high in the structure
> than are the psychoses which tend to cluster in populations lower in
> the stratification system.

The interpretation of the research still leaves a definite casual relationship unspecified: Does mental illness cause social standing, or the reverse? In an attempt to gather data that would yield more specific knowledge, Catalano and Dooley (1977) found that stressful life events and mood were significantly correlated with economic change. Stressful life events seemed to be related to more of the economic measures, and the economic variable "unemployment rate by region" seemed to be the best predictor variable. The unique character of this study was that the sample was noninstitutionalized and the economic indices were by region rather than by state or nation.

In a review of studies that attempted to establish a relationship between economic change and mental disorder, Dooley and Catalano (1980) report that a large majority of the studies of this type found an inverse relationship to social-economic status and mental disorder. They conclude that the studies reviewed provided support, of varying degrees, for the following hypotheses: that mental disorder increases with (a) undesirable economic change, (b) desirable economic change, or (c) change per se.

A second review, by Liem and Liem (1978), likewise focused on the question of social class and mental illness. After a review of Faris and Dunham (1939) and Dunham (1969), in which the latter reports findings contradicting the former, Liem and Liem conclude that "the weight of existing evidence strongly indicates that social class is related in important ways to mental disorder." On the other hand, they remind the reader that the social system is very complex and has varying effects upon its members, and that the conclusion that social class and mental disorder stand in a one-to-one relationship is a hasty one.

The significance of the above studies for Blacks is that, regardless of other variables, social class is related to mental disorder. The critical point here is that Blacks are heavily represented in the lower social class, which is overrepresented in populations receiving mental health treatment. It is in the interest of Black Americans to search for resources that will change their lives; it is equally important to think in terms of social resources rather than in terms of traditional mental health resources.

Treatment

Just as models for etiological development are scarce, so are those for treatment. Fairweather, Sanders, Maynard, Cressler, and Beck (1969) turned their attention to the hospitalized patient population. Hollinghead and Redlich (1958) had noted that discharge from a state mental hospital was a rare event. As a matter of fact, treatment was simply custodial care. In the decade that followed, based on new maintenance strategies and increased service needs, discharge became a more realistic treatment goal. Fairweather et al. found that a substantial number of the discharged population were unable to function in the community and had to be readmitted to the hospital. The old policy that made discharge almost impossible actually hindered the success of the new one. Patients had become socialized to the hospital system, which did not call for the same behavioral patterns as community living. These researchers hypothesize that employment is a critical factor for keeping ex-patients in the community and restoring them to full citizenship.

With this in mind, Fairweather et al. proceeded to develop a treatment program in which the patient was removed from the hospital, put to work in a meaningful way, and given responsibility for making decisions affecting his or her personal and work life. The setting for the program was an abandoned motel, referred to as a "community-lodge." Initially, the treatment included professional supervision but excluded traditional use of psychotherapy. Small group meetings were held on a regular basis to discuss problems in living and working. The professional supervision was eventually replaced by a graduate student and finally by a resident member of the program. The program was so successful in keeping ex-patients in the community and employed that the lodge program has been adopted as a standard intervention for patients throughout the country.

Cowen (1973) recognized the importance of the theoretical framework to ensuing treatment. He states that

> the future of MH rests as much with its conceptual stance as with any other simple factor. The term "conceptual stance" is used simplistically rather than rigorously to connote a loose network of guiding views and interlocking assumptions about how disordered behavior comes about and how best to cope with it. Such a stance permits policymakers to hierarchize and select from a vast array of prospective approaches; it is thus an orienting framework for making allocations in a private resource system [Cowen, 1973, p. 428].

This quote captures an understanding of the power of concepts, but, equally important, it gives a glance at the direction that psychological interventions have adopted. Cowen refers to policymakers allocating resources from a finite pool. Treatment in the traditional sense meant psychotherapy, in which a cure or relief was sought for the individual. The expanded approach centers on environmental and social change, resulting in the overall reduction of the rate of mental illness. Social status reflected by income, education, and occupation became legitimate outcome measures for human service workers.

Ryan's (1971) critique of social policy and social programming is an example of how this perspective could be applied to explanation. He claims that the treatments implemented by liberals during the War on Poverty era were misguided. Rappaport (1977) and Seidman (1978) have referred to this as an error in logical typing. Liberals identified the inadequacy in the social system to provide proper resources; however, the programs they designed ultimately blamed the victim. The issue of educational opportunity, for example, was not handled by simply upgrading the schools—instead the Head Start Program (a program of varying success), which centered on improving children, was chosen.

At that time, and even today, these theories and data are mixed blessings for Blacks. First of all, because the findings suggest that members of the lower socioeconomic classes are more likely to suffer from mental disorders, and because Blacks have always been overrepresented in the lower class, they gave a certain approval to these studies. Second, the underlying message in the research was that the "patient" was not the one source of the observed problem. Instead there was a great possibility that social systems that are powerful and that control needed resources of all kinds prevent people from functioning in appropriate and productive ways. Third, the findings simply reflected something that Black leaders had known for some time; however, when members of the status quo began to say these things they met with more acceptance. Blacks felt that this was another example of not being recognized. Nonetheless, the focus change from person to system meant that issues regarding mental health could be expanded.

Social Issues of Significance to Blacks

The question of how Black Americans are doing has its answer in social indices. In reviewing these data, the absolute gains in social standing are celebrated because they indicate an improvement in status for a number of people; however, if gains relative to the mainstream have not occurred, then little change has actually taken place. In the following section social indicators such as population changes, health, earnings and unemployment, and education will be presented for Blacks and, when possible, compared across race. The improvement of Blacks' status in each of these areas indicates a greater access to and involvement with physical and social resources.

Beginning in the late 1950s, the plight of Black Americans received much public attention, and in the 1960s it became a focal point for national priorities. In 1954 the Supreme Court, in Brown v. the Board of Education of Topeka, Kansas, ruled that dual educational systems were unconstituional. That original ruling has been appealed in numerous ways throughout the years, but its most significant impact was seen in the series of rulings that followed—rulings that all had the purpose of equalizing opportunities for Black Americans. These were acts to structure the agents of social control to be more open. They were an attempt to change the rules of the game.

Of equal importance was the 1955 bus boycott in Montgomery, Alabama. The city's Black population of 50,000 waged a year-long protest against racial discrimination in public transportation. Although the major concession, "the right to sit anywhere on public transportation," may at this point in history seem trivial, it served as a mobilizing force for Blacks throughout the country to actively demand equal rights and privileges in this country. The Montgomery incident provided a leader and an awareness of the power that could be mustered through organization. A commitment to social change that lasted for a decade and a half was made by Blacks, as individuals and as a people, and by the federal government. The programs and actions that grew out of that period have been hailed as a great successful experiment by some and as an embarrassing failure by others.

Following is a brief review of census data that will present the increase in numbers of Black Americans over the last two decades. It is significant to note that this is primarily an urban population, and when the cities are beset with social problems, Blacks are more likely to suffer than anyone else. Wealth is the next category that is considered. Here the illusion of the converging wage differential is discussed. Health is the next area in which the statistics show gains and losses. The final area is that of education. These areas then become the focal point of social intervention and change.

Population

The impact of public policy and social programming is better understood if one begins by reviewing general population figures. Furthermore, the comparison between Blacks and Whites in specific areas causes one to question the claims of relative gains for Blacks. In 1960, 10 percent of the American population was Black (18.8 million). By 1970 there were 22.5 million Blacks, and in 1980 that figure had grown to 26.4 million. This represented 11.1 and 11.7 percent of the total population, respectively. The majority of Black Americans live in the urban South. The trend, however, has been movement away from these regions. In the late 1700s, of course, 91 percent of Blacks lived in the South; by 1960, 60 percent resided there, and in 1975, 52 percent. The last two decades have seen a slowdown in the southern outmigration of Blacks.

Black Americans represent a sizable segment of the larger population, and as the social climate changes and becomes more hostile to human well-being, they stand to share less and less of the resources associated with a quality existence.

Wealth

The second area of review is that of income, earnings, and wealth. Income and earnings are monetary rewards given in exchange for work. This is to be distinguished from wealth, which is an accumulation of assets used to determine worth. While the Census Bureau reports the earnings of the population, there is a growing concern among labor economists that wealth plays a significant role in a person's status.

In 1959 the data for income are reported for Blacks and other races together. The median family income was $3,233 for Blacks, and for Whites it was $5,835. Blacks' and other races' median family income was 55 percent of that of Whites. By 1970 median family income is reported for Blacks alone: It was $6,279, and $10,236 for Whites. In 1970 the median family income for Blacks was 61 percent of that for Whites. Although the data on Blacks alone for 1960 are not available, a comparison between the two measurement points clearly represents a gain in family income. The median income for Black families in 1979 was $11,609 and for Whites it was $20,438. In 1979 Black median income was 57 percent of that of Whites, which is a trend back to 1959.

Willhelm (1970) reported that in 1963 a Negro who had spent some time in college earned less than a White male with an eighth-grade education, while a Negro college graduate earned slightly more than a White high school graduate. In the last several years economists have been reporting that the wage differential between Blacks and Whites is narrowing, and in 1972 it had completely disappeared. However, Lazear (1979) cautions that the gap still exists, especially if other forms of compensation are considered. One of the premises of his research is that even though two individuals are currently at the same wage level, they do not have the same real income if one is on a track that will yield him or her a higher yearly earning at age 30 than the other will earn at age 30. The unit of measurement should be wage growth rather than observed wage. Lazear found that the component of "on-the-job training" was different for Blacks and Whites and, while actual wages for young workers were about equal, experience was not. Furthermore, down the line the White workers with greater experience enjoyed greater earnings. Thus the differential still exists.

Rumberger (1981) investigated the relationship of wealth on earning power. He found that family wealth had a direct effect on White males' earnings. It also accounted for other factors, such as school, that are in turn related to earnings. For Black males there was no effect of parent wealth on earnings. Rumberger suggests that this simply reflects the lower status of Black parents compared to White parents.

The conclusion, then, is that Blacks have experienced tremendous gains as compared with themselves. On the other hand, when compared to Whites as a group and even as counterparts, there continues to be a great difference in immediate and long-range earning and subsequent purchasing power. In a supposedly free-market society this causes real problems. Prices are set to accommodate those who can pay. When a large portion of the population, which Whites represent, has considerably more money and wealth than other portions, the lower-income subpopulation cannot purchase the necessary goods and services to maintain their quality of life.

It would not be reasonable to discuss earnings and avoid unemployment. This tends to be a social variable that weakens the individual and her or his social network and community. Not only do individuals suffer when employment is low, but whole towns and cities have been known to die with the loss of employment. In 1960 the overall rate of unemployment for men was 5.4 percent. For White males that was 4.8 percent and 10.7 percent for Blacks. Blacks were more than twice as likely to be unemployed as Whites. By 1970 Black males' unemployment rate was 7.3 and that of White males was 4.0. At this point a relative gain was made for the Black unemployed. Nine years later a reversal of both the absolute and relative gain was observed: Black males had a 10.3 percent unemployment rate and White males 4.4 percent.

Health

Lunde (1981) reviewed the quality of health in America over a ten-year period. He compared indices of health by country, race, sex, age, and income. Although he predicts that Americans can anticipate increased improvement in health and health care throughout the 1980s, he found that there were definite differences among Blacks and Whites and other minorities, and the poor and nonpoor. He concludes:

In the 1980's, a focus on the problems related to the poor and minorities can create a further narrowing of gaps and can raise the general level of health of the nation [Lunde, 1981].

The infant mortality rate, for instance, among Blacks and other minorities in 1960 was 43.2 per 1000 live births, compared to 21.7 in 1977. This represents a substantial decrease of 21.5 in infant deaths over 17 years. The rate of White infant mortality was at a much lower rate to begin with and did not have as far to drop; however, it went from 22.9 in 1960 to 12.3 in 1977. While there is cause to rejoice and acknowledge that, within racial groups, progress is being made, infant mortality continues to have a greater affect on Black families than on White families. At the life expectancy end of the scale the relationship between Blacks and Whites is the same. Life expectancy for Blacks (and other minorities) from 1900-1975 rose 119 percent, from 33 to 70 years. During the same period for Whites, life expectancy increased 56 percent, from 47.6 to 74 years. Again, the percentage increase among Blacks is overwhelming and may serve as an indication that drastic changes in the quality of health and health care of Black Americans are occurring. On the other hand, there is still a real difference in actual years of life. The point becomes clearer when life expectancy is broken down by race and sex. Life expectancy for Black women is 74.5 years and for White women, 78.3 years; for Black men, 65.5 years and for White men, 70.6 years. In general, women tend to live longer than men, but both Black women and men can expect a shorter life span than White women and men.

In addition to infant mortality rates and life expectancy, causes of death from selected diseases show a definite difference by race. The trend of deaths caused by major cardiovascular diseases, diseases of the heart, and cerebrovascular diseases from 1950 to 1977 has been down. Similar to the changes in infant death and life expectancy, this trend has been in a positive direction, but Blacks continue to suffer more from these ailments than Whites. Malignant neoplasms of digestive organs and peritoneum deaths have shown a moderate decline. Malignant neoplasms of the respiratory system and diabetes mellitus are disorders that have taken a greater toll on human life. Malignant neoplasms of the respiratory system

have become more troublesome for Blacks. Lunde (1981) suggests cigarette smoking and carcinogenic properties of the urban environment as
possible causes.

One may simply conclude that Black Americans are experiencing better
health and health care overall. From this several assumptions regarding the
improvement of availability and quality of health care services for Blacks
can be made. At the same time, however, we must keep in mind the fact
that all is not well. Second-class status for Blacks continues in the health
domain.

Education

Education has always been a matter of concern for Black Americans. It
has been the way that one generation passes down to the next information
that is important for survival and participation in society. Education is as
much a socialization process—learning of social rules—as it is an intellectual
one (Coleman, 1959; Inkeles, 1966). For one reason or another, Blacks
have been denied equal access to educational opportunities. In terms of
mental illness, there are fewer psychiatric admissions among the population with some college and fewer still among those completing college.
Ashenfelter and Ham (1979) found that schooling, not the actual wage
rate, accounted for higher yearly earnings. Their explanation is that
schooling reduces the likelihood of becoming unemployed. Education is a
decision tool in society. Therefore, a change in the rate of participation in
the educational system would be a welcome achievement for Blacks.

In 1961 there were 44.4 million White children between the ages of 5
and 19. This is generally the period in which most education occurs.
Unless an individual performs well during these years it is highly unlikely
that he or she will continue on to higher education. Of that 44.4 million,
89 percent were enrolled in school. Actually, the 5-year-olds and the
18-19-year-old category had far fewer enrollments (U.S. Department of
Commerce, 1962). At the same time, there were 6.9 million Black children
between the ages of 5 and 19, and 86 percent were enrolled in school.
When students reached the age of 16 the enrollment rates for both groups
tended to decrease, but there was a substantial difference between races:
84.5 percent of White children at age 16 were enrolled in school, as
opposed to 76.8 percent of Black 16-year-olds. By 1978, 89 percent of the
White children between 5 and 19 years old were enrolled in school, while
90 percent of Black children of the same age were enrolled. During this
time, 91.2 percent of Blacks ages 16 and 17 were enrolled in school,
compared to 89.1 percent of Whites in that age group.

College enrollment is an especially significant measure of progress for Blacks in education. In 1961, 4.9 percent of the 18-34-year-old Black population was enrolled in college. As might be expected, the bulk of these students, 9.2 percent, were of the 18-24-year-old category. In 1978, 17 years later, 11 percent of the larger group (18-34-year-olds) were enrolled in college; 15 percent of that group were 18-24-year-olds. The 6.1 percent gain in college enrollment for Blacks between 18 and 34 is close to the 6.2 percent gain for the same group of Whites over the same time period. Blacks have imporved their actual participation in education and have maintained their relative standing with regard to college enrollment; however, a different picture is presented when quality is considered. Black children score 10 percent below the national mean in reading and science. Likewise, they fail to meet the national average in job knowledge and skills (National Center for Education Statistics, 1979). Edelman and Smith (1980) report that for every 100 high school graduates, 26.1 students drop out. The number of Black students dropping out is asonishing. For every 100 Black students who graduate, 49.6 drop out, compared to 23.3 White students.

Summary

The areas of health, earnings and unemployment, and education have been chosen as indicators of the status of Blacks. In none of these areas have the changes between Blacks and Whites been sufficient enough to say that the society is moving in a way that Blacks are sharing more equally in its resources. Healthwise, in 1977 infant mortality for Blacks had just reached the level that it had been for Whites in 1960. The encouraging sign is that the rate is dropping. Respiratory illnesses continue to plague Blacks. The causes for such disorders are believed to lie in cigarette smoking and the urban environment. The latter is especially significant to Blacks, given that they tend to live in urban settings. At the midpoint of the twenty-year span between 1960 and 1980, the median income of Blacks, in a small way, edged closer to that of Whites, but by 1979 it had begun to return to the 1961 spread.

According to *Current Population Reports* (U.S. Department of Commerce, 1962, 1979), Blacks have increased their relative gain during the years of mandatory education, and have made no change at the college level. Tragically, dropping out seems to be an acceptable way of dealing with education for many Black children. All in all, over the last twenty years, Blacks have been able to maintain their educational status. They are not necessarily worse off nor are they appreciably better off.

Levels of Intervention

The provision of mental health services for Black Americans by either the private or public sector has historically been ignored or at best overlooked. The precedent for such a position is entangled in the attitudes and practice of government representatives and theoretical reasoning of the helping professions. Gary (1978) notes that social organization and concominant services are created for the acknowledged members of a society. In the case of the Black American, the Constitution of 1787 designated them to be nonpeople. For purposes of tax assessment and legislative representation, Blacks' legal status was that of three-fifths of a person. In other words, it took five Black slaves to equal three White persons. There was no attempt to recognize Black slaves as people because that would have entitled them to all *rights* and *privileges* of citizens. No thought was given to mental health services for Blacks.

Mental health professionals at the time devised their own rationale for maintaining a position that excluded Blacks from receiving services. In the mid-nineteenth century, it was a common opinion that the "uncivilized races" (for example, Native Americans and slaves) had much less or almost no mental illnesses as compared to Whites. Prudhomme and Musto (1973, p. 30) report that

> psychological theorists asserted that the constitution of the civilized was initially more sensitive, more liable to creativity and unfortunately, to insanity. The lower races, the uncivilized, were less emotionally sensitive and were thereby protected from the stories of progress. Therefore, the American Indian and Black slave, and various other apparently sluggard groups gave evidence of their retardation through an almost embarrassing lack of insanity, the presence of which thus became considered as a sign of progress.

For close to one hundred years now, the mental health concerns of the Black American have been of little interest to anyone other than the Black American. By constitutional law Blacks were legally excluded from any right to service. Even more astonishing was the fact that the scientific community proposed that there was little reason for concern because Blacks were not advanced enough to be subject to mental illness. Finally, the delivery system at the time structured the Black mental patient out of the mainstream of service.

The legal exclusion of Blacks from mental health services is one of many racist policies that prevented them from enjoying the same equality of life as Whites. Gary (1978, p. 27) says:

> Mental health problems are those conditions affecting a significant number of Black people in ways which they consider undesirable, and there is a strong commitment through social action to changing the situation or condition so that a significant number of individuals can become, or remain, functioning members of their community.

When environmental characteristics such as social class, social systems, and public policy are adopted as the causes of mental illness, this creates an even greater risk for the health of Blacks. Because Blacks are under-represented in the upper social economic classes, are excluded from powerful and influential positions in the larger social system, and are rarely found among policymakers, there is little opportunity to have their interests reflected. This helps to create an environment that tends to be hostile and leads to unfulfilled expectations.

How then are services to be defined and delivered? Watzlawick, Weakland, and Fisch (1974) have developed a theory of change—the issue of how anything can be modified—in which the resolution of a problem can be of two types. There is change in which the relationship of the members of a system stays the same; this is called "first-order change." Then there is change in which the relationship of one member to the next is different; this is "second-order change." The mental health system, for example, has responded to an increase in service demand by training more human service workers in the old tradition. Often this means that the person orientation continues to be the training strategy of choice, and people receiving service are subject to the traditional doctor-patient roles. Even though the individual may improve his or her behavior in this situation, the chances that the relationship between the patient and the problem source will be altered is minimal. Patients, in effect, learn how to cope. In a second-order change the conceptualization of the problem is different and the role of the therapist changes. The patient can be a major actor in developing the intervention and the therapist may serve as a consultant. The Fairweather et al. (1969) intervention was of a second-order type.

Essential to this strategy is the ability to reframe the question. Rather than being concerned with mental health services, the question that needs be considered is: What social changes are likely to promote the involvement and participation of Black Americans as full and equal citizens? Poverty, for example, approached through welfare payments to the recipient maintains the individual's status in the system. On the other hand, employers and unions can become more aggressive in pursuing an economic policy of full employment. The latter of these two is an example of a second-order change. One caution here is that second-order change assumes systems to be dynamic. A change that is one-time second order will, over a long period, eventually become first order. The introduction of the welfare system was at one time an innovative way to ensure that needy people were provided for. As time passed, however, these people continued to be needy and their relationship to other members of the system was unchanged. Finally, it should be understood that there may be times when a first-order change is preferred to a second-order change.

What Changes Are Called For

Social change to effect the mental health of the Black community in the way that Gary (1978) suggests is best accomplished with social interventions directed at the different levels of the social order. These levels begin with the individual and go through the society. Rappaport (1977) identifies four corresponding sources of strategies and techniques for social intervention: (a) individual, (b) interpersonal, (c) organizational, and (d) institutional. There are numerous examples of individual and interpersonal intervention. They are the more traditional one-to-one therapies, family therapy, interpersonal communication training, and group therapy. Thus, when performed in a way that increases awareness and capacity to work effectively against injustice, traditional interventions may ultimately contribute to social change. Organizational and social analysis, on the other hand, are interventions with which the human service worker is less familiar.

At the organizational level, Rappaport (1977, p. 165) says:

> Because a great deal of behavior is under the control of the social structures of organizations, these structures and techniques for changing them are the key to solution of social problems.

Behavior under the control of the organization can be illustrated by the following example. The National Black Child Development Institute (1980) reports that declining tax bases in large cities with substantial minority populations have necessitated severe budget cuts. They note that in New York, for example, this coincides with an increasing school dropout rate (45 percent). While no real cause and effect relationship can be established, it is clear that some inner-city schools are unable to meet the needs of their students. Such fiscal limitation makes it impossible for the organization to realize its mission. Without adequate funding, educational organizations will be unable to acquire the resources needed to perform as expected.

In moving to the next level, Rappaport says that the real key to social change rests in the attitudes, values, goals, and political-economic ideology and social policy of which the institutions are composed. His distinction between institutions and organizations is that an organization implements the values and goals formulated by the institution. An institution sets policy that is reflective of its constituency's values and goals. At this level the tactics emphasize power, autonomy, and self-control. Rev. Jesse Jackson's Operation Push in Chicago is an example. His orientation is one of economic independence, the use of power and influence, and attention to improving individual worth.

Change strategies at these four levels are a comprehensive way for attacking the social condition and racism that continues to limit the well-being of Black Americans.

Recommendations

The very first change that must occur is at the policy level. The nation must develop an economic policy that is sensitive to human life. At the 1979 hearings of the House Committee on the Budget, Harvey Brenner (1979) testified that, based on the 1970 population, a 1 percent increase in unemployment was associated with 36,887 deaths, 920 suicides, 648 homicides, 495 deaths from cirrhosis of the liver, 4,227 state mental hospital admissions, and 3,340 state prison admissions. If the actual 1.4 percent increase in unemployment is translated into cost to society, then suicides cost $63 million dollars; state prison admissions, $210 million; homicides, $434 million; and cardiovascular diseases, $1.3 billion. This testimony indicates that the nation pays a heavy price for a slight downward change in the economy. The National Black Agenda for the '80's has recommended that the federal government stop using unemployment to fight inflation. They have also called for a policy of full employment. This is a major recommendation and it demands that Black Americans take the political process seriously. Williams and Morris (1981) reviewed the voter turnout of Blacks in the 1980 national election and found that 61 percent of registered Blacks voted. This is compared with a 52 percent turnout for the nation as a whole. They say that this is the fifth consecutive presidential election in which turnout declined. Surprisingly, the largest nonvoting segment of the population is that of the poor and disadvantaged. A concentrated effort to move Blacks into public office is one of the more significant items on the agenda.

The second recommendation involves education. Since schooling has been found to be highly related to yearly earnings, public education is in need of support. Black children seem to be especially at risk because support of all kinds is being channeled out of public school education. Blacks should be encouraged to organize and participate in parent-teacher organizations and local education boards. In this same area the National Black Child Development Institute has raised a question about the overwhelming number of Black children placed in the educable mentally retarded class (EMR). Black children represent 41 percent of all EMR students, while only constituting 17 percent of the entire student population. Although the decisions are typically made by trained professionals, school districts may need the services of child advocates in making these decisions. Because there is a need caused by the shortage of funds, many more Black parents have to volunteer their services to their local schools. By being involved with the schools, Black parents and their representatives can have input into the form and quality of educational services to be delivered.

Income is one of the areas in which creative ways of using influence and power must be developed. While affirmative action programs continue to exist, they have lost a considerable amount of influence. A renewed interest in the purpose behind that idea is called for. A call on unions, especially trade and construction unions, to be responsive to the needs of Black workers as well as their White workers is in order. In addition, the implementation of an aggressive plan by Black businesses to invest in Black-controlled enterprises that can compete in the lucrative high-technology field is needed.

What of changes at other levels? Problems of racism and conflicting cultural orientations in individual and group interventions have received a degree of overdue attention. However, the basic commitment underlying this chapter is to speak on behalf of other needed reforms--social change of a kind that can bring widespread enhancement of Black mental health. It is a matter of the greatest importance, particularly in the political climate of the 1980s, that we reaffirm our recognition of these factors and our commitment to work for greater social responsibility and service.

References

Ashenfelter, O., & Ham, J. Education, unemployment and earnings. *Journal of Political Economy*, 1979, 87, 99-116.

Brenner, M. H. Appearance before the Committee on the Budget, House of Representatives. 96th Congress, First Session, 1979.

Caplan, N., & Nelson, S. D. On being useful: The nature and consequences of psychological research on social problems. *American Psychologist*, 1973, 28(3), 199-211.

Catalano, R. A., & Dooley, D. C. Economic predictors of depressed mood and stressful life events. *Journal of Health and Social Behavior*, 1977, 18, 292-307.

Coleman, J. S. Academic achievement and the structure of competition. *Harvard Educational Review*, 1959, 29(4), 1959.

Cowen, E. L. Social and community interventions. *Annual Review of Psychology*, 1973, 24, 423-472.

Dooley, D., & Catalano, R. Economic change as a cause of behavioral disorder. *Psychological Bulletin*, 1980, 87, 450-468.

Dunham, W. H. City care and suburban fringe: Distribution patterns of mental illness. In S. C. Plog & R. B. Edgerton (Eds.), *Changing perspectives in mental illness*. New York: Holt, Rinehart & Winston, 1969.

Edleman, M. W., & Smith, P. V. *Portrait of inequality: Black and White children in America*. Washington, DC: Children's Defense Fund, 1980.

Fairweather, G. W., Sanders, D. H., Maynard, H., Cressler, D. L., & Beck, D. S. *Community life for the mentally ill: An alternative to institutional care*. Chicago: Aldine, 1969.

Faris, R.E.L., & Dunham, H. W. *Mental disorders in urban areas: An ecological study of schizophrenia and other psychoses*. Chicago: University of Chicago Press, 1939.

Gary, L. E. Mental health: A challenge to the Black community. Philadelphia: Dorrance, 1978.

Hollingshead, A. B., & Redlich, R. C. *Social class and mental illness: A community study*. New York: John Wiley, 1958.

Jaco, E. G. *The social epidemiology of mental disorder: A psychiatric survey of Texas*. New York: Russell Sage Foundation, 1960.

Inkeles, A. Social structure and the socialization of competence. *Harvard Educational Review*, 1966, 36(3), 265-283.

Lazear, E. The narrowing of Black-White wage differential is illusory. *American Economic Review*, 1979, (69)4, 553-564.

Leighton, D., Harding, J., Macklin, D., Macmillan, A., & Leighton, A. *The character of danger*. New York: Basic Books, 1959.

Liem, R., & Liem, J. Social class and mental illness reconsidered: The role of economic stress and social support. *Journal of Health and Social Behavioral*, 1978, 19(2), 139-156.

Lunde, A. S. Health in the United States. *Annals of the American Academy of Political and Social Science*, 1981, 453, 28-69.

Meyers, J. K., & Bean, L. L. *A decade later: A follow-up of social class and mental illness*. New York: John Wiley, 1967.

Murphy, R. J. Stratification and mental illness: Issues and strategies for research. In S. C. Plog & R. B. Edgerton (Eds.), *Changing perspectives in mental illness*. New York: Holt, Rinehart & Winston, 1969.

National Black Child Development Institute. *The status of Black children in 1980.* Washington, DC: Author, 1980.

National Center for Education Statistics. *The condition of education* (1979 ed.). Washington, DC: U.S. Department of Health, Education and Welfare, 1979.

Prudhomme, C., & Musto, D. F. Historical perspectives on mental health and racism in the United States. In C. V. Willie, B. M. Kramer, & B. S. Brown (Eds.), *Racism and mental health.* Pittsburgh: University of Pittsburgh Press, 1973.

Rappaport, J. *Community psychology: Values, research and action.* New York: Holt, Rinehart & Winston, 1977.

Rumberger, R. W. *The inheritance of earnings and wealth.* Columbus: Center for Human Resource Research, Ohio State University, 1981.

Ryan, W. *Blaming the victim.* New York: Random House, 1971.

Seidman, E., Justice, values and social science: Unexamined premises. In R. Simond (Ed.), *Research in law and sociology: An annual compilation of research.* Greenwich, CT: JAI, 1978.

Srole, L., Langner, T., Michael, S., Opler, M., & Rennie, T.A.C. *Mental health in the metropolis: The Midtown Manhattan Study.* New York: McGraw-Hill, 1962.

U.S. Department of Commerce, Bureau of the Census. *Current population reports.* Washington, DC: Government Printing Office, 1962.

U.S. Department of Commerce, Bureau of the Census. *Current population reports.* Washington, DC: Government Printing Office, 1979.

Watzlawick, P., Weakland, J., & Fisch, R. *Change.* New York: Norton, 1974.

Willhelm, S. M. *Who needs the Negro.* Cambridge, MA: Schenkman, 1970.

Williams, E. N., & Morris, M. D. The Black vote in a presidential election year. In National Urban League (Ed.), *The state of Black America.* Washington, DC: National Urban League, Inc., 1981.

9

Asian and Pacific Americans

Herbert Z. Wong

San Francisco Richmond-Maxi Center
and
National Asian American Psychology Training Center

The Asian and Pacific American population has grown dramatically in recent years. Between 1970 and 1980 this group increased by 128 percent, from 1.5 million to 3.5 million (Kim, 1981). This represents the largest proportional increase of any ethnic minority population in the United States during that period. Growth in the major urban areas has been particularly striking; for example, looking at major cities using EEOC district boundaries (U.S. Department of Commerce, 1981), Asian and Pacific Americans constitute 25 percent of the population of San Francisco, 17 percent of Los Angeles, 17 percent of San Jose, 13 percent of San Diego, 12 percent of New York City, 10 percent of Denver, 9 percent of Chicago, 9 percent of Seattle, and 7 percent of Philadelphia.

A large segment of this population is made up of immigrants or refugees. A total of 98 percent of all Indochinese, 90 percent of all Koreans, 70 percent of all Filipinos, and 60 percent of all Chinese residents of the United States are newly arrived and face language barriers, culture shock, unemployment and underemployment, role and status reversal, intergenerational conflicts, and lack of community support systems. Compounding these problems unique to the immigrants are the general sources of emotional distress and concern affecting other Americans.

At present the most vulnerable and high-risk Asian immigrants are Indochinese refugees. However, they are only part of the larger whole of Asian and Pacific Americans who continue to be visible and distinct because of commonalities in culture, life experience, and racial background. Despite these similarities, even larger differences exist within this group because of national background and adaptation, assimilation, and community development in the United States.

Unfortunately, the degree and significance of the mental health needs of Asian and Pacific Americans largely have been ignored or misunderstood, and the service and programmatic responses have often been piecemeal and uncoordinated (Lee, 1979; Sue & Kitano, 1973; Wong, 1981). The President's Commission on Mental Health (1978) notes that the general delivery of mental health services has been inappropriate and ineffective, even beyond the general shortcomings of community mental health (Chu & Trotter, 1974). In this chapter, the state of the art is reviewed with respect to the delivery of mental health services for Asian and Pacific Americans. Following the definition of this ethnic minority group, a brief review of the service and research literature is provided. A model for viewing mental health services is presented, and individual, group, and system issues for the delivery of mental health services to Asian and Pacific Americans is highlighted. Finally, recommendations are made with respect to models for mental health service delivery.

Asian and Pacific Americans Defined

The phrase "Asian and Pacific Americans" is actually a contraction of two terms, "Asian Americans" and "Pacific Island Peoples." It is borrowed from the convention developed by the Special Population Subpanel on the Mental Health of Asian and Pacific Americans of the President's Commission on Mental Health (1978). Although used throughout this chapter, "Asian and Pacific Americans" is in fact a convenient summary label for a very heterogeneous group. There certainly is not universal acceptance of this labeling convention, but for practical purposes it has been adopted frequently, with occasional variations (for example, "Asian/Pacific Americans," "Pacific/Asian Americans"). It represents the self-designation preferred by many Asian and Pacific people in the United States, particularly in preference to "Oriental."

"Asian and Pacific Americans" refers to a constellation of people from a number of ethnic and cultural backgrounds who had, in the past, been designated simply as "other" (Yoshioka, Tashima, Chew, & Murase, 1981; Wong, 1979). At least 32 distinct ethnic and cultural groups might meaningfully be listed under this designation: Bangladeshi, Belauan (formerly Palauan), Bhutanese, Burmese, Chamorro (Guamanian), Chinese, Fijian, Hawaiian, H'mong, Indian (Asian or East Indian), Indonesian, Japanese, Kampuchean (formerly Cambodian), Korean, Laotian, Malaysian, Marshallese (of the Marshall Islands, which include Majuro, Ebeye, and the U.S. missile range, Kwajalein), Micronesian (of the Federated States of

Micronesia, which include Kosrae, Ponape, Truk, and Yap), Nepalese, Okinawan, Pakistani, Filipino, Saipan Carolinian (or Carolinian from the Commonwealth of the Northern Marianas), Samoan, Singaporian, Sri Lankan (formerly Ceylonese), Tahitian, Taiwanese, Tibetan, Tongan, Thai, and Vietnamese. Morishima, Sue, Teng, Zane, and Cram (1979) provide a more formal definition, that Asian and Pacific Americans (AAPA) constitute

> at least the following: (1) the descendents of immigrants from China, Japan, Korea, the Philippines, Southeast Asia (Thailand, Vietnam), East Asia (Tibet, Ryukyu Islands), and Oceania (Samoa, Guam); (2) immigrants from those areas in Asia; and (3) children of "mixed" marriages where one of the parents was Asian American. . . . Given the diversity of languages, norms, mores and immigrant/American born [status], it is evident that to [label these peoples AAPA] implies a homogeneity which is lacking. Aggregation into one category is similar to aggregating the Irish, the Poles, the Swedes, and the Italians into one group—European—ignoring the vast language and cultural differences.

Morishima et al.'s definition excludes individuals from Asia and/or the Pacific Islands who reside in the United States with an intention of returning to their "homelands"; for example, business persons, visitors, diplomatic personnel, and those on student visas.

Thus, marked between-group differences exist among the various Asian and Pacific ethnic groups. As previously noted, individuals within these groups differ in a vast number of ways, and it is important to recognize the full extent of these differences, since any particular constellation of factors defines a specific subpopulation with its own needs for service. Dimensions of difference include: (1) area of residence in the United States, (2) generational status in the United States (first, second, third generation, and so on), (3) degree of acculturation, (4) native-language facility, (5) degree of identification with the "home" country and/or region of self or parents' origin, (6) education (number of years in Asia, in the United States, and elsewhere), (7) age, (8) family composition and degree of family intactness/dispersion with accompanying motivation for the particular family constellation, (9) social-political identification, (10) embeddedness in the local formal network (such as family associations, churches) and informal network (such as Saturday-night mahjong get-togethers), (11) religious beliefs and value orientations, (12) economic status and financial standing, (13) comfort and competence with the English language, and (14) perception of choice in emigrating to the United States.

The pooling of separate Asian and Pacific Island groups under the label of "Asian and Pacific Americans" also emerged out of political necessity. Merging these 32 ethnic groups into a collective entity allowed for sufficiently large numbers for meaningful representation in the political arena.

In its development one can see this aggregate minority group as an ever-emerging mosaic of diverse constituencies. Groups are added and removed based on self-definition and needs for self-determination. To the extent that its members find enough commonalities in experiences, goals, needs, and visions, the collective is strengthened. To the extent that specific groups pursue individual goals and identities and otherwise accentuate differences, the collective is weakened. Thus this alliance of diverse constituencies is at once a rallying point for action and an arena for division struggle when common goals or visions to guide collective action are lacking. In the past decade the pursuit of adequate mental health and other human services has provided a focus and opportunity for unified, collective action.

State of the Knowledge

Morishima et al. (1979), in the *Handbook of Asian American/Pacific Islander Mental Health Research,* present a review of 1500 selections from the mental health literature to 1977, and note the following general trends: (1) research on Asian and Pacific Americans has increased geometrically in the past six to seven years; (2) most research has, however, focused primarily on Chinese and Japanese populations; (3) many reports tend to be highly repetitive in their themes, particularly in analyzing and criticizing popular stereotypic beliefs; (4) the reports of findings are often in hard-to-obtain journals or periodicals; and (5) the recent literature is more data based and substantial, while previous reports tended to be more rhetorical.

From the 400 articles and essays selected as specifically relevant to AAPA mental health, several conclusions were drawn that square with informal impressions from the field. First, mounting evidence has made it clear that mental health distress and disorder have bypassed no minority population, and certainly not Asian and Pacific Americans (Morishima et al., 1979; Tsai, Teng, & Sue, 1981; Special Populations Subpanel, 1978; Kim, 1978; Bourne, 1975; Morales, 1974; Watanabe, 1973; Berk & Hirata, 1973; Cordova, 1973; Nakagawa & Watanabe, 1973; Harding & Looney, 1974; Sue, 1977; Sue, Sue, & Sue, 1975; Kuramoto, 1971; Kitano, 1969;

Duff & Arthur, 1967; Jew & Brody, 1967; Ball & Lau, 1966; Ikeda, Ball, & Yamamura, 1962; Kimmich, 1960; Yap, 1958).

Researchers and practitioners have had to disprove and counter popular stereotypes of AAPA and the widespread belief that AAPA do not suffer the discrimination and disadvantages associated with other minority groups. On the contrary, research shows that AAPA, particularly recent immigrants, youth, and elderly, are extremely vulnerable to severe stress and a variety of life crises, and are at great risk to mental and emotional disorder (Lin, Tazuma, & Masuda, 1979; Liu, Rahe, Looney, Ward, & Tung, 1978; Aylesworth, Ossorio, & Osaki, 1978; Morishima et al., 1979; Murase, 1977; Hoang, 1976; Brown, Stein, Huang, & Harris, 1973; Ayabe, 1971; Sue & Frank, 1973; Sue & Sue, 1971; Fong & Peskin, 1969; Meredith & Meredith, 1966; Fenz & Arkoff, 1962).

Second, research studies show that Asian and Pacific Americans tend to (1) underutilize the more traditional existing mental health services (San Francisco Community Mental Health Services, 1982, 1977; Hatanaka, Watanabe, & Ono, 1975; Brown et al., 1973; Sue & McKinney, 1975; Sue & Sue, 1974; Quisenberry, Lummis, & Berry, 1972; Kitano, 1969; Jew & Brody, 1967); (2) drop out after initial contact or terminate prematurely in such existing service settings (Sue, 1977; Sue & McKinney, 1975); and (3) endure stress for a long time, only coming to the attention of the mental health system at the point of acute breakdown and crisis (Sue, 1977; Hoang, 1976; Sue & McKinney, 1975; Sue & Sue, 1974; Brown et al., 1973; Berk & Hirata, 1973). An interpretation that can be placed on Asian and Pacific Americans' not using mental health services, or prematurely terminating if they do, is that services are not responding to their needs. That is, to the extent that patients are not satisfied, find the services unresponsive, or find little help in treatment, they may discontinue, and they may also discourage others from seeking help.

Also, the evidence seems to show that rather than being unusually low, the projected need of AAPA for mental health services may be greater than the norm, because of several factors. These include the long history of previously untreated and undetected mental health problems within any Asian and Pacific American community because of a lack of appropriate and responsive resources, the changes that face growing immigrant populations in adjusting to the United States (the stress of personal, familial, and social change compounded by cultural and language barriers), and the larger societal problems of racism and social, economic, and political inequities. In this light, studies showing low service utilization by Asian and Pacific Americans are best interpreted as indicating lack of adequate resources and services, rather than lack of need.

Third, the evidence available indicates that services specifically designed by and targeted to Asian and Pacific Americans increase utilization (Special Populations Subpanel, 1978; Kim, 1978; Wong, 1977; Sue & McKinney, 1975; True, 1975; Hatanaka et al., 1975). About two dozen such programs are found in urban cities with large numbers of Asian and Pacific Americans (such as San Francisco, Los Angeles, Seattle, Oakland, New York, Boston, San Diego, Denver, and Honolulu). Other programs of this type include the Indochinese refugee mental health projects initiated and sustained in fiscal years 1978 and 1979 by the Department of Health, Education and Welfare under the Special Project Grant Programs.

Several studies have demonstrated that service utilization is greatly enhanced in programs specifically targeted for Asian and Pacific Americans. For example, Sue and McKinney (1975) report that with the start of the Asian Counseling and Referral Services in Seattle, the number of Asian and Pacific American clients in one year was at least equal to the total reported by eighteen other community mental health centers serving the same area over a three-year period. Wong (1977) reports that after the establishment of a mental health center specifically designed to serve Asian and Pacific Americans in San Francisco, more Asian clients were seen in the first three months of operation than had been seen in the previous five years by the Department of Psychiatry of a public health hospital mandated to provide services to this same catchment area. True (1975) reports similar findings for the Asian Community Mental Health Services in Oakland.

Measures believed to counteract low utilization of mental health services include community outreach, community participation in decision making, and bilingual and culturally sensitive therapists (Kim, 1978; True, 1975; Sue & Wagner, 1973). However, the mere presence of Asian American personnel in a general mental health system does not appear to improve Asian and Pacific American underutilization significantly (Wu & Windle, 1980).

Given that AAPA will utilize specifically designed and targeted services, what happens to them in treatment, and what seems to be effective? On this subject, there is a virtual vacuum of empirical research (Morishima et al., 1979; Sue & Morishima, in press). However, since special services *are* used, it can be hypothesized that whatever factors are related to success do capitalize on ethnic, linguistic, and cultural similarities between clients and therapists, reducing the dropout rate and facilitating treatment continuity and ongoing care.

Conceptual Model for Viewing Services

A goodness-of-fit model, involving the client/consumer needs and the mental health services/resources, is proposed to clarify individual, group, and systems-level issues in the delivery of mental health services to Asian and Pacific Americans. Client outcomes (such as improved psychological functioning, continuation in treatment, satisfaction with services, and the like) can be viewed as a function of the goodness of fit between the client's needs and the resources of the mental health system. From this perspective, the lack of success in service delivery noted in this review is attributable to a poor fit between client systems and service systems.

Both clients and services are part of larger systems. The client system may include the individual, his or her family, groups to which the client and family may belong, and other progressively encompassing structures. The mental health system includes a counterpart to each client: the individual provider, the service unit, the agency, the service program, and so on. We will use this model in reviewing existing mental health service efforts for Asian and Pacific Americans, and will propose new alternatives for the future. First, we will identify existing reviews and recommendations for service delivery.

A variety of efforts and strategies have been employed to improve client-service fit. The President's Commission on Mental Health (1978) offers 67 recommendations for improving mental health services, research, and training, and for moving toward a better fit between needs and resources. The commission's report is the single best source of comprehensive recommendations for improving services to Asian and Pacific Americans.

Other major sources of recommendations also exist. Means to improve the fit between the client system and the service delivery system were a major concern in three recent national mental health research and service priority-setting conferences funded by the National Institute of Mental Health (NIMH). These were titled (1) "Pacific Island Conference: Prioritization of Mental Health Services Development for the Pacific Islanders" (Tseng & Young, 1981); (2) "Research Priorities for Mental Health Services for Asian/Pacific Islanders" (Owan, 1980); and (3) "Community-Involved Research for Pacific/Asian American Minority Groups" (Park, 1980). Other sources of recommendations are (1) the four AAPA core discipline caucuses (psychiatry, psychology, psychiatric social work, and psychiatric nursing) at the national conference on "Training of Psychiatrists, Psychologists, Psychiatric Social Workers, and Psychiatric Nurses for Ethnic Minority Communities" sponsored by Howard University

(1980); (2) key national consultants at the "Minority Mental Health Services Conference" sponsored by the Western Interstate Commission on Higher Education–WICHE (1980); (3) the two national consultations to ADAMHA by the Asian and Pacific Americans Consultation Group (Shon, 1980) and the Indochinese Refugee Consultation Group (Nguyen, 1980); (4) the Social and Human Service Panels at the "Asian/Pacific American National Leadership Conference: 1980–A Decade of Progress for Asian/ Pacific Americans" sponsored by the U.S.-Asia Institute (1980); and (5) testimony before the Civil Rights Commission on "Civil Rights Issues of Asian and Pacific Americans: Myths and Realities" (Lee, 1979; Shon, 1979).

Several strategies come into focus in this body of recommendations and from other literature. These will be considered first at individual and group levels, and then at larger systems levels.

Individual and Group-Level Factors

Belief Systems About Mental Health and Mental Illness

As noted by Lee (in press), western-trained providers attend to intrapsychic influences on behavior, whereas AAPA use such psychological explanations only rarely. For example, Chinese Americans believe that mental health is achieved through the exercise of willpower and the avoidance of morbid thoughts (Lum, 1974). Sue, Wagner, Ja, Margullis, and Lew (1976) found similar results for Japanese and Filipino Americans, for whom good mental health was perceived as being a result of the avoidance of morbid thoughts. Lee (in press) notes a wide range of common etiological beliefs among Chinese Americans, including: organic disorders, supernatural intervention, genetic vulnerability or hereditary weakness, physical or emotional exhaustion caused by situational factors, metaphysical factors such as the imbalance between yin and yang, fatalism, and character weakness. Such differences in belief systems about health and illness by clients often necessitate special efforts on the part of the provider to ensure acceptability of services.

Stigma and Shame

As noted by Shon and Ja (in press), "The concepts of 'shame' and 'loss of face' involve not only the exposure of one's actions for all to see, but also the withdrawal by the family, the community, and the society of their confidence and support." In the seeking of mental health services, not only personal shame but also personal and family stigma come into play. Community education and communication efforts as well as client outreach efforts (such as services in the home) have been instrumental in reducing stigma and shame in AAPA clients.

Family Structure and Reactions to Mental Illness

In eastern cultures the family rather than the individual is considered the unit of focus and identity. AAPA clients tend to view themselves as members of an extended family with strong emphasis on family obligations, mutual dependency, and collective responsibilities and decision making. As noted by several authors (Kim, 1982; Lee, in press; Shon & Ja, in press), the family structure and the family's reaction to mental illness may have much greater impact on any family member seeking and continuing with mental health treatment than the individual's inclination to pursue treatment. Consideration of the AAPA family has been noted as critical in ensuring client participation.

Patterns of Help Seeking

For reasons related to their more holistic view of health and other cultural traditions, AAPA clients tend to exhibit patterns of help seeking that emphasize self-help and natural community resources as alternatives to mental health services. These include physical health care and other human services instead of, or as a pathway to, mental health services (Lin et al., 1979; Leong, 1982; Lee, 1982); family and friends, herbalists, acupuncturists, and other indigenous healers are all utilized both before and concurrent with mental health treatment.

Lee (1979, in press), using data from clinical case materials from the mental health treatment of Chinese Americans, traces the pathway of service alternatives, programs, and agencies. Over a dozen alternatives were tried and repeated before use of the mental health system. AAPA clients may use family and relatives, willpower and self-action, social service providers (such as teachers of English as a second language, or translators), instructive readings, informal friendship networks, herbalists, other indigenous healers/helpers (such as martial arts masters), ministers and priests, providers in a health clinic, general practitioners, or specialists in medicine. Mental health services are likely to be the last alternative tried. The ability of mental health providers and programs to identify and collaborate with the full range of caregivers is critical to effective referral, entry, and continuation in treatment. Consultation and education activities with referral sources are also important (Lum, 1981; Lew & Zane, 1981).

Cultural-Specific Models and Practice of Health Care

There are differences not only in help-seeking behaviors, but also in underlying models of health care. Specific community models can include traditional and folk healing methods (for examples, see Kleinman & Lin, 1981; Tseng & Young, 1981); perception of specific western practices as effective or ineffective (such as the Vietnamese view of injection as more effective than oral ingestion of medication); and expectations about the roles, functions, and treatment practices of providers.

Community Support, Linkage, and Acceptability

For AAPA populations, the community provides the arena for interaction and exchange; thus it is not uncommon to see in large urban cities the variety of Chinatowns, Japantowns, Koreatowns, and Manilatowns that exist. Since mental health concerns and mental illness are still quite stigmatizing to the individual (and the family), the community's reaction to them plays a critical role in whether clients seek and continue treatment. Program planners and providers must engage community members and leaders in developing support for and acceptability of mental health services within the AAPA community. Ongoing education and community information programs have been found to be effective in this regard (Lum, 1981; Lew & Zane, 1981).

Degree of Acculturation

Several studies (Conner, 1974; Kikumura & Kitano, 1973; Masuda, Matsumato, & Meredith, 1970; Meredith & Meredith, 1966) have noted the greater similarity to Caucasian personality characteristics and the adoption of White American values by Asian and Pacific Americans who have become more assimilated or acculturated into mainstream America. The greater the assimilation, acculturation, or biculturality, the more likely that such individuals will find western-oriented mental health services acceptable and appropriate. Lee (in press) has indicated four variables that are related to acculturation: years in the United States, country of origin (more western-like countries of origin make for easier transitions), professional affiliation and status, and age at immigration. To the extent that individuals remain unassimilated, special efforts must be made via such channels as mental health education and information programs and pretherapy orientation to ensure a good match between expressed needs for services and the actual mental health services available. Especially for recent immigrants and refugees, the request for mental health services may be instigated by some third party—a school counselor, a family court, or a public health nurse, for example. An accurate assessment must be made of the client system as to degree of acculturation and extent of receptivity and understanding of mental health treatment.

Religion

No one religion or philosophical system, western or eastern, can be said to dominate the Asian and Pacific American population. Both western religions (such as Judaism, Catholicism, Protestantism) and eastern religions (Buddhism, Hinduism, Taoism, Confucianism) are practiced, depending on the degree of assimilation and acculturation to the West. In some religions priestly functions and roles are associated with a self-disclosing, confessional quality inherent in verbal therapies. However, in other eastern religions the qualities of endurance, self-sacrifice, and personal suffering are admired and fostered. Strong belief in such qualities results in a stance completely at odds with the verbal expressiveness of western modes of treatment. Thus the client's religious belief system can have a significant effect on the client's view of and participation in mental health services.

Language

In arenas of work in which small nuances of speech can carry major differences in surplus meaning and connotation, language is clearly an important consideration. If a provider does not speak the language (or the particular dialect) of the client, the client-provider gap can be tremendous. The gap can be widened by differences in socioeconomic class, educational level, sociopolitical identification (such as mainland China versus Taiwan), age and sex, generational status in the United States, and vocational-professional standing. Linguistic, structural, and lexiconal variations in the different Asian and Pacific American languages provide the native speaker (most often the client) with subtle but specific cues about the provider and the nature of the treatment relationship. Few alternatives exist in the mental health treatment of monolingual or English-limited clients to language proficiency on the provider's part. The use of a translator for services may be necessary, but this only provides rough approximation to the expressed meanings of the client. Language gaps represent one of the most difficult barriers to adequate services for Asian and Pacific Americans.

Cost

Recent immigrants and refugees are usually not covered by medical insurance or other third-party benefits. At the same time, cultural values governing obligation and self-sufficiency may result in conflict within families over participation in financially assisted services in which fees are not collected. Moreover, for many AAPA immigrants who may want to achieve permanent legal status as residents in the United States, participation in a government-supported service, usually Medicaid or Medicare, may be at odds with their goal, because immigrants must be family sponsored, and therefore not in receipt of federally sponsored benefits. Effective and sensitive handling of issues of cost determination and ability to pay constitutes a significant element in successful service delivery.

Perceived Responsiveness of Services

It is important for the actions of "gatekeepers" in the mental health setting to convey a sense of acceptance and willingness to help. For AAPA, the perception of responsiveness is enhanced by various measures: (1) an acceptable name for the facility, (2) the general appearance and upkeep of the facility and waiting areas, (3) bilingual assistance on the first telephone call, (4) friendliness of reception personnel, (5) a pre-first-session confirmatory telephone call, (6) a postsession follow-up telephone call, (7) willingness of providers to assist in other functions besides mental health services (such as translation services), (8) the taking of a more informal and less professional role, and (9) willingness of the provider to share information about him- or herself. Larsen (1978), in a study of intake practices, found that the use of confirming telephone calls at the Richmond Maxi-Center in San Francisco, with 50 percent AAPA clients, produced a failed-to-show rate for first appointments of less than 10 percent. This compares favorably with rates that were double and triple this figure at two other outpatient facilities that did not follow similar practices. One of the clearest indicators of responsiveness for monolingual or English-limited AAPA clients on encountering the mental health system is a staff that can speak to them in their primary language. To improve perceived responsiveness, an effective procedure is client-flow/client-entry system evaluation to identify practices associated with varying utilization.

Location and Knowledge of Facilities

Kim (1978), in her study of Chinese, Japanese, Korean, and Filipino Americans in the Chicago area, found that for a significant number of AAPA, especially immigrants and women, a primary reason for not seeking help was not knowing where to go. AAPA lack of knowledge of service facilities can be corrected by public service announcements, community education, advertisement, and other public relations activities. Problems related to location, given the need to serve a dispersed population, are not so easily overcome. For example, Sue and Morishima (in press) note that in the Seattle area, AAPA clients may have to travel over 100 miles before they can use the Chinese Information and Service Center or the Asian Counseling and Referral Services. In Los Angeles, clients have similar or greater kinds of travel distances in the use of the Asian/Pacific Counseling and Treatment Center. The problem is even greater for residents in the Pacific Islands, where services may be more than 600 miles away (Tseng & Young, 1981). Another barrier for AAPA is that of the catchment or service area restrictions limiting who can be served. Since many AAPA are spread much wider than one catchment or service area, their participation in one specialized AAPA mental health program, with its concentrated resources, is problematic.

Hours of Operation and Client/Family Work Schedules

AAPA, especially recent immigrant and refugee families, tend to have extended work hours (sometimes two or more jobs) and multiple family members at work. Very few can get release time to utilize mental health services during normal office hours. In order to ensure accessibility, flexible scheduling—usually around father's day off for families—and evening or weekend hours may be necessary.

Broader System-Level Factors

Community Orientation

Services that are to be highly utilized and effective tend to be community based, with strong linkages, positive credibility, and good reputations with the particular AAPA community and its networks. Providers tend to be known within, or are members of, the ethnic community. Although sometimes affiliated with major institutions, they are more likely free-standing and physically located in or near the particular AAPA community. AAPA community members are active on the governing or advisory boards of such programs, and there is often a sense of pride within the community about the existence of the facility.

Longitudinal and Developmental Orientation

The program or agency and its personnel are historical presences in the community. They have positive "track records," and their motivations, attitudes, skills, and performance are known and accepted. Commitment to the program and its services is high. There is review and evaluation of the present and past and a planned perspective toward future services. AAPA community members are part of this history and expect to be part of the future.

Outreach Orientation

Requiring clients to come to the agency for services is deemphasized. Rather, services are provided, within cost constraints and clinical appropriateness, in the home or in more familiar settings, such as churches, schools, and community centers. Staff members are not penalized for such work by making it lower in status—for example, by assigning paraprofessionals to outreach and more credentialed clinicians to "therapy." Rather, outreach is considered vital and highly skilled work. Also, community members perceive providers to be a part of their community, its events, and its activities.

Human Resource Orientation

A spirit of mutual teaching and learning pervades the environment in which service providers explore with and learn from peers and subordinates, and always seek to enhance their skills. No clinician necessarily knows the varied, diverse, and complex world of AAPA populations, and an open learning-growing environment contributes toward the development of programs in which staff are viewed as resources for the organizations. Activities to enhance the ability of the community members to help each other (such as community education forums) and to share with staff (such as training workshops) are encouraged.

Treatment-Systematic Approach

Services are planned, organized, implemented, and evaluated not as the sum of the various program parts and individuals that make up those programs, but as a coordinated and continuous delivery system. Thus ethnic personnel are not added in a piecemeal fashion; rather, selection of staff and program elements is made in terms of their contribution toward the total mission of the agency in providing mental health services.

Critical Mass

A certain minimum number of ethnic staff and of clients appears necessary for a successful program. The actual number depends on kind of staff (professional field, ethnicity) and kind of programs (inpatient, partial day, outpatient, preventive). Programs that merely add single "minority specialists" do not appear to have as much impact (Wu & Windle, 1980).

Multidisciplinary Support

Programs that tend to show shared support and decision making across disciplines in services, planning, and other programmatic functions appear more effective. For AAPA communities, with the limited number of mental health professional human resources available, multidisciplinary support is a necessity.

Community Network Orientation

Services and programs are organized as a part of the total community network of human services to an AAPA community. Great emphasis is put on collaborative and cooperative relationships among service programs. Interagency referrals and resource sharing are encouraged.

Indirect Benefits

Programs and agencies organized around programs that have some preventive and indirect services (consultation, mental health education, and information, community organization and program technical assistance) appear to have their direct clinical services enhanced. Staff and programs are organized around prevention as well as direct services; interest in indirect service programs is shared by the majority of the staff.

Recommendations and Conclusions

As noted earlier, the report of the Special Populations Subpanel on Mental Health of Asian and Pacific Americans (1978) provides the single best source for comprehensive recommendations on mental health services for this population. Rather than repeat those recommendations, I refer the interested reader to that report. I would like, however, to note specific strategies or models by which mental health programs have been improved for AAPA. Murase (1977), Sue (1977), and Wong (1977) provide the following kinds of strategies: (1) augment existing mental health services, personnel, and programs with additional AAPA resources (personnel, programs, activities, satellite centers); (2) create a parallel service program specifically for AAPA clients; (3) create a special umbrella AAPA organization containing multiple service programs to include mental health services; and (4) support and fund AAPA community coalitions and consortiums to establish mental health services for a particular AAPA community.

Lee (in press) suggests a model service organization that has been found consistent with Chinese Americans (and other AAPA populations): (1) provide mental health services in conjunction with primary health care; (2) provide mental health services in conjunction with other human services (such as child care, employment, and legal services); (3) provide mental health services in a neighborhood-based multiservice center; and (4) provide mental health services in community mental health centers, with perhaps a specific satellite to serve AAPA clients in particular.

In this chapter, the state of the art with respect to the provision of mental health services to Asian and Pacific Americans was reviewed. For political and other reasons the Asian and Pacific American population is a result of a collective of over 32 distinct ethnic and cultural groupings. With such heterogeneity and diversity inherent in the groups that make up this collective, uniformity in terms of mental health service provision and programs would be counterproductive, if not impossible. Rather than providing concrete examples of different kinds of mental health services for this diverse population, I have chosen instead to present a model for conceptualizing the mental health service system and the client consumer/ user system. Individual, group, and system-level factors were then presented so that the goodness of fit between the client and the service system might be improved for AAPA populations. It is hoped that careful consideration of these factors will lead to improved mental health services for Asian and Pacific Americans.

References

Aoki, B. *Role preparation of Asian American clients for psychotherapy.* Paper presented at the annual convention of the Western Psychological Association, Los Angeles, August 1981.

Ayabe, H. L. Deference and ethnic differences in voice levels. *Journal of Social Psychology,* 1971, 72, 181-185.

Aylesworth, L. S., Ossorio, P. G., & Osaki, L. T. *Stress and mental health among Vietnamese in the United States.* Chicago: AAMHRC Research Report, 1978.

Ball, J. C., & Lau, M. P. The Chinese narcotic addict in the United States. *Social Forces,* 1966, 45, 68-72.

Berk, B., & Hirata, L. Mental illness among the Chinese: Myth or reality? *Journal of Social Issues,* 1973, 29, 149-166.

Bourne, P. G. The Chinese student—acculturation and mental illness. *Psychiatry,* 1975, 38, 269-277.

Brown, T. F., Stein, K., Huang, K., & Harris, D. Mental illness and the role of mental health facilities in Chinatown. In S. Sue & N. Wagner (Eds.), *Asian Americans: Psychological perspectives.* Ben Lomond, CA: Science and Behavior Books, 1973.

Chin, R. *Montreal Chinese: Studies of personal and cultural identity. A report on the Chinese Canadian community in Montreal.* Boston: Author, 1976.

Choi, G. *Clinical issues encountered in treating Asian American families.* Paper presented at the annual convention of the Western Psychological Association, Sacramento, April 1982.

Chu, F., & Trotter, S. *The madness establishment: Ralph Nader's study group report on the National Institute of Mental Health.* New York: Grossman, 1974.

Connor, J. W. Acculturation and changing need patterns in Japanese-American and Caucasian-American college students. *Journal of Psychology,* 1974, 93, 293-294.

Cordova, F. The Filipino-American: There's always an identity crisis. In S. Sue & N. Wagner (Eds.), *Asian Americans: Psychological perspectives.* Ben Lomond, CA: Science and Behavior Books, 1973.

Duff, D. F., & Arthur, R. J. Between two worlds: Filipinos in the U.S. Navy. *American Journal of Psychiatry,* 1967, 123, 836-843.

Fenz, W., & Arkoff, A. Comparative need patterns of five ancestry groups in Hawaii. *Journal of Social Psychology,* 1962, 58, 67-89.

Fong, S.L.M., & Peskin, H. Sex role strain and personality adjustment of Chinaborn students in America: A pilot study. *Journal of Abnormal Psychology,* 1969, 74, 563-567.

Harding, K., & Looney, G. Problems of Southeast Asian children in a refugee camp. *American Journal of Psychiatry,* 1974, 134, 407-411.

Hatanaka, H. K., Watanabe, B. Y., & Ono, S. The utilization of mental health services in the Los Angeles area. In Ishikawa & N. Archer (Eds.), *Service delivery in Pan Asian communities.* San Diego: Pacific Asian Coalition, 1975.

Hoang, T. A. *Mental health needs of Indochinese refugees: A survey.* San Francisco: International Institute, 1976.

Ikeda, K., Ball, H. V., & Yamamura, D. S. Ethnocultural factors in schizophrenia: The Japanese in Hawaii. *American Journal of Sociology,* 1962, 68, 242-248.

Ito, J. *Asian cultural values and family structure.* Paper presented at the annual convention of the Western Psychological Association, Sacramento, April 1982.

Jew, C. C., & Brody, S. A. Mental illness among the Chinese: I. Hospitalization rates over the past century. *Comprehensive Psychiatry,* 1967, 8, 129-134.

Kikumura, A., & Kitano, H.H.L. Interracial marriage: A picture of the Japanese Americans. *Journal of Social Issues,* 1973, 29, 67-81.

Kim, B.L.C. *The Asian Americans: Changing patterns, changing needs.* Urbana, IL: Association of Korean Christian Scholars in North America, 1978.

Kim, G.C.C. Asian-Americans: No model minority. *Social Work,* 1973, 18, 44-53.

Kim, S. C. *A conceptual analysis of the family systems approach as applied to Asian American families.* Paper presented at the annual convention of the Western Psychological Association, Sacramento, April 1982.

Kim, Y. K. *Asian and Pacific Islander population in the United States.* Washington, DC: Bureau of the Census, 1981.

Kimmich, R. A. Ethnic aspects of schizophrenia in Hawaii. *Psychiatry,* 1960, 23, 97-102.

Kitano, H. Japanese-American mental illness. In A. Plog & M. Edgerton (Eds.), *Changing perspectives in mental illness.* San Francisco: Holt, Rinehart & Winston, 1969.

Kleinman, A., & Lin, T. Y. (Eds.). *Normal and deviant behavior in Chinese culture.* Hingham, MA: Reidel, 1981.

Kuramoto, F. H. What do Asians want? An examination of issues in social work education. *Journal of Education for Social Workers,* 1971, 7, 7-17.

Larsen, D. L. *Enhancing client utilization of community mental health outpatient services.* Unpublished doctoral dissertation, University of Kansas, 1978.

Lee, E. Mental health services for the Asian Americans: Problems and alternatives. In *Civil rights issues of Asian and Pacific Americans: Myths and realities.* Washington, DC: Government Printing Office, 1979.

Lee, E. *Social cultural aspects of working with Chinese American families.* San Francisco: National Asian American Psychology Training Center Videotaped Library, 1982.

Lee, E. A social systems approach for assessment and treatment practices for Chinese American families. In M. McGoldrick, J. K. Pearce, & J. Giordano (Eds.), *Ethnicity and family therapy.* New York: Gilford Family Therapy Series, in press.

Leong, C. *Asian Americans and somatization.* Paper presented at the annual convention of the Western Psychological Association, Sacramento, April 1982.

Leung, A. *Asian American families in therapy: Some potential recommendations and alternatives.* Paper presented at the annual convention of the Western Psychological Association, Sacramento, April 1982.

Lew, W. M., & Zane, N. *Treatment issues with Chinese children and families.* Paper presented at the annual convention of the Western Psychological Association, Los Angeles, April 1981.

Lin, K. M., Tazuma, L., & Masuda, M. Adaptational problems of Vietnamese refugees: I. Health and mental health status. *Archives of General Psychiatry,* 1979, 36, 955-961.

Lin, T., & Lin, M. Service delivery issues in Asian-North American communities. *American Journal of Psychiatry,* 1978, 135, 454-456.

Liu, W. T. *Transition to nowhere: Vietnamese refugees in America.* Nashville: Charter House, 1979.

Liu, W. T., Rahe, R. H., Looney, J. G., Ward, H. W., & Tung, T. M. Psychiatric consultation in a Vietnamese refugee camp. *American Journal of Psychiatry,* 1978, 135, 185-190.

Lum, R. *Issues in the study of Asian American communities.* Paper presented at the annual convention of the Western Psychological Association, San Francisco, April 1974.

Lum, R. *Evolution of a community-based Asian prevention mental health service: Conceptual and practical issues in development.* Paper presented at the annual convention of the Western Psychological Association, Los Angeles, April 1981.

Masuda, M., Matsumoto, G. H., & Meredith, G. M. Ethnic identity in three generations of Japanese Americans. *Journal of Social Issues,* 1970, 81, 199-207.

Meredith, G. M., & Meredith, C.G.W. Acculturation and personality among Japanese-American college students in Hawaii. *Journal of Social Psychology,* 1966, 68, 175-182.

Morales, R. *Makibaka: The Phillipino American struggle.* Los Angeles: Mountainview, 1974.

Morishima, J., Sue, S., Teng, L. N., Zane, N., & Cram, J. *Handbook of Asian American/Pacific Islander mental health research.* Rockville, MD: National Institute of Mental Health, 1979.

Murase, K. Delivery of social services to Asian Americans. In National Association of Social Workers (Ed.), *Encyclopedia of social work.* Washington, DC: Author, 1977.

Nakagawa, B., & Watanabe, R. *A study of the use of drugs among the Asian-American youth of Seattle.* Seattle: DPAA, 1973.

Nguyen, T. D. *Indochinese refugee consultation report to the Alcohol, Drug Abuse, and Mental Health Administration (ADAMHA).* Rockville, MD: ADAMHA, 1980.

Owan, T. *Research priorities for the Asian/Pacific in mental health service development.* Rockville, MD: NIMH, 1980.

Park, P. *Community involved research for Pacific/Asian American minority groups. Final Report.* Amherst: University of Massachusetts, 1980.

President's Commission on Mental Health. *Report to the President of the President's Commission on Mental Health.* Washington, DC: Government Printing Office, 1978.

Quisenberry, W. B., Lummis, W. S., Jr., & Berry, R. P. *1970 statistical report.* Honolulu: Department of Health, State of Hawaii, 1972.

San Francisco Community Mental Health Services. *Chinese bilingual mental health task force preliminary report.* San Francisco: Department of Public Health, 1977.

San Francisco Community Mental Health Services. *Report of the task force on residential services.* San Francisco: Department of Public Health, 1982.

Shon, S. P. The delivery of mental health services to Asian and Pacific Americans. In *Civil rights issues of Asian and Pacific Americans: Myths and realities.* Washington, DC: Government Printing Office, 1979.

Shon, S. P. *Asian and Pacific American consultation report to the Alcohol, Drug Abuse, and Mental Health Administration (ADAMHA).* Rockville, MD: ADAMHA, 1980.

Shon, S. P., & Ja, D. Y. Asian families. In M. McGoldrick, J. K. Pearce, & J. Giordano (Eds.), *Ethnicity and family therapy.* New York: Gilford Family Therapy Series, in press.

Special Populations Subpanel on Mental Health of Asian and Pacific Americans. Report. In *Report to the president of the President's Commission on Mental Health,* Vol. 3: *Task Panel Reports.* Washington, DC: Government Printing Office, 1978.

Sue, D. W., & Frank, A. A typological approach to the psychological study of Chinese and Japanese college males. *Journal of Social Issues,* 1973, 29, 129-148.

Sue, S. Community mental health services to minority groups: Some optimism, some pessimism. *American Psychologist,* 1977, 32, 616-628.

Sue, S. *Mental health in a multi-ethnic society: Person-organization match.* Paper presented at the annual convention of the American Psychological Association, Toronto, September 1978.

Sue, S., & Kitano, H. Stereotype as a measure of success. *Journal of Social Issues,* 1973, 29, 83-98.

Sue, S., & McKinney, H. Asian Americans in the community mental health care system. *American Journal of Orthopsychiatry,* 1975, 45, 111-118.

Sue, S., & Morishima, J. *Asian American mental health: Knowledge and directions.* San Francisco: Jossey-Bass, in press.

Sue, S. & Sue, D. W. Chinese-American personality and mental health. *Amerasia Journal*, 1971, 1, 36-48.

Sue, S., & Sue, D. W. MMPI comparisons between Asian-American and non-Asian students utilizing a student health psychiatric clinic. *Journal of Counseling Psychology*, 1974, 21, 423-427.

Sue, S., Sue, D. W., & Sue, D. W. Asian Americans as a minority group. *American Psychologist*, 1975, 30, 906-910.

Sue, S., & Wagner, N. N. (Eds.). *Asian-Americans: Psychological perspectives.* Palo Alto, CA: Science and Behavior Books, 1973.

Sue, S., Wagner, N., Ja, D., Margullis, C., & Lew, L. Conception of mental illness among Asian and Caucasian students. *Psychological Reports*, 1976, 38, 703-708.

True, R. H. Mental health services in a Chinese American community. In Ishikawa & N. Archer (Eds.), *Service delivery in Pan Asian communities.* San Diego: Pacific Asian Coalition, 1975.

Tsai, M., Teng, L. N., & Sue, S. Mental health status of Chinese in the United States. In A. Klienman & T. Y. Lin (Eds.), *Normal and deviant behavior in Chinese culture.* Hingham, MA: Reidel, 1981.

Tseng, W. S., & Young, B.B.C. *Prioritization of mental health services development for the Pacific Islanders. Workshop report.* Honolulu: John A. Burns School of Medicine, University of Hawaii, 1981.

U.S. Department of Commerce, Bureau of the Census. *1980 census of population and housing.* PHC 80-V Series. Washington, DC: Government Printing Office, 1981.

Watanabe, C. Self-expression and the Asian American experience. *Personnel and Guidance Journal*, 1973, 51, 390-396.

Western Interstate Commission for Higher Education (WICHE). *Minority mental health conference report.* Boulder, CO: Author, 1980.

Wong, H. Z. *Demographic and socio-economic characteristics of the Chinese population, implications and concerns of the Chinese communities for the 1980 census.* Paper presented to the Subcommittee on the Census, U.S. House of Representatives, San Francisco, 1979.

Wong, H. Z. Contextual factors for the development of the National Asian American Psychology Training Center. *Journal of Community Psychology*, 1981, 4, 289-292.

Wong, H. Z. *Community mental health services and manpower and training concerns of Asian Americans.* Paper presented to the President's Commission on Mental Health, San Francisco, June 1977.

Wu, I H., & Windle, C. Ethnic specificity in the relationship of minority use and staffing of community mental health centers. *Community Mental Health Journal*, 1980, 16(2), 156-168.

Yap, P. M. Hypereridism and attempted suicide in Chinese. *Journal of Nervous and Mental Disease*, 1958, 127, 34-41.

Yoshioka, R. B., Tashima, N., Chew, M., & Murase, K. *Mental health services for Pacific/Asian Americans* (2 vols.). San Francisco: Pacific Asian Mental Health Research Project, 1981.

Zane, N. *Rational restructuring with Asian American clients.* Paper presented at the annual convention of the American Psychological Association, Los Angeles, August 1981.

PART III

DIRECTIONS FOR CHANGE

10

Psychotherapy with the Underserved

Recent Developments

Enrico E. Jones
David R. Matsumoto
University of California, Berkeley

Community Psychology and Psychotherapy:
Rapprochement?

The terms "underserved" and "disadvantaged" are used here as synonymous with the term "lower socioeconomic status," which is generally taken to include both Class IV and Class V individuals on the Hollingshead Index of Social Position (Hollingshead & Redlich, 1958). These two classes are sometimes described as the "working class" and the "poor," respectively. Within community psychology there is a perspective that holds that the intrapsychic, interpersonal, and behavioral problems of the disadvantaged derive from economic and reality-based difficulties, and that their amelioration is not to be sought in traditional forms of mental health interventions, but in social and political action. From this point of view mental health care is at best a palliative; at worst it detracts from recognizing the true source of the problem. The patient is not sick, society is, it is argued, and "blaming the victim" (Ryan, 1971) for difficulties caused by a social order that distorts his or her life locates the problem incorrectly, and leads to misguided and ultimately futile attempts at intervention. The locus of the problem is instead the social context or system—the reality of social stress, economic disadvantage, and oppression is self-evident. This is the context in which mental health interventions must occur and, as a result, will often fail. The individual who may have in fact benefited substantially from psychotherapy is forced to return to a pathogenic environment of poverty and community disorganization. This perspective emphasizes the psychological damage of oppression, and advocates broad social reform as the only ultimate cure for psychological problems that invariably spring from being disadvantaged. According to this view, social action is seen as the vehicle for psychological health, and social change is seen as a necessary precondition for lasting personal change.

An important contribution of the social change perspective within community psychology has been the shift of focus away from the individual and the tendency to locate the source of all psychological disorders within the person. It has alerted us to the fact that traditional treatment models can contribute to the avoidance of the social issues that are involved in the individual's malaise about him- or herself, and can in this sense contribute to the maintenance of the status quo. This perspective has addressed and in part has corrected an imbalance that existed in traditional conceptions of psychopathology and its treatments by formally acknowledging the impact of socioeconomic issues and discrimination on deprived youth, poor Whites, poor Blacks, blue-collar workers, and the rural poor, and by championing the notion of the prevention of mental disorders.

There are, however, some important limitations inherent in this point of view. One shortcoming has been its rejection of, or at least antagonism toward, more traditional forms of mental health interventions. Psychotherapy that improves the functioning of the individual does not necessarily adapt him or her to the existing social order, preempting his or her desire for social change. On the contrary, individuals may indeed become more effective in focusing on the insufficiencies of their social environment, and become increasingly effective in reaching out in some way to change their condition. The real dilemma is that too many individuals in fact defeat themselves in reaching out for desirable and proper social objectives. The social change perspective tends to diminish the importance of individuals asserting what control they can over their personal existence, however limited this control might be by external social forces. It overlooks the possibility that individuals may externalize their problems and fail to assume responsibility for dysfunctional patterns of behavior that, if changed and corrected, could result in greater personal efficacy and satisfaction in living despite an unfavorable social context that is resistant to change.

This leads us to a related issue—the systems change perspective's rather strong propensity toward a kind of social reductionism; that is, the notion that all psychological problems derive, in some way, from social conditions in every instance. Only if emotional disturbance were present exclusively among the lower social classes could it be linked directly and solely to economic factors or to social context. While it is unquestionably true that economic deprivation is one factor contributing to psychological disturbance among the disadvantaged, it is not the only stress. The fact that people from all social classes and ethnic backgrounds can experience psychological difficulties suggests that other factors clearly contribute to their etiology (Siassi & Messer, 1976). This view, then, neglects to take into account that individuals from disadvantaged backgrounds can suffer from psychological disorders that are associated only minimally with social conditions.

Yet another issue is the problem of short-term strategies. While a longer-term goal for improving the psychological health of the disadvantaged must include social change, there remains the problem of treating the underserved who are in psychological distress now, whatever the presumed etiology of their difficulties, and existing forms of mental health care can clearly contribute here. What is needed, in short, are not only social intervention strategies, but also psychological therapies to deal with problems of psychological (cognitive and emotional) structure (Jones & Korchin, 1982).

If the ideological rigidity that has sometimes characterized the debate between proponents of the systems change perspective and apologists for traditional treatment approaches could be overcome, and some of the arguments outlined above were conceded, then it is possible to arrive at the conclusion that there is no essential antagonism between the systems change approach, with its emphasis on prevention, and the psychological therapies. One could indeed arrive at the opinion that, in principle, a rapprochement between the two orientations is possible. But, it might be responded, even if a rapprochement is possible in the abstract, in reality the concepts, institutions, and practices developed by the mental health establishment are ill adapted to the problems and needs of the underserved, and traditional approaches to psychotherapy are inadequate for the economically disadvantaged.

Clinical lore has long held that the economically disadvantaged are less suited for psychotherapy, which requires of the client the capacity for introspection, the ability to articulate ideas and feelings freely, and a certain amount of psychological-mindedness. The literature is replete with statements describing the lower socioeconomic status (SES) client as holding different expectations about treatment and wanting action-oriented treatments that involve medication, direction, and advice. For these and other reasons it has until recently been commonly assumed that such clients achieve less successful outcomes in psychotherapy, even if they manage to negotiate successfully the obstacles of lack of availability of treatments, expense, and negative therapist attitudes that frequently bar their entry into treatment. The following discussion will challenge some of these assumptions, and will suggest that lower-SES clients are better risks for expressive psychotherapies than commonly acknowledged, that treatment outcomes can be successful with such clients, and that specific procedures can be employed in the treatment of this type of client to promote more favorable outcomes.

The Underserved Client

Changing Attitudes Toward Psychotherapy

During the 1950s and 1960s, research findings repeatedly showed that the economically disadvantaged held more negative attitudes toward, and were significantly less sophisticated about, mental health services and psychotherapy than the middle class (Lorion, 1978). The poor were found to be less certain about the effectiveness of mental health treatments, more concerned about the stigma and negative connotations of being in treatment, less ready to discuss personal information and emotional issues, and less likely to seek psychological treatment when other avenues of aid proved of no help (Hollingshead & Redlich, 1958; Brill & Storrow, 1960; Reiff & Scribner, 1964; Riessman, 1964).

Over the past decade, however, there appears to have been an important shift in the attitudes of the underserved toward mental health services, and more recent studies of treatment attitudes have questioned the extent of SES-related differences. A large-scale study by Kadushin (1969) as well as other investigations (Calhoon, Dawes, & Lewis, 1972) found very few social class differences. Lorion (1974) found that lower-SES clinic applicants expressed the same level of confidence about the effectiveness of psychotherapy as middle-class applicants, saw little stigma in seeking treatment, and stated a willingness to talk about personal issues. Lorion (1978) cautions that these data do not necessarily mean that SES differences in treatment attitudes have disappeared entirely over the years. Nevertheless, it is evident that the attitude of the underserved toward mental health care has changed. This shift is perhaps partially attributable to the greater availability of mental health services to these populations (Sue, 1977; Edwards, Greene, Abramowitz, & Davidson, 1979), and the community mental health movement's emphasis on educating the public about mental health and available services. In part this shift can also be attributed to the recent tremendous popularization and penetration of psychological concepts into the cultural life of our society, a social movement whose importance has not yet been fully realized, and that has had an impact even among society's economically disadvantaged.

Expectations of the Underserved About Psychotherapy

The ideology of community mental health centers and the programs and services they provide is closely tied to meeting the needs and expectations of diverse populations. Treatment expectations are an important issue for those who plan and provide services in community mental health centers. Client expectations about the nature of therapy and appropriate role behaviors for therapy have been shown to influence the duration of treatment and attrition rates (Overall & Aronson, 1963), patient perceptions of outcome (Wynne, 1981), and level of patient comfort and involvement in the therapeutic process (Lorion, 1978). It is a fairly widely held assumption that client treatment expectations differ by social class. It is presumed that the discrepancy between client expectations and actual experience of treatment is related to the higher dropout rate among lower-SES therapy patients. Heitler (1976), for example, has argued that widely discrepant role expectations between lower-class patients and psychotherapists make the establishment of a therapeutic alliance difficult.

Research findings on this subject are, however, far from conclusive. Again, early studies seem to support the assumption of class differences in treatment expectations. In Overall and Aronson's (1963) original study of this issue, 40 economically disadvantaged clients were given questionnaires regarding their expectations before their initial interviews; after the interview they were given another questionnaire concerning their reactions to what actually occurred in the interview. The results indicated that these clients expected therapists to assume an active, medical role in the interview, that the actual conduct of the therapists during the interview was less active and medically oriented than the clients expected, and that the degree of discrepancy between client expectations and their perceptions of what actually occurred was significantly related to whether the client returned for treatment. Williams, Lipman, Uhlenhuth, Rickels, Covi, and Mock (1967), in a study of treatment expectations that employed the same questionnaire, found significant differences across social class among a large sample of therapy clients, and similarly concluded that lower-SES clients expect a more active, supportive, medically oriented therapist than do middle-class clients.

Other studies have, however, established conflicting findings. Goin, Yamamoto, and Silverman (1965) hypothesized that most lower-class patients would expect help in the form of active advice, reassurance, and support in a few sessions, rather than from treatment centered around the long-term development of introspection and self-understanding. The reactions of Class IV and V clients at the Los Angeles County General Hospital were observed as they were given treatment congruent or incongruent with their expectations. A total of 52 percent of the clients indicated their wish to solve their problems by talking about their feelings and past life, that is, they wanted insight therapy; 48 percent wanted active help, either in the form of advice (34 percent) or medication (14 percent). The majority (60 percent) expected their needs to be met in 10 or fewer treatment sessions. Only 25 percent expected more than 25 sessions. Those clients who expected advice and received it did not stay in treatment longer than those who expected advice and did not get it. The fact that patients whose expectations about therapy were incongruent with the nature of the treatment did not terminate sooner than those whose expectations were congruent contradicts findings of studies cited earlier.

It is of special interest, too, that in this study 52 percent of lower-SES clients wanted insight therapy. It should not come as too great a surprise if middle-class clients displayed a similar range in terms of the nature of their treatment expectations. And, indeed, subsequent studies appear to bear out this supposition. Lorion (1974) found that social classes no longer differ in treatment expectations, and that similar percentages of lower-SES and middle-class clients anticipate active, supportive, problem-solving therapists. Balch, McWilliams, Lewis, and Ireland (1978), in a study of a sample of almost 300 outpatients in a community mental health center, similarly found no differences in treatment expectations across social class, though they did find that a substantial number of clients, regardless of SES, expected a directive, advice-oriented interchange.

It appears, then, that the pretherapy expectations of the economically disadvantaged have, like their mental health attitudes, undergone an important change in recent years, and that the assumption that lower-SES clients have a particular and commonly shared set of expectations is no longer valid. While it is certainly true that some lower-SES clients will hold uninformed or incongruent expectations, it now appears that a similar proportion of their middle-class counterparts do so as well.

The Underserved and Treatment Outcome

SES and Continuation in Psychotherapy

The phenomenon of early termination or premature dropout among economically disadvantaged patients has long been noted by concerned workers in the field, and has served as a cornerstone for the argument that traditional forms of psychotherapy are inadequate for this sort of client. Early studies have generally shown some relationship between length of treatment and social class position (Imber, Nash, & Stone, 1955; Cole, Branch, & Allison, 1962; Gibby, Stotsky, Miller, & Hiler, 1953). Once again, however, more recent studies have reported data that is more equivocal about this relationship. Feister and Rudestam (1975), for example, found a relationship between client SES and early termination in one clinic, but not in a hospital-based community mental health center, while Albronda, Dean, and Starkweather (1964) found no significant relationship between social class and premature termination. Sue, McKinney, Allen, and Hall (1974) report a weak correlation between SES and treatment duration that disappeared when patient ethnicity was controlled. Wold and Sanger (1976) discovered that continuation in group psychotherapy for two or more years was correlated with SES only if lower-SES clients were also chronically unemployed, and that unemployment was also significantly associated with diagnoses of schizophrenia and relatively severe depression. They suggest that the idea that expressive therapies are not appropriate for the economically disadvantaged may apply more specifically to those patients whose ego functioning or coping capacities are sufficiently impaired to prevent them from holding jobs. The two most recent studies of this issue (Edwards et al., 1979; Schmidt & Hancey, 1979) also found no differences between social classes and treatment duration. Indeed, the latter study demonstrates that lowered treatment costs encourage the economically disadvantaged to use mental health facilities, and suggests that social-environmental costs are more important in class-related differences to seek therapy, and to remain in therapy, than such oft-cited variables as inappropriate expectations, educational level, or value conflict.

It appears, then, that the relationship between SES and early termination is not entirely straightforward. What can be concluded safely on the basis of research evidence is that the economically disadvantaged client is less likely to drop out of therapy now than his or her counterpart twenty years ago. This change can undoubtedly be attributed at least in part to the concerted effort on the part of community mental health centers to provide low-cost services to the underserved client (Sue, 1977).

It should be pointed out here that the meaning of early termination is itself not altogether clear. The assumption is usually made that a certain amount of contact with a therapist must be made to achieve progress. It is for this reason that early termination is usually viewed as a failure in psychotherapy, even though there are few data evaluating outcomes in such cases (Garfield, 1978). The few studies of this issue have found that the relationship between successful outcome and length of treatment is not linear. Cartwright (1955), for example, discovered two groups of improved patients: One group was composed of short-term clients, and the other of successful long-term clients. Within each group the number of interviews and success ratings were positively related. Cartwright also, however, identified a "failure zone," a period when potential long-term clients dropped out of therapy. In short, he, as well as others (Taylor, 1956; Rosenthal & Frank, 1958), found that optimum time in treatment produces a bimodal distribution. It has been hypothesized (Jones, 1974) that brief successful cases and longer successful cases differ in the kinds of problems presented by the client, and that short-term clients have mainly situational problems, while longer-term clients have more enduring personality difficulties. In view of the rediscovery by community psychology of the relationship of psychological health to social and environmental circumstances, it seems reasonable to conjecture that the economically disadvantaged client may sometimes have significant reality problems that brief contact with a therapist can be helpful in resolving. While some lower-SES clients who drop out of treatment early may in fact be considered treatment failures, not all early terminators can be confidently classified as such. Dropout rates, then, are not the clear and precise index of treatment effectiveness that critics—who use this statistic as evidence of the inadequacy of traditional forms for the underserved—would have us believe.

Can the Economically Disadvantaged Achieve Successful Therapy Outcomes?

Actual studies of psychotherapy outcomes with the economically disadvantaged that formally assess treatment outcomes (rather than merely relying on dropout rates as an index of outcome) have not been done frequently. Most studies have failed to find SES differences among successful patients, and have generally reported that outcome and social status characteristics are independent (Katz, Lorr, & Rubenstein, 1958; Brill & Storrow, 1960; Cole et al., 1962; Albronda et al., 1964). Lorion (1973) has arrived at the conclusion that while SES sometimes correlates with attrition rates, it does not correlate with available treatment outcome data. A fine study by Lerner (1972) convincingly documents the potential efficacy of dynamically oriented psychotherapy with low-income patients, demonstrating the positive impact of therapy with ghetto residents as reported not only by therapist and patient, but also by independent behavioral ratings. In a similar vein, a report on treatment outcomes with blue-collar workers at the Columbia Psychoanalytic Clinic (Terestman, Miller, & Weber, 1974) showed that although the dropout rate for these patients was higher than in the middle-class comparison group, those who continued in therapy had comparable success rates. Two recent large-scale studies, one conducted in a consortium on community mental health centers (Edwards et al., 1979) and the other at a military hospital (Schmidt & Hancey, 1979), also failed to demonstrate any difference in success rates across social class. In short, *there is virtually no actual, formal therapy outcome study that shows lower rates of success among the economically disadvantaged.*

These outcome findings do not, of course, indicate that all low-income patients can be treated successfully with traditional psychotherapies. They do, however, demonstrate the invalidity of assuming that psychotherapy is a vain venture for such clients. As Terestman et al. (1974) point out, sociological or psychological stereotypes about the economically disadvantaged are highly unreliable predictors of patient characteristics and of therapeutic outcome. Within the subgroup that shares the "underserved" label are individuals with a wide range of problems, personality types, and attitudes toward therapy. The image of the lower-SES client as more fearful of therapy, more pessimistic and passive, and wanting authoritarian direction and quick and concrete results rather than introspective talk may in fact apply to some; it certainly, however, does not represent all. Moreover, as we have pointed out earlier, these same characteristics can probably be found among a substantial number of middle-class clients. What is important is to be able to identify those economically disadvantaged clients who can benefit from traditional forms of therapy; at the same time, those who are unable to benefit from expressive therapies must be identified and provided with alternative psychotherapy and behavior change methods.

Patient Preparation for Psychotherapy

An important development in recent years has been the invention and implementation of techniques for preparing or socializing clients for psychotherapy. Most approaches involve some type of pretraining or orientation to ready psychologically ingenuous clients for the kind of activity required of them in psychotherapy, how the therapist is likely to behave, and how much time is likely to be required before they may experience some improvement, and to help clients anticipate certain events that may occur during the course of therapy, such as resistance or strong feelings about their therapist.

Orne and Wender (1968) have developed a clinical interview method of patient preparation termed "anticipatory socialization." This technique, which can be applied by either an intake interviewer or the therapist in the initial phase of treatment, aims to provide a rational basis for the patient to help him or her accept psychotherapy as a means of overcoming personal difficulties, to clarify the role of patient and therapist, and to provide a general outline of the course of therapy, especially the antici-pation of negative transferences. Hoehn-Saric, Frank, Imber, Nash, Stone, and Battle (1964) developed a similar technique called the "role induction interview," an informal intake interview during which the prospective client is encouraged to interrupt and ask questions. Psychotherapy is described by the interviewer as a way of learning to deal more effectively with problems; it is explained that the therapist may not talk very much, but would listen carefully and try to understand the client's thoughts and feelings; it would be up to the patient, however, to find his or her own way to handle problems and make decisions. The client is then urged to talk freely to the therapist, to describe his or her fantasies and daydreams, and to express feelings, especially any feelings about the therapist. In short, the role induction interview helps clarify what will go on in treatment, assures the patient that therapy will be helpful, and dispels unrealistic hopes as a way of avoiding disillusionment. The role induction interview has been shown to increase useful in-therapy behavior as well as to promote significantly better outcomes (Frank, 1978).

Strupp and Bloxom (1973) compared the effects of a role induction interview with a role induction-type film that was presented to prospective clients. Compared with a control group, important advantages were observed among the prepared patients, who at termination rated them-selves as more satisfied with their interpersonal relationships, showed greater understanding about the nature of psychotherapy, and perceived themselves as benefiting more from treatment. The two preparation techniques appeared to have somewhat different impacts, with the interview method better conveying specific information about how the patient should behave in treatment, and the film increasing clients' motivation to begin and involve themselves in the treatment process.

Yet another method of patient preparation employs an extratherapy intervention (Warren & Rice, 1972), and has been shown to reduce attrition rates and to train clients successfully to participate more productively in the therapy process. This approach involves a series of half-hour sessions outside of therapy concurrent with the early therapy hours, during which the client is encouraged to discuss any problems or concerns he or she may have about the therapy or therapist; attempts are then made to teach the patient how to derive benefits more effectively from the treatment process.

Unfortunately, from the standpoint of this discussion, the studies described above did not specifically focus on client socioeconomic status. Heitler (1973), however, conducted an investigation expressly aimed at assessing the effectiveness of a preparatory technique in readying lower-class clients for psychotherapy. In a sample of 48 lower-SES patients in group psychotherapy, he found that prepared patients communicated and engaged in self-exploratory efforts more frequently. Prepared patients were also rated by their therapists as more involved in treatment, as having more hopeful prognoses, and as generally having established more effective therapeutic alliances.

The evidence suggests that patient preparation techniques of the kind described here can significantly improve the mental health treatment experiences of the disadvantaged (Heitler, 1976), and that some sort of pretreatment preparation, if made available to lower-SES clients on a regular basis, should improve treatment duration and outcome rates. Indeed, Lorion (1978) finds the evidence of the positive impact of preparatory procedures "too overwhelming to ignore." We, too, consider the appearance of preparation techniques an extremely important recent development in the field. Preparatory techniques are relatively simple and easily conducted (they do not, for example, require the kind of training necessary to conduct psychotherapy), and obviously cost-effective. Still, it may be important to restate here a recurrent theme of this discussion: While preparation techniques can undoubtedly benefit lower-SES clients, the majority of the studies involving pretreatment training demonstrate that such approaches can likewise be beneficial to the middle-class client.

The Technique

The patient preparatory techniques that have been described attempt to alter the prospective patient, his or her expectancies, and other therapy-readiness characteristics in order to more adequately fit the patient role. Rather than focusing on the presumed deficiencies of lower-SES patients, another point of view can be assumed—that is, that traditional methods of expressive psychotherapy require modification. That is to say, rather than making the patient fit the therapy, it is possible to attempt to alter or reformulate psychotherapy so that it corresponds more closely with the presumed characteristics of the patient. Several researchers and clinicians have suggested somewhat informal, unsystematic modifications to traditional methods such as flexibility in scheduling, nonverbal contact, and role playing (Gould, 1967; Baum & Felzer, 1964; Riessman & Scribner, 1965) as helpful in treating the lower-SES client.

Goldstein (1973, 1981) has developed a more formal, structured method of therapy, which he contends is highly effective with traditionally underserved groups. This approach to treatment, termed "Structured Learning Therapy," derives conceptually from contemporary cognitive-behavioral therapies, and is couched in the language of behaviorist psychology. Its major components include modeling, role playing, performance feedback, and transfer of training. The patient is provided with specific, detailed, frequent, and vivid displays of adaptive behavior or of specific skills in which he or she is deficient (modeling); given opportunity and encouragement to rehearse or practice such modeled behavior behaviorally (role playing); provided with positive feedback, approval, or reward for successful enactments (performance feedback); and asked to engage in the kinds of behavior that increase the probability that the behaviors taught in therapy will be used in other settings (transfer of training; Goldstein, Gershaw, & Sprafkin, in press).

In this approach, patients are called "trainees," and each potential problematic behavior or deficiency is reconceptualized as a "skill"; treatment is usually conducted in groups of 6-12 people who share similar skill deficiencies. Each skill is differentiated into a number of different behavioral steps, and a series of audiotapes have been developed in which actors expertly depict the various steps of the skill. Discussion follows, and trainees' statements about difficulties in behaving effectively in this particular skill area are used as material for realistic role playing. After the trainees have described their skill problems, as well as the real persons involved in them, role playing is begun.

After completion of the role play, there is a feedback period to inform the trainee how well the skill's steps were followed and in which fashion the client departed from them, and to provide encouragement to try out the role-play behaviors in real life. Transfer of skills to real-life situations, a crucial element in this treatment approach, is attempted through over-learning (repetition of the skill, practice sessions), stimulus variability (for example, having trainees role play a given skill across several relevant settings), and through real-life reinforcement by creating external or environmental support by involving staff, relatives, and friends who can encourage and reward trainees as they practice their new skills.

There is a good deal of research evidence that demonstrates the effectiveness of Structured Learning Therapy with populations with whom classic expressive therapies have not been notably successful: geriatric patients, child-abusing parents, aggressive or disturbed adolescents, and other traditionally underserved populations (Goldstein, 1981). This is not to say that more structured, behaviorally oriented treatments are a more appropriate approach to treatment for lower-SES clients in general. As we have already emphasized, there are clearly many clients from underserved groups who can and do benefit from traditional therapies. Nevertheless, it is important to identify those who cannot, and provide them with alternative forms. Structured Learning Therapy is one of the most fully evolved of these alternative approaches, and is of proven effectiveness. Still, it is important to hold in check generalized assumptions about the lower-class client's wishes and expectations, and not simply assume that a more behaviorally oriented training approach is the treatment of choice. And, once again, it is important to realize that many middle-class patients may likewise benefit from the kinds of modifications in therapy technique represented by Structured Learning Therapy.

The Therapist

Attitudes Toward the Underserved

There is a good deal of evidence that therapists' attitudes and expectations significantly affect the effectiveness of psychotherapy for the economically disadvantaged client. During the 1950s and early 1960s, reports consistently reflected psychotherapists' discomfort and discouragement about treating lower-SES patients. Such clients were often considered inappropriate for therapy, and treating them was sometimes considered hopeless because of these patients' alleged hostility and suspicion; in comparison, middle-class clients were considered easier to handle, more acceptable, and more understandable (Hollingshead & Redlich, 1958; Schaffer & Myers, 1954). One report characteristic of that epoch is Brill and Storrow's (1960) study, which attempted to evaluate psychological-mindedness, and hence suitability for psychotherapy, in relation to social class. Through an analysis of data collected at an intake interview, the researchers found that lower SES was significantly related to lower "estimated" intelligence, to a tendency to see the presenting problem as physical rather than emotional, to a desire for symptomatic relief rather than "overall" change, and to a lack of desire for psychotherapy. They also report that the interviewer tended to react less positively to the lower-class client, and viewed him or her as less treatable than his or her middle-class counterpart. The study seemed to validate the assumption that lower-class clients are frequently not suitable candidates for psychotherapy, and to support therapists' stereotypes of lower-SES clients.

This study and others like it (see Auld & Myers, 1954; Myers & Roberts, 1959; Affleck & Garfield, 1961) are a manifestation of the curious circularity to the thinking then prevalent about clients from underserved groups. Lower-SES clients were less likely to be seen as "good" patients, were diagnosed less hopefully (Haase, 1964), tended to evoke less positive responses on the part of therapists, and, probably as a result of these factors as well as others, were less likely to be accepted for treatment than middle-class therapy candidates (Schaffer & Myers, 1954). It should come as no great surprise, then, that when they were actually treated they were seen as less improved. It seems that a self-fulfilling prophecy was created in which unfavorable therapist attitudes toward the disadvantaged frequently led to negative treatment outcomes (Jones, 1974).

There is some evidence that reports of the sort cited above probably reflect a bias against the economically disadvantaged client, which mediated to a certain degree the differences observed between lower-SES and middle-class patients (Lee & Temerlin, 1970). Lerner (1973), for example, found that therapists who scored higher on a Democratic Values Scale (a measure of the extent of respect or valuing of individual autonomy) were more effective in working with lower-class and more severely impaired patients, and also displayed greater interest in treating them. Moreover, more "democratic" therapists tended to achieve better therapeutic results even when the severity of patient disturbance was held constant (Lerner & Fiske, 1973). In a similar vein, Yamamoto, James, Bloombaum, and Hattem (1967) observed that therapists who scored low on an ethnocentricity measure tended to treat ethnic minority clients in proportion with White clients, while more ethnocentric therapists less often saw minority group clients in treatment.

There is growing evidence, however, that professionals in the field are beginning to display fewer biases, and are now increasingly less likely to hold negative stereotypes about clients from underserved groups. Newer reports indicate that more clinicians are expressing the conviction that lower-class patients are more psychological-minded (Goin et al., 1965) and verbally expressive (Riessman, 1964; Gould, 1967), and are generally better therapy risks (Riessman & Scribner, 1965) than has been assumed in the past.

A relatively recent study (Del Gaudio, Stein, Ansley, & Carpenter, 1976) designed to examine therapists' attitudes toward case histories of patients with differing social class backgrounds appears to bear out the supposition of changing attitudes among psychotherapists. In this study a sample of therapists rated each of eight case histories of psychiatric outpatients on five dependent variables: likability, comfort, interest in treating, interest in friendship, and prognosis. Within the case histories the patient's social class, diagnosis, and insight level were systematically varied. As expected, patient diagnosis and insight level were significantly related to prognosis and interest in treating the person. Therapists also reported that they would be more comfortable with, and indicated more interest in becoming friendly with, neurotic, high-insight patients. But more to the point of this discussion, the study indicates relatively little evidence for the salience of social class in determining therapists' attitudes.

One explanation offered for these results is that the verbal-conceptual ability of patients and their greater emotional well-being may have always been more important factors in determining therapists' attitudes than social class status. Anther plausible alternative explanation for the relatively minor impact of patient social class is that fewer therapists today are biased against lower-class patients than was the case in earlier years. Certainly these findings stand in marked contrast to those of an analogous study by Haase (1964), in which similar ratings of case histories by therapists revealed a clear and systematic bias against the lower-SES client. Koscherak and Masling (1972) provide additional support for the notion that therapist attitudes toward traditionally underserved groups are changing in a study that suggests that community-oriented psychologists tend to evaluate middle-class patients less favorably than lower-class patients. If this is in fact a valid assertion, such a shift in attitudes among mental health workers sheds light on a parallel set of findings that shows there is currently little racial prejudice among clinicians in comparison to that so strongly evident in the past (Jones, in press; Benefee, Abramowitz, Weitz, & Armstrong, 1976; Bloch, Weitz, & Abramowitz, 1980; Merluzzi & Merluzzi, 1978).

It appears that the movement for social change of the past decades has had an impact, the extent of which is not fully appreciated, on the mental health field, not only in terms of the shifting emphasis of government agencies and programs toward the needs of special populations, but also in terms of a genuine growth of sensitivity toward clients from underserved groups among workers in the field. We consider these recent developments to constitute sufficient grounds for a cautious optimism about the improved effectiveness of psychological therapies for economically disadvantaged clients in the future.

Preparation and Training for
Treating the Disadvantaged Client

The impact of therapists' attitudes on the success or failure of psychotherapy with the disadvantaged is evident. In fact, the therapist, and not the patient or the technique, is probably the crucial target in efforts to improve treatment with the disadvantaged (Lorion, 1978). Given this fact, there are a number of possibilities for increasing therapist effectiveness with such clients. One such possibility is the more careful selection of those therapists who work with lower-class clients. Several writers (Rogers, Gendlin, Kiesler, & Truax, 1967; Karon & Vendenbos, 1977) have commented that the therapist must be particularly skillful and sensitive if he or she is to involve the lower-SES client in treatment. The idea that a high level of therapeutic skill is required for such clients is supported by more than one study. Baum, Felzer, D'Zmura, and Shumaker (1966) observed that therapists who were more secure and clinically experienced, and who had undergone personal therapy themselves, established better relationships with lower-class clients and had lower dropout rates with such patients than other therapists. Similarly, Hughes (1972) found that White therapists who had undergone personal therapy had better outcomes in therapy with non-White clients than therapists who had not. Terestman et al. (1974) also made the important finding that therapists' therapeutic skill, as judged by their teachers, was significantly related to success in treating blue-collar workers. In light of these findings, it is particularly unfortunate that lower-SES clients are still more likely to be treated by less well-trained and less experienced psychotherapists (Sue, 1977).

Another possibility for improving therapist effectiveness with the economically disadvantaged client is to attempt more formally to alter the therapist's potentially negative set at the beginning of treatment by employing procedures that enable therapists to recognize and resolve their stereotypic view about the poor. Baum and Felzer (1964) report a procedure in which therapists were educated about client lifestyles, needs, and expectations, and staff conferences were devoted to openly discussing therapists' reluctance to work with lower-SES clients, as well as differences in communication styles and possible changes in treatment approaches. These procedures had the beneficial effect of lowering the attrition rate among poor clients.

Another approach to therapist preparation, one that parallels the patient preparation procedures described earlier, has been tested successfully by Jacobs, Charles, Jacobs, Weinstein, and Mann (1972). Their study attempted to examine the relative efficacy of simultaneously orienting both the therapist and the lower-SES client before the first treatment session. A group of 120 therapy applicants were randomly assigned to 4 different treatment groups: (1) "prepared" patients to be seen by "prepared" therapists; (2) "nonprepared" patients seen by "prepared" therapists; (3) "nonprepared" patients seen by "nonprepared" therapists; and (4) "prepared" patients seen by "nonprepared" therapists. If the patient was to be prepared, he or she was given a 15-minute orientation for treatment after a regular screening interview. The orientation involved a discussion with the client about such issues as the differences between seeing their family doctor or surgeon and seeing a psychiatrist, the use of medication, the exploration of feelings and interpersonal relationships, and the like. Therapist preparation involved a 15-minute orientation focusing on the difficulties lower-SES clients may experience in exploring their feelings, in accepting the concept of psychological motivation, and in tolerating delay in receiving immediate help. Nonprepared therapists were not formally oriented to SES-relevant issues.

Treatment effectiveness was evaluated on a number of different indices. Prepared therapists retained disadvantaged patients in treatment significantly longer than nonprepared therapists, and were more likely to perceive their patients as improving whether patients had been prepared or not. Nonprepared patients seen by nonprepared therapists demonstrated the least improvement, and were also significantly more likely to have their treatment experience limited to evaluative sessions only. Prepared patients seen by prepared therapists achieved the most successful outcome.

This study underscores the fact that negative expectations and treatment biases of therapists (as well as of patients) are in fact reversible, and by using relatively simple procedures. Indeed, one of the remarkable aspects of this study is the extent of the impact of such a brief therapist preparation procedure. It could well be that the strong psychological orientation shared by most psychotherapists is in some sense antagonistic to general biases and stereotypic thinking, and that if therapists are given the opportunity to focus on the problems of treating disadvantaged clients, along with some support and encouragement, they can become effective service providers to the disadvantaged. In view of this, it is encouraging that there has been in recent years an increased emphasis on special training programs to prepare mental health professionals to provide treatment to underserved groups; the President's Commission on Mental Health (1978), for example, has advocated strong support for programs of clinical service and professional training for such populations. There has been a growing consciousness, both in society at large as well as among mental health professionals and supporting government agencies, about the special needs of underserved groups, which has made more possible the potential benefits of psychotherapy to more people. There is no question that psychotherapy is becoming less and less an exclusively middle-class enterprise.

Conclusion

This review of recent research and literature bearing on psychotherapy with underserved populations suggests that there have been significant new developments in this area of abiding interest to mental health workers. It appears that long-held assumptions concerning the attitudes and expectations of lower-class clients about treatment require important modification. The most recent data demonstrate that there is in fact no unified set of attitudes and expectations about therapy that are held in common by disadvantaged clients, and that their view of psychological therapies no longer differ greatly from those of the middle class. Moreover, the traditional view that lower-SES clients are less likely to benefit from expressive psychotherapy, an opinion that has never been founded solidly on an empirical base, has consistently failed to be verified by research over the past decade. There are indications, too, of a gradual corresponding shift in therapists' attitudes toward the underserved, characterized by a reduction in negative biases and stereotypes, a greater willingness to treat such clients, and greater optimism about the potential effectiveness of psychotherapy with such groups. The time has arrived to focus away from socioeconomic status per se; it is a mere proxy variable that fails to inform adequately about an individual's views of psychotherapy, about personality and psychological conflict, and about aspirations and goals in therapy. What is now needed is a concentration on the actual impediments to successful therapeutic work, including the development of specific procedures aimed at better preparing clients for the experience of psychotherapy, the modification of therapist attitudes about work with such clients, and the development of alternative treatment techniques that could allow a broader range of traditionally underserved populations to benefit from psychotherapy.

References

Affleck, D., & Garfield, S. Predictive judgments of therapists and duration of stay in psychotherapy. *Journal of Clinical Psychologyy*, 1961, 17, 134-137.
Albronda, H. F., Dean, R. L., & Starkweather, J. A. Social class and psychotherapy. *Archives of General Psychiatry*, 1964, 10, 276-283.
Auld, F., & Myers, J. K. Contributions to a theory for selecting psychotherapy patients. *Journal of Clinical Psychotherapy*, 1954, 10, 56-60.
Balch, P., McWilliams, S., Lewis, S., & Ireland, J. Clients' treatment expectations at a community mental health center. *American Journal of Community Psychology*, 1978, 6, 105-113.
Baum, O., & Felzer, S. Activity in initial interviews with lower-class patients. *Archives of General Psychiatry*, 1964, 10, 345-353.
Baum, O., Felzer, S., D'Zmura, T., & Schumaker, E. Psychotherapy, dropouts and lower socioeconomic patients. *American Journal of Orthopsychiatry*, 1966, 36, 629-635.
Benefee, L., Abramowitz, S., Weitz, L., & Armstrong, S. Effects of patient racial attribution on black clinicians' inferences. *American Journal of Community Psychology*, 1976, 4, 263-273.
Bloch, P. M., Weitz, L. J., & Abramowitz, S. I. Racial attribution effects on clinical judgments: A failure to replicate among white clinicians. *American Journal of Community Psychology*, 1980, 8, 485-493.
Brill, N. Q., & Storrow, H. A. Social class and psychiatric treatment. *Archives of General Psychiatry*, 1960, 3, 340-344.
Calhoon, L. G., Dawes, S., & Lewis, P. M. Correlates of attitudes towards help-seeking in outpatients. *Journal of Consulting and Clinical Psychology*, 1972, 38, 153.
Cartwright, D. S. Success in psychotherapy as a function as a function of certain actuarial variables. *Journal of Consulting Psychology*, 1955, 19, 357-363.
Cole, N. J., Branch, C. H., & Allison, R. Some relationships between social class and the practice of dynamic psychotherapy. *American Journal of Psychiatry*, 1962, 118, 1004-1012.

Del Gaudio, A., Stein, L., Ansley, M., & Carpenter, P. Attitudes of therapists varying in community mental health ideology and democratic values. *Journal of Consulting and Clinical Psychology,* 1976, 44, 646-655.

Edwards, D. W., Greene, L. R., Abramowitz, S. I., & Davidson, C. V. National health insurance, psychotherapy, and the poor. *American Psychologist,* 1979, 34, 411-419.

Feister, A. R., & Rudestam, K. E. A multivariate analysis of the early dropout process. *Journal of Consulting and Clinical Psychology,* 1975, 43, 528-535.

Frank, J. D. Expectation and therapeutic outcome–The placebo effect and the role induction interview. In J. D. Frank, R. Hoehn-Saric, S. D. Imber, B. L. Liberman, & A. R. Stone (Eds.), *Effective ingredients of successful psychotherapy.* New York: Brunner/Mazel, 1978.

Garfield, S. Research on client variables in psychotherapy. In S. Garfield & A. Bergin (Eds.), *Handbook of psychotherapy and behavior change.* New York: John Wiley, 1978.

Gibby, R. G., Stotsky, B. A., Miller, D. R., & Hiler, E. W. Prediction of duration of therapy from the Rorschach test. *Journal of Consulting Psychology,* 1953, 17, 348-354.

Goin, M. K., Yamamoto, J., & Silverman, J. Therapy congruent with class linked expectations. *Archives of General Psychiatry,* 1965, 13, 133-137.

Goldstein, A. P. *Structured learning therapy: Toward a psychotherapy for the poor.* New York: Academic, 1973.

Goldstein, A. P. *Psychological skill training.* Elmsford, NY: Pergamon, 1981.

Goldstein, A. P., Gershaw, N. J., & Sprafkin, R. P. Structured learning therapy: Background, procedures and evaluation. In D. Larson (Ed.), *Giving psychology away: Innovative programs for mental health training and delivery.* In press.

Gould, R. E. Dr. Strangeclass: Or how I stopped worrying about the theory and began treating the blue-collar worker. *American Journal of Orthopsychiatry,* 1967, 37, 78-86.

Haase, W. The role of socioeconomic class in examiner bias. In F. Riessman, J. Cohen, & A. Pearl (Eds.), *Mental health of the poor.* New York: Macmillan, 1964.

Heitler, J. B. Preparation of lower-class patients for expressive group psychotherapy. *Journal of Consulting and Clinical Psychology,* 1973, 41, 251-260.

Heitler, J. B. Preparatory techniques in initiating expressive psychotherapy with lower-class, unsophisticated patients. *Psychological Bulletin,* 1976, 83, 339-352.

Hoehn-Saric, R., Frank, J. D., Imber, S. D., Nash, E. H., Stone, A. R., & Battle, C. C. Systematic preparation of patients for psychotherapy: 1. Effects of therapy behavior and outcome. *Journal of Psychiatric Research,* 1964, 2, 267-281.

Hollingshead, A. B., & Redlich, F. C. *Social class and mental illness.* New York: John Wiley, 1958.

Hughes, R. *The effects of sex, age, race and social history of therapist and client on psychotherapy outcome.* Unpublished doctoral dissertation, University of California, Berkeley, 1972.

Imber, S. D., Nash, E. H., & Stone, A. R. Social class and duration of psychotherapy. *Journal of Clinical Psychology,* 1955, 11, 281-294.

Jacobs, D., Charles, E., Jacobs, T., Weinstein, H., & Mann, D. Preparation for treatment of the disadvantaged patient: Effects of disposition and outcome. *American Journal of Orthopsychiatry,* 1972, 42, 666-674.

Jones, E. E. Social class and psychotherapy: A critical review of research. *Psychiatry*, 1974, 37, 307-320.

Jones, E. E. Psychotherapists' impressions of treatment outcome as a function of race. *Journal of Clinical Psychology*, in press.

Jones, E. E., & Korchin, S. J. Minority mental health: Perspectives. In E. E. Jones & S. J. Korchin (Eds.), *Minority mental health*. New York: Praeger, 1982.

Kadushin, C. *Why people go to psychiatrists*. New York: Atherton, 1969.

Karon, B. P., & Vandenbos, G. R. Psychotherapeutic technique and the economically poor patient. *Psychotherapy: Theory, Research, and Practice*, 1977, 14, 169-180.

Katz, M. M., Lorr, M., & Rubinstein, E. A. Remainer patient attributes and their reaction to subsequent improvement in psychotherapy. *Journal of Consulting Psychology*, 1958, 22, 411-413.

Koscherak, S., & Masling, J. Noblesse oblige effect: The interpretation of Rorschach responses as a function of ascribed social class. *Journal of Consulting and Clinical Psychology*, 1972, 39, 415-419.

Lee, S., & Temerlin, M. D. Social class, diagnosis, and prognosis for psychotherapy. *Psychotherapy: Therapy, Research, and Practice*, 1970, 7, 181-185.

Lerner, B. *Therapy in the ghetto: Political impotence and personal disintegration*. Baltimore: Johns Hopkins University Press, 1972.

Lerner, B. Democratic values and therapeutic efficacy: A construct validity study. *Journal of Abnormal Psychology*, 1973, 82, 491-498.

Lerner, B., & Fiske, D. W. Client factors and the eye of the beholder. *Journal of Consulting and Clinical Psychology*, 1973, 40, 272-277.

Lorion, R. P. Socioeconomic status and traditional treatment approaches reconsidered. *Psychological Bulletin*, 1973, 79, 263-270.

Lorion, R. P. Patient and therapist variables in the treatment of low-income patients. *Psychological Bulletin*, 1974, 81, 344-354.

Lorion, R. P. Research on psychotherapy and behavior change with the disadvantaged: Past, present and future directions. In S. L. Garfield & A. E. Bergin (Eds.), *Handbook of psychotherapy and behavior change*. New York: John Wiley, 1978.

Merluzzi, B. H., & Merluzzi, T. V. Influence of client race on counselors' assessment of case materials. *Journal of Counseling Psychology*, 1978, 25, 399-404.

Myers, J. K., & Roberts, B. H. *Family and class dynamics in mental illness*. New York: John Wiley, 1959.

Orne, M., & Wender, P. Anticipatory socialization for psychotherapy: Method and rationale. *American Journal of Psychiatry*, 1968, 124, 88-98.

Overall, B., & Aronson, H. Expectations of psychotherapy in lower socio-economic class patients. *American Journal of Orthopsychiatry*, 1963, 33, 421-430.

President's Commission on Mental Health. *Report to the president of the President's Commission on Mental Health*. Washington, DC: Government Printing Office, 1978.

Reiff, R., & Scribner, S. Issues in the new national mental health program relating to labor and low-income groups. In F. Riessman, J. Cohen, & A. Pearl (Eds.), *Mental health of the poor*. New York: Macmillan, 1964.

Riessman, F. *New approaches to mental health treatment for labor and low income groups: A survey*. New York: National Institute of Labor Education, 1964.

Riessman, F., & Scribner, S. The underutilization of mental health services by workers and low-income groups: Causes and cures. *American Journal of Psychiatry*, 1965, 121, 798-801.

Rogers, C. R., Gendlin, E. T., Kiesler, D. J., & Truax, C. B. *The therapeutic relationship and its impact.* Madison: University of Wisconsin Press, 1967.

Rosenthal, D., & Frank, J. D. The fate of psychiatric clinic outpatients assigned to psychotherapy. *Journal of Nervous and Mental Disease,* 1958, 127, 330-343.

Ryan, W. *Blaming the victim.* New York: Random House, 1971.

Schaffer, R., & Myers, J. R. Psychotherapy and social stratification. *Psychiatry,* 1954, 17, 83-93.

Schmidt, J. P., & Hancey, R. Social class and psychiatric treatment: Application of a decision-making model to use patterns in a cost-free clinic. *Journal of Consulting and Clinical Psychology,* 1979, 47, 771-772.

Siassi, I., & Messer, S. B. Psychotherapy with patients from lower socio-economic groups. *American Journal of Psychotherapy,* 1976, 30, 29-40.

Strupp, H., & Bloxom, A. Preparing lower-class patients for group psychotherapy: Development and evaluation of a role induction film. *Journal of Consulting and Clinical Psychology,* 1973, 41, 373-384.

Sue, S. Community mental health services to minority groups. *American Psychologist,* 1977, 32, 616-624.

Sue, S., McKinney, H., Allen, D., & Hall, J. Delivery of community mental health services to black and white clients. *Journal of Consulting and Clinical Psychology,* 1974, 42, 794-801.

Taylor, J. W. Relationship of success and length in psychotherapy. *Journal of Consulting Psychology,* 1956, 20, 332.

Terestman, N., Miller, D., & Weber, J. Blue collar workers at a psychoanalytic clinic. *American Journal of Psychiatry,* 1974, 131, 261-266.

Warren, N. C., & Rice, L. N. Structuring and stabilizing of psychotherapy for low-prognosis clients. *Journal of Consulting and Clinical Psychology,* 1972, 39, 173-181.

Williams, H. V., Lipman, R. S., Uhlenhuth, E. A., Rickels, K., Covi, L., & Mock, J. Some factors influencing the treatment expectations of anxious neurotic outpatients. *Journal of Nervous and Mental Disease,* 1967, 145, 208-220.

Wold, P., & Sanger, J. Social class and group therapy in a working class population. *Community Mental Health Journal,* 1976, 12, 335-341.

Wynne, M. *Client and therapist expectations related to the outcome of crisis intervention therapy with black clients.* Unpublished doctoral dissertation, University of California, Berkeley, 1981.

Yamamoto, J., James, Q. C., Bloombaum, M., & Hattem, J. Racial factors in patient selection. *American Journal of Psychiatry,* 1967, 124, 630-636.

11

Service System Models for Ethnic Minorities

Nolan Zane
Pacific Asian Mental Health Research Project
Stanley Sue
Felipe G. Castro
University of California, Los Angeles
William George
University of Washington

For well over two decades great concern has been expressed over the delivery of mental health services to ethnic minority individuals and communities (see Torrey, 1970; Karno & Edgerton, 1969; Sue, 1977; Mollica, Blum, & Redlich, 1980). This concern has stimulated two major developments. First, there has been a greater understanding of the types of problems that exist in attempting to deliver effective services to ethnic minority groups. These problems include the lack of bilingual/bicultural mental health personnel, the failure to take into consideration the cultural backgrounds and community dynamics of clients, and the infrequent application of innovative intervention approaches for nonmainstream Americans. Second, knowledge about these problems has resulted in efforts to develop certain conceptual strategies for more appropriate service delivery systems, a task advocated by the President's Commission on Mental Health (1978).

While obtaining knowledge of problems and generating developmental strategies for service delivery are important processes in the eventual implementation of ethnically responsive programs, it seems wise to exam-

AUTHORS' NOTE: This work was supported by NIMH Grant MH 32148, Kenji Murase, Principal Investigator.

ine core principles that can be derived from such conceptualizations. Thus the purpose of this chapter is twofold: (1) to formulate core or guiding principles that underlie many mental health service delivery systems for ethnic minority groups and (2) to identify certain service system models that exemplify the successful operationalization of such principles into practice.

In the ethnic mental health literature, many investigators have proposed various conceptual schemes for the design and reorganization of service delivery systems embedded within minority communities. For example, Cuellar (1980) underscores the necessity of making changes at all four levels of the social structure—namely, the individual, the family, the organization, and the community or social system—when examining approaches to the intervention and resolution of Hispanic problems and needs. Undoubtedly, this comprehensive approach to intervention applies to any community mental health system regardless of the type of community it purports to serve. Yee and Lee (1977) have suggested that effective service delivery approaches for ethnic minorities should enhance cultural identity. Weidman (1973) has introduced the role of the culture broker as a key element in effective service delivery to various cultural groups. The culture broker is a clinically oriented social scientist from the particular culture being served. This person would mediate between the clinical and community systems using his or her expertise based on the integration of social science and cultural perspectives.

Apart from recommendations for ethnic minorities in general, others have proposed alternatives specifically designed for a particular ethnic minority group. King (1981) delineates five criteria for consideration when delivering services to Black communities: (1) the setting must be accessible; (2) service agents must be catalysts for facilitating change; (3) recipients must be addressed in the context of the kinship network; (4) the mode of delivery must address the conception of time; and (5) evaluation should involve the interaction of the family and the agency.

Kahn et al. (1975) urge the sole use of indigenous personnel, both professional and paraprofessional, as the ultimate goal for systems of service delivery to Native Americans. Others have emphasized the need for more collaboration between traditional healers and non-Indian mental health personnel (Attneave, 1974), greater community control of service programs (Ostendorf & Hammerslag, 1977), and more involvement of social networks in treatment interventions (Murdock & Schwartz, 1978). The latter consists of having family or clan members help the individual client or family make certain transitions, encourage family cohesion, and serve as adaptive coping role models.

In their review, Padilla, Ruiz, and Alvarez (1975) have recommended that innovative programs for the Spanish-speaking/surnamed (SSS) population incorporate many of the following features: (1) treatment services that address the nature of specific social problems that plague the SSS; (2) use of some combination of (a) community consultation as a preventive measure, (b) crisis intervention as the primary mode of treatment, and (c) "back-up" treatment with individual, group, family, and drop-in therapies; (3) validation research to guide effective program development; (4) community representation in the program's administration; and (5) adoption of a business model approach (such as use of the advertising media to disseminate information concerning available services) to attract clientele.

With regard to services for Asian Americans, Murase (1977) indicates that a culturally relevant social service has many of the following structural and organizational characteristics: (1) location of delivery site within the community itself; (2) involvement of a broad cross section of the community in decisions concerning the service programs; (3) employment of fully bilingual and bicultural staff; (4) cultivation and utilization of existing indigenous formal and informal community care/support systems; and (5) development of intervention methods that (a) recognize the family as an integral part of treatment, (b) establish a more active, supportive, directive, and highly personalized therapeutic relationship, (c) focus on survival-related, task-oriented services to facilitate the engagement process, (d) consider the possible conflict between the concept of "face" and the "confessional" character of the therapeutic situation, (e) differentiate between cultural behavioral tendencies and pathology, (f) reevaluate the self-determination construct, (g) allow for flexibility in session duration and schedule, and (h) acknowledge the therapeutic function of a familiar and predictable cultural milieu.

From this modest survey of the literature it becomes apparent that certain guiding principles and rationales for the development of effective and responsive service delivery systems to ethnic minority communities have received thoughtful attention and elaboration. However, the question remains whether such concepts have been developed into a coherent model of service delivery that, in turn, has directed the design of a viable service delivery system for a particular ethnic minority community.

Guiding Principles for Effective Service Delivery

Although the specific policies considered to be crucial for the development of an effective service delivery system vary depending on the particular ethnic minority community involved, the literature tends to converge on a set of core principles that can be implemented to guide such development efforts. Four of the six principles presented are similar to those proposed by Baker (1974) as characteristic of the "human service ideology" but are particularly oriented toward ethnic minority concerns. The following principles can be considered as an interrelated set of essential conceptual components of any responsive service delivery model for ethnic minorities:

(1) *Match or fit of services* to the particular needs and help-seeking patterns of the client population with a particular emphasis on addressing the impact of social problems (such as alcohol abuse, truancy, unemployment) on adaptive psychological functioning.

(2) *Integration and linkage of relevant services,* namely, mental health services with other health related and social services.

(3) *Efficient utilization of services,* primarily by focusing on primary prevention efforts that incorporate natural support systems.

(4) *Comprehensive services* at the four levels of intervention individual, family, organizational, and social system levels.

(5) *Community control* by means of advisory board and administration representation and service accountability.

(6) *Knowledge development and utilization* with an emphasis on promoting the adoption and implementation of innovative service system models.

This review will examine each of the principles in terms of their implications for service delivery, the specific service system problems involved in implementation, and the actual service system models that have succeeded in operationalizing such principles. Despite the independent treatment of these principles, the close interrelationships between each of them cannot be underemphasized. For instance, one cannot discuss match or fit of services without considering service linkage issues. However, for heuristic clarity each principle will be discussed separately to highlight the various programmatic features each service system model exemplifies.

Match or Fit of Services

Frequently, it has been found that services delivered from a traditional clinic setting have focused on issues and problems that held little relevance for the needs of the minority clientele (Brown, Stein, Huang, & Harris, 1973). These services often were delivered in a manner that conflicted with or failed to capitalize on the typical help-seeking patterns found in the community. The match or fit principle posits that both the content and process of services should be culturally relevant and culturally functional. For ethnic minorities culturally relevant service content involves particular attention to the ways in which social problems in the current living situation affect the client's mental health. This focus implies the employment of interventions that affect not only the immediate, more tangible social problems, such as unemployment, language barriers, and immigration regulations, but the broader social and political realities in which these problems are embedded. In other words, interventions must facilitate the development of coping skills (on the individual level), supportive relations (on the family and neighborhood levels), program policies (on the organization level), and social action (on the social/community system level) to ameliorate the adverse consequences of racism.

Process matches entail the delivery of services in a manner that is (1) congruent with the client's world view, (2) supportive of culturally acceptable help-seeking behaviors, and (3) compatible with the natural support systems within the community. Besides the logical attraction of the match principle, client-system matches may facilitate positive outcomes because they enhance perceptions of control (Sue, 1978). An impressive array of studies have found that perceived control or noncontrol has effects on behavior and emotion (Seligman, 1975). The perception of noncontrol or learned helplessness may result in (1) poor motivation, apathy, and passivity; (2) cognitive disruption and the subsequent failure to learn that events can be controlled; and (3) emotional disturbance such as anxiety, depression, and withdrawal. Thus the enhancement of the perception that what happens to oneself (outcomes) is affected by what one does (actions) mitigates against the development of motivational, cognitive, and emotional disturbances that may disrupt effective coping and problem-solving behavior.

To increase the fit between clients and the service delivery system, Sue (1978) has identified three strategies for change. The first alternative involves finding the right service for the person. This strategy is based on the assumption that appropriate services are available somewhere. The primary task is to make a wide range of services accessible basically involving effective referral and public knowledge of services. In general, the former has been plagued by impermeable catchment area boundaries and poor linkage among mental health and other health-related services. Despite the President's Commission on Mental Health's (PCMH, 1978) recommendations to have greater flexibility in delineating catchment area boundaries by using waivers of boundaries where it would best serve the needs of natural communities and those requiring services and to encourage cross-catchment-area program sharing to facilitate the delivery of high cost and/or specialized services, the catchment area will remain the basic unit for the development of community mental health service systems. The utility of the catchment area concept deserves critical review particularly when applied to ethnic minority communities. Frequently, catchment area boundaries fail to accommodate the structure of natural communities and create unnecessary barriers for both those who need and those who provide care (PCMH, 1978). The use of the waiver to make barriers more permeable appears to be a "band-aid" measure. In its implementation report on the PCMH recommendations, the Health, Education and Welfare (HEW) Task Force (1978) did not propose any specific guidelines for waiver use. If waivers are to be at all effective, specific criteria for waiver acceptance must be established along with recognized procedures for maximum community input in these decisions. It is not surprising that the service system models with successful service linkage operations tend to exist within one catchment area (see Lefley & Bestman, 1982; Delgado & Scott, 1979).

This problem becomes more acute when a service system attempts to reach ethnic communities widely dispersed across a certain geographical region. For example, in San Francisco the Asian/Pacific population is concentrated in three different catchment areas. In this case catchment area boundaries have impeded the efficient delivery of certain highly specialized services such as bilingual/bicultural inpatient services to monolingual clients.

The public's lack of knowledge about available services compounds the establishment of accessible services within and across catchment areas. Miller (1981) found that of the programs and services offered within one catchment area the clinical staff correctly identified 84 percent and the clerical staff correctly identified 73 percent. However, the general public sample only correctly identified 45 percent of the available services. Considering that the findings pertain to services within a catchment area, they suggest that public awareness of services across catchment areas is poor. Interestingly, when asked to indicate services that needed development in the future, both the client and general public samples listed public information groups as important. However, such groups were not so designated by any of the advisory board, administrator, or clinical staff samples. Not only does the public have little knowledge of services, but this problem is exacerbated by the apparent lack of interest in educating the community about programs and services that exist. Because of these problems in knowledge dissemination and catchment area crossover, the task to make a wide range of appropriate services available to clients with particular needs remains very difficult and infrequently used.

The second approach is to change the person to fit the service. Preparing clients for services (explaining the services, giving information on the process of treatment, correcting stereotypes of treatment, or other forms of pretherapy intervention) may facilitate a better person-mental health service match. Orne and Wender (1968) have developed the "anticipatory socialization interview" to educate clients who have had little experience or understanding of psychotherapy. The interview includes an explanation of the process and rationale behind traditional (psychodynamic) expressive psychotherapy, a discussion of client and therapist roles throughout the process, and the consideration of possible resistances that may develop. Extensive history taking is recommended to facilitate rapport building.

Although proposed to increase the potential efficacy of traditional psychotherapy with lower socioeconomic status and ethnic minority clients, the method can also be hazardous if it is carried to the extreme of denying cultural differences and of implying that there exists but one standard helping process for psychological change and progress. In an example of an effort to minimize these problems, Aoki (1981) has offered several alterations to the typical socialization interview to account for the cultural nuances of the Asian American experience. The therapist must minimize the egalitarian nature of the therapeutic learning process with many Asian American clients who seek an "authoritative guide" in solving their problems. A discussion of immediate survival-related as well as the typical planning of long-term personality-related goals will facilitate engagement. As the therapist moves from an active to a more nondirective, reflective role, the transition is presented to the client as a planned, intentional change. In this way the therapist has not relinquished the roles of authority and expert. An open discussion of the client's disillusionment that could occur regarding the helpfulness of therapy and of the client's possible feelings of shame over seeking help outside the family adds credibility to the psychotherapist and helps the client sustain the relationship, increasing the likelihood that he or she will return for subsequent sessions. Because the expression of negative feelings toward significant others is often considered unacceptable, indirect methods (nonverbal symbolic gestures, fantasies, dreams, letters) are utilized to process affects without discussing them openly in the beginning of therapy.

Implicit in the application of socialization interviews and other pre-therapy methods is the assumption that traditional modes of psycho-therapy require little modification to be optimally effective with ethnic minority clients. The validity of this notion varies depending on such factors as the acculturation level, presenting problem, previous therapy experience, language capability, and mental ability of the client. In many cases with ethnic minorities subtle modifications prove insufficient and drastic changes are required, which leads us to the third and final approach to achieving a client-system match.

To change services to accommodate persons from diverse cultures is the most innovative and responsive but also the most complicated and difficult alternative. It implies system flexibility, multiethnic and multilingual mental health personnel, an organizational structure dictated by community needs rather than by bureaucratic precedent or roles, extensive knowledge, and, more important, experiences relevant to ethnic groups, and the integration of new forms of intervention. The first step in modifying services to maximize fit requires a way of accounting for the social and political realities of the minority experience in the clinical conceptualization of a case.

McFadden (1976) has offered a conceptual method for examining the Black experience in clinical assessment. In his framework each therapeutic issue has three primary dimensions, the cultural-historical, the psycho-social, and the scientific-ideological. The first dimension refers to cultural heritage and knowledge passed from one generation to another and to personal experiences linked to the individual's status as a member of a minority culture. The second dimension refers to intrapsychic issues. The third dimension refers to actual observed behaviors or attitudes regarding one's relationship with the external environment. McFadden conceptualizes Black experiences as gradually progressing from the cultural-historical dimension into the psychosocial dimension into the scientific-ideological dimension. For example, the dynamics of slavery (cultural-historical) may influence a Black client's psychological security (psychosocial), which influences logic-behavioral chains (scientific-ideo-logical). These chains correspond to the person's perception of a behavior and its logical or adaptive value in a situation.

Regardless of the validity of certain aspects of the model (such as the unidirectional flow of the psychological dynamics), it represents an effort to develop a heuristic device that allows clinicians to integrate the influence of culture into their case conceptualizations. Despite the awareness of ethnic-specific issues, normative behaviors, and coping styles, few explicit conceptual strategies (that is, models of assessment) have emerged to guide the incorporation of such knowledge into an integrated understanding of the minority client. Just as the advent of family systems theory resulted in the effective implementation of family therapy approaches, viable system changes to match minority client needs are largely contingent on the development of conceptual models that can be used as cognitive thinking tools to do a sensitive, comprehensive assessment of the minority client and his or her specific cultural milieu. Equally important is the explicit delineation of traditional models of assessment to examine value biases and erroneous assumptions that could lead to misinterpretations of minority client behavior. Some promising developments include critiques of traditional models for the assessment of family systems (Kim, 1982) and irrational belief patterns (Zane, 1981) with respect to Asian Americans.

The most frequently adopted model for organizational changes to increase match is the professional adaptation model as described by Padilla et al. (1975). Basically, the model incorporates only slight variations from the traditional community mental health model, with the major change involving professionals and paraprofessionals who "adapt" their clinical skills, service orientation, and language skills to the specific requirements for serving the ethnic minority population. Usually these adaptations translate into placement of the center within the community and the hiring of bilingual/bicultural personnel, the majority of whom are paraprofessionals who originate from the target population. There tends to be a greater emphasis placed on prevention efforts, on short-term, crisis-oriented, problem-focused treatment, and on more community input into program policy. However, the basic service structure, program priorities, and staff-client roles essentially resemble those of the traditional community mental health center. Unchanged features may include adherance to the 50-minute session, placement of clients on a waiting list, reliance on office-based outpatient therapy as the primary treatment mode, and focus on diagnosed problems with little attention to the direct problems of food, housing, employment, and so on. As an alternative service system the professional adaptation model represents a conservative and, typically, a center's first rudimentary step toward the development of responsive services.

More innovative service delivery models involve major changes in service system structure and program priorities. Programs based on these models frequently capitalize on a major cultural feature or a culturally acceptable attitude or practice to engage and treat clients. The barrio service center model organizes its services around a critical feature of many Hispanic communities, the concurrent need for mental health and basic economic services (Padilla et al., 1975). The model emphasizes the "social broker" role, in which staff help clients obtain jobs, bank loans, and other economic services in addition to providing counseling in the community. Abad, Ramos, and Boyce (1974) describe a clinic primarily serving Puerto Rican residents. Besides providing typical outpatient services (such as walk-in coverage, psychiatric evaluations, individual, group, and family therapy, and referral services) the clinic offers home visit and transportation services. A major role of the bicultural/bilingual staff centers on that of "intermediary between Spanish speaking clients and other agencies" (Abad et al., 1974, p. 592). Treatment may focus on numerous problem situations that are not "clinical" in nature.

The Chinatown Child Development Center (CCDC) has reorganized services around an educational model to make the delivery of mental health services more acceptable to immigrant Chinese families (Chan-sew, 1980). Traditionally, the Chinese culture places a high value on education and considers it to have great utility for survival and upward mobility. CCDC programs capitalize on these attitudes by offering mental health services in the context of educational experiences. The continuum from preventive to clinical mental health services is presented as a progression from general to more intensive education. The chronic shortage of appropriate child-care facilities in Chinatown provides the motivation for parents to enroll their children in either the Drop-In or After School program, both of which charge no fees. Participation in these educational programs enables the clinic to screen each child for existing or potential mental health problems and to provide feedback about the child's progress to parents. The on-site mental health education program enhances continuity of service by offering parents classes and activities that address not only mental health concerns but also basic economic, language, and legal problems faced by immigrant families. The group experiences embedded within this program frequently facilitate the development of supportive networks among parents. Because of the educational child-care programs, the frequency of interaction between staff and parents is much higher than at most clinics, resulting in the enhancement of cooperative, trusting relationships. Such relationships reduce the resistance to subsequent referrals for diagnostic evaluations and outpatient treatment.

Thus far, the models discussed with respect to the match or fit principle have focused on the individual client or family as the basic unit of service. The design of service systems to accommodate community needs at the other two levels of intervention, the organizational and social system levels, implicates the fourth principle (comprehensive services), which basically is an elaboration of Sue's third alternative to achieve match at all four levels of intervention.

Integration and Linkage of Services

The intimate relationship between mental health and other health or social service problems is an ecological reality for most ethnic minority groups and directly influences their conceptualization of mental health difficulties (Harwood, 1981). Mental health is considered to be an element in the total welfare of the individual. Frequently, psychological problems gain expression in terms of other health or social difficulties such as physical or work/study complaints. For example, Kleinman (1980) and Tung (1980) have noted that somatization is the common mechanism for coping with psychological difficulties such as depression in the Chinese and Southeast Asian cultures, respectively. Consequently, effective service linkage can enhance treatment effectiveness by concurrently affecting interrelated problems in living. It also embodies an approach that reflects the manner in which ethnic minority individuals conceptualize mental health problems.

Lawrence (1975) identified three types of interorganizational linkage patterns: consultative, confederated, and federated. The consultation model is commonly found where there exists a shortage of mental health specialists (Schulberg, 1977). Due to the professional human resource problems within ethnic communities, most ethnic service systems have this type of linkage pattern. Consultation agreements tend to be inconsistently implemented and are constrained by fiscal limitations (that is, third-party insurers do not include consultation as a reimbursable service). In essence, the burden of establishing service linkages falls on individual staff members, with little emphasis on a systems approach to network development. The resultant pattern of system coordination is one of nonuniform agency relationships, with some being of a close collaborative nature while others involve only infrequent individual case referrals.

In response to the National Institute of Mental Health's requirement that mental health centers establish affiliation agreements with local resources to ensure continuity of care, confederated linkages have emerged. Within such system arrangements there are formal, specified patterns of personnel, client, or information exchange, but the participating agencies retain their functional autonomy. Although the establishment of confederated linkages requires extensive interagency negotiations, such costs in time and effort are often offset by savings in startup costs and operating demands needed to establish separate clinics in several geographical locations. The Worcester Youth Guidance Center's Hispanic Program has succeeded in circumventing many problems in service delivery through collaborative agreements with two health and social service centers serving high concentrations of Hispanics in Worcester, Massachusetts (Delgado & Scott, 1979). Placement of mental health personnel in these host agencies helped destigmatize the use of mental health services and enabled the provision of many services in the home. In another formalized collaborative arrangement with the local court and a youth service agency, the Hispanic program helped develop a foster parent program for children referred from juvenile court (Delgado, 1978). In addition, the program provided support and consultative services to the foster parents once children were placed in their homes. In this manner intervention efforts were applied prior to the full development of problems in these potentially high-risk situations.

In terms of comprehensiveness of service connections, the federated linkage model provides the structure for maximizing agency collaboration. Under this model, agencies are components of a larger system whose central authority can prescribe operating policies and practices for all member programs. Using this approach, the South Cove Community Health Center has provided mental health services as part of a low-cost, comprehensive general health care program for Boston's Chinatown and South Cove area residents. According to Lee (1979), the programmatic and geographic integration of mental health services with other health services yields the following advantages: (1) easier and quicker referrals with less patient "loss" between referring agencies and caregivers; (2) better coordinated care of patients with multiple problems as facilitated by the ready access to allied caregivers, a common record system, and a common administrative hierarchy; (3) reduction in health care delivery problems through the improvement of patient-provider relationships by means of mental health staff input into the management of behaviorally difficult patients and of health staff use of their ongoing relationships with patients to facilitate the acceptance of mental health services; and (4) increased appreciation of emotional problems by general health staff as a result of frequent informal contacts between health and mental health personnel located in the same setting. In addition, the health center maintains confederated linkages with the three agencies (the public elementary school, a day care center, and an elderly residential project) that share the same complex.

Although the federated model appears to be most effective and efficient in the development of coordinated service linkages, certain structural and dynamic conditions of an ethnic community may limit its application. First, the wide geographic dispersal of ethnic communities mitigates against the development of multiservice centers. In contrast, the South Cove Community Health Center basically serves Boston Chinatown, which is the fourth largest Chinese community in the United States. Second, the degree to which there exists consensus among members as to the community's aspirations may affect efforts to establish a federated system. The implementation of a major project such as a comprehensive multiservice center requires a sustained, concerted, collective effort on the part of the community. The South Cove Community Health Center was an outgrowth of seven years of community planning and development. The pursuit of common goals by the community reflects its high degree of integration (Mann, 1978). Parsons (1951) has identified two fundamental dimensions of integration: the coordination among the community's working parts or processes and the distinctiveness or integrity of the social system in relation to other systems in its environment. Thus ethnic communities that have poor internal coordination and problems of a boundary-maintenance nature may find it difficult to summon the resources and commitment necessary for the federated approach. In these cases confederated linkages may actually serve the community more effectively.

Efficient Utilization of Services

In an overview of the projected federal program and policy changes under the proposed block grant program, the director of the National Institute of Mental Health indicated, "It behooves us to identify cost-effective programs because the current legislative climate is to reduce Federal spending on many social and health programs" (ADAMHA News, 1981). The combination of funding cutbacks and the resultant cost-effective focus places an even greater demand than before on ethnic community agencies to deliver services in the most efficient manner. The emphasis on maximizing impact with minimal cost involves two processes that are frequently in opposition. Powerful, effective interventions often incur high costs as a result of the extensive organizational development and human resource effort needed to implement such projects.

To circumvent these problems certain agencies have adopted primary prevention strategies that encourage the use of natural helping resources within the ethnic community. Conceptually, primary prevention efforts based on natural support systems appear cost-effective for the following reasons. First, they enhance the coping potential of individuals and groups, which decreases their susceptibility to the development of mental health problems. Second, the resultant reduction in incidence and prevalence as well as in the severity of mental disorders decreases the need for the more costly clinical interventions. Third, the utilization of natural support systems makes use of that which the community already possesses, reducing the need for further resource development. Finally, the incorporation of systems that people would naturally use when seeking help facilitates case-finding and outreach efforts, thereby conserving some time and energy normally applied to increasing accessibility and availability of services. Despite the conceptual appeal of this approach, its cost-effectiveness requires empirical validation. This is not a simple matter. Heller, Price, and Sher (1980, p. 286) have noted that the evaluation of primary prevention interventions is "a complex undertaking with conceptual ambiguities and methodological difficulties which impede the systematic collection of evidence." Moreover, cost-effectiveness requires not only that interventions be effective but that they only be applied when less costly and simpler interventions have proven ineffective. Thus cost-effectiveness implies two principles, intervention efficacy and effort conservation.

Muñoz (1980) has adopted a prevention model proposed by Christensen, Miller, and Muñoz (1978) to promote the utilization of natural Hispanic support systems. He addresses the two principles of cost-effectiveness by incorporating into the model an evaluation methodology that regulates the extensiveness of the prevention services. Muñoz indicates that educational programs focused on preventive mental health issues hold particular relevance for many Latinos whose families have reinforced the values of learning more, becoming more educated, and increasing control over their own lives. This emphasis on learning to be more self-efficacious facilitates the acceptance of mental health services delivered in the form of education rather than of therapy. While the strategy increases effective outreach efforts to people who want information and advice, it does not forestall treatment to Latinos whose problems require more extensive clinical intervention.

The approach specifies three levels of intervention: prevention, treatment, and maintenance. Within each level, six types of mental health agents perform various functions in the delivery of mental health services. Besides professionals, the strategy uses five adjuncts: (1) paraprofessionals, (2) partners (nontrained voluntary helpers), (3) peer clients, (4) communicative paraphernalia (such as mass media, tapes), and (5) printed material.

These agents are listed in decreasing order of training sophistication and implementation cost. Through adjuncts the model utilizes natural support systems at every level to make optimum use of available personnel found in Latino communities. Because adjunctive agents are less expensive but more available to the community, their use prior to professional intervention for certain problems and certain people embodies a cost-effective approach to service delivery. In other words, service delivery proceeds in a systematic hierarchical fashion guided by evaluation outcomes. If evaluation finds a certain adjunct to be more effective or as effective as professionals or other more expensive adjuncts, there exists no need to invoke the more extensive and sophisticated procedures. Finally, the clear delineation of each agent's functions and procedures at the three intervention levels establishes an empirical base for the determination of provider status. For example, whether or not a person can qualify as a paraprofessional or a partner-companion will depend on the outcomes that the person obtains at the preventive, treatment, and maintenance levels. This competency-based approach to personnel development also enhances cost-effectiveness.

In summary, this model incorporates the following features that would facilitate the efficient utilization of resources in many ethnic minority communities: (1) a teaching orientation in the presentation of preventive mental health issues and interventions; (2) the basic evaluation-controlled strategy of delivering less costly and more available interventions, followed, if needed, by increasingly more costly and more extensive clinical efforts; (3) the employment of adjuncts in prevention, treatment, and maintenance to make optimal use of natural support systems; and (4) an outcome-oriented approach to determine personnel qualification.

One adjunctive agent in the Muñoz model involves the use of peer clients. Peer clients represent a rich but as yet undeveloped community resource for service delivery. Besides increasing mental health human resource potential, the peer client role may have a therapeutic effect on the peer client's own psychological functioning. According to Goldberg (1972), the client must experience three roles in the ameliorative process. Clients commonly see themselves in the role of a patient, one who is sick, disabled, and unable to help others. Alternatively, they assume the role of student, a person who perceives him- or herself as having few or no psychological problems. Rather, the person seeks therapy to learn about the therapeutic process and to promote his or her own psychosocial development. The third and least recognized role is that of a healer. As a healer the client makes an attempt to cope with his or her own problems and tries to help and assist others. The recognition and appreciation of such helping efforts enhances the client's sense of self-worth and interpersonal relatedness.

The experience of discovering that one can be effective in helping others and that such efforts are appreciated may be the most basic therapeutic feature in treatment. According to Bandura (1977), self-efficacy expectations—the belief that one can successfully execute the behavior required to produce certain desired outcomes—affect both the initiation and persistence of coping behavior. In addition, he contends that personal mastery experiences are especially powerful in the enhancement of perceived self-efficacy. By performing the role of healer, clients can engage in many activities that result in these crucial personal mastery experiences. Unfortunately, most mental health agencies have failed to incorporate the client healer role into their treatment programs.

The Laurel Center in Maryland has designed a program to provide clients with the opportunity to demonstrate their particular skills and abilities in the process of helping others (Goldberg & Kane, 1974). The services in-kind program allows clients to compensate the center for services rendered them by delivering services in-kind to others. For example, one client paid for marital and individual counseling services by serving as a cotherapist in a play therapy group. Other clients who received marital counseling tutored students having problems in school. Some clients who were housewives provided child-care and transportation services for other mothers. The most in-kind services delivered were of a secretarial nature. These contributions have furnished many auxiliary services to the agency, which, like many other community-based organizations, operates with a limited budget for support personnel. Notwithstanding its economic value, the primary function of giving services in-kind is seen as therapeutic. During sessions, therapist and client discuss the specific compensatory service and incorporate it into the client's treatment plan. Despite certain problems in implementation (state and county health systems resistance, staff resistance, systematizing the assignment of services, and supervision of services), the services in-kind program appears to be a feasible approach for service delivery expansion and resource conservation worthy of inclusion in many ethnic minority mental health programs.

Comprehensive Services

There has been an increasing awareness of two primary social conditions that are associated with mental health difficulties. First, it has become apparent that many psychological disorders have their etiological and developmental bases in deep-rooted and interrelated social problems (such as racism, poverty, and overcrowding). Second, the sources of these problems emanate from the respective social structures of groups, organizations, communities, or larger social systems. Recognition of the larger social environment as an important part of the treatment context has stimulated service programs to expand the scope of intervention to include not only the individual but the family or group, the organization, and the social system as appropriate foci for change. The degree to which services are delivered in a comprehensive fashion determines to a great extent the efficacy of such interventions. This is especially true for many ethnic minority communities burdened by the social consequences of economic and political inequities.

The emphasis on affecting the broader ecological context reflects a relatively new ideology that is just beginning to gain extensive consideration in terms of program design and theory development (see Snow & Newton, 1976). Consequently, few working models exist to guide the formulation and operation of a systematic approach to comprehensive service delivery. For most agencies, including those serving ethnic minority populations, the individual client, the client group, and the family remain as the basic units of service. Occasional attempts to intervene at the organizational and social system levels usually occur at the personal initiative of one or several staff members. The absence of a programmatic approach to change organizational and social system conditions such that they enhance mental health constitutes one of the major gaps in the delivery of services to ethnic minority communities. As La Follette and Pilisuk (1981, p. 221) have noted, "The community movement in mental health presents the mental health advocate with a major decision. Will we retreat behind more manageable forms of treatment for mental illness and the now legitimate ancillary community services, or will we push the frontiers of service into areas which our community approaches have exposed as vital to the emotional well-being of our clients?"

Already some pioneering efforts have emerged. Most of these models rely on a core individual or team of individuals to deliver services at each level of intervention. This generalist approach to comprehensive service delivery probably reflects the natural evolutionary expansion of service responsibilities for agency staff. Whether this approach is more or less cost-effective than a specialist orientation in which certain staff only work at certain levels remains a matter for empirical inquiry.

Using an approach that emphasizes social systems reform and ethnic accountability, the University of Miami-Jackson Memorial Medical Center Community Mental Health Program (CMHP) has provided proactive and reactive mental health services to a low-income, multiethnic catchment area within inner-city Miami (Lefley & Bestman, 1982). The area contains five ethnic groups, Bahamian, Black American, Cuban, Haitian, and Puerto Rican, as well as an elderly Anglo American population. At the core of the CMHP are seven teams, one team for each ethnic population and two geriatric teams to serve elderly Anglo Americans and elderly Blacks. Each ethnic team employs professional and paraprofessional personnel whose cultural background matches that of the ethnic community served. The director of each team is a culture broker. As previously indicated, the culture broker is a social scientist with expertise in the culture being served and, in most cases, of the same ethnicity. The combination of professional qualifications with culturally relevant personal experiences allows the culture broker to exert influence in both the community and the mental health network as well as on the relationship between these two systems.

In practice, directors and team members share the culture broker role. Besides providing highly accessible and culturally responsive preventive, treatment, and aftercare services to individuals and families, the teams act as social change agents to alter environmental conditions that may contribute to mental health problems. Some teams may initiate or coordinate projects that bolster existing resources or supply new resources for the community. Others will design and implement action research to obtain empirical support for needed services or programs. They may organize the community and/or advocate on its behalf for changes in agencies found lacking in culturally appropriate services. Teams also have advised residents on how to induce these agencies to rectify certain neighborhood problems. They have developed support systems for both preventive and aftercare purposes. They have established linkages between consumer groups and appropriate agencies.

Prior to these social action efforts, each team conducted an extensive community entry program involving advisory board selection and utilization (in terms of assisting in personnel selection and suggesting needs of the area), key informant and indigenous leadership contact, and comprehensive multimodal needs assessment (empirically derived survey questionnaires, block mapping and observation to assess availability of community resources, reanalysis of census data to determine ethnic clustering and need patterns, and so on). Using this data base, each team established an accessible, multiservice "mini-clinic" with confederated linkages to other community agencies and to the area's two psychiatric hospitals.

Several examples of social action projects demonstrate the CMHP's effectiveness in producing change at various levels of the community social structure. The Cuban team, in collaboration with other ethnic interest groups, successfully procured $450,000 of Community Development Project funds for the area. It also has developed a crime prevention program for predelinquents in public housing projects. The Puerto Rican team initiated a project to start a community school. The project represented the first collective action effort taken by all the Latino groups in the largely Puerto Rican area. The Bahamian team, in conjunction with another community agency, organized an innovative summer employment program for low-income Black teenagers. Rather than employ teenagers in typical summer jobs such as janitorial and recreational assistants, the program consisted of training in office procedures, viewing films on mental health and social services, recreation, and field experience involving participation in a community needs assessment survey. Upon discovering that 70 percent of its clients were illegal aliens with multiple needs but with questionable eligibility for public benefits, the Haitian team helped conduct two advocacy projects for the Haitain community. One resulted in the changing of school admission requirements to enroll Haitain children of illegal alien parents. The other helped Haitian illegal aliens obtain social security cards in order to qualify for the concomitant welfare benefits.

Several features of the Miami model merit mention as potentially key factors in any attempt to achieve service comprehensiveness by addressing social system concerns as well as individual ones. First, the team approach to social system intervention can foster the necessary emotional and intellectual support to sustain concerted advocacy and organizing efforts in the face of social system inertia or resistance. Often the complicated and arduous task of initiating social system reform appears less intimidating and more feasible when seen from a collective perspective as opposed to an individualistic one.

Second, a detailed needs assessment of the community can enhance the efficiency of system change projects. Frequently, advocacy projects fail because they are too broadly focused or inappropriately targeted. Besides helping to minimize these problems, a community needs assessment may exert a beneficial iatrogenic effect on staff. A training issue often overlooked is whether or not indigenous mental health personnel actually have embraced the human service ideology (Zane, 1982). The reorientation of professionals trained under the traditional, individual-focused clinical model is a related matter that has received more attention in the field. However, the assumption that, once trained, indigenous personnel can totally suspend traditional culturally ingrained beliefs about mental illness (for example, the stigma of being mentally ill, illness caused by an

individual's transgressions) in favor of mental health concepts has proven
to be a naive one. Both of these factors can operate to increase staff
resistance to the adoption of innovative interventions, particularly those of
a social action nature. A comprehensive needs assessment scrutinizes the
role of environmental factors in the development and maintenance of
psychological difficulties. Social stressors, social systems, and social
resources become more of the foreground in the conceptualization of
mental health problems. Consequently, in the process of obtaining information for a needs assessment both indigenous and nonindigenous staff
may develop a perspective that is more in accordance with the human
service approach.

Third, the indirect positive effects of collective action often have
received little attention. Social action projects increase the availability of
direct services (Lefley & Bestman, 1982). In addition, community
development helps assure the longevity of a mental health program.
Community organization efforts demonstrate the program's utility to the
community as an important resource. More significantly, the organization
of the community into a potent advocate force can generate the necessary
local support for continued public funding of the agency. Considering the
current scarcity of public funds for mental health, effective lobbying on
the part of local constituents is a political necessity. The potential economic benefits indirectly accruing from social action interventions cannot
be underemphasized. Many agency administrators still see their primary
responsibilities as involving the management of direct and ancillary services. Redefinition of the administrator role to incorporate collective
advocacy concerns will not only increase service comprehensiveness, but
will expand the supportive base needed for the economic survival of the
program.

Finally, it must be recognized that lowering environmental stress
actually does improve psychological functioning. Frequently this premise
is not taken seriously and receives less consideration than the traditional
psychodynamic assumption that improved intrapsychic functioning is
required before a client can significantly change environmental conditions.
This intrapsychic focus persists in the face of literature indicating that
mental health problems are lower in well-organized communities (Leighton, Harding, Macklin, Macmillan, & Leighton, 1963). Lefley (1979) has
provided evidence supporting the social problem orientation to psychological adjustment. She found a significant relationship between the level of
success in attaining environmental goals (finding jobs, locating appropriate
social and medical services, obtaining financial benefits) and therapeutic

outcome as defined by symptom reduction, level of functioning at home or work, quality of interpersonal relationships, and the client's success in utilizing therapeutic resources. Until the social problem approach to psychological amelioration gains the widespread acceptance that it merits, the development of comprehensive services will remain a socially desirable but inconsistently attained objective for many mental health programs serving ethnic minority populations.

Community Control

A widely accepted notion in community mental health is the value of community participation in the planning of service delivery programs. This proposition holds particular relevance for ethnic minority communities, because often there has existed a clear disparity in values and goals between program administration and citizens. A community advisory group can help align agency goals and operations with community needs by establishing program policy, advocating for client interests and safety, evaluating services, and consulting on community dynamics and problems (Morrison, 1976; Silverman & Mossman, 1978).

In practice, the response to community control has been less enthusiastic. Chu and Trotter (1974, p. 83) indicate: "By and large community advisory boards have been added after the fact, few of them with any real fiscal control, policy making power, or program responsibility." Their study examined only publicly supported community mental health centers developed in response to federal and state legislation. In contrast, alternative mental health agencies that originated more from organized community efforts than from governmental directives have had more local involvement in the decision and policymaking process of programs (La Follette & Pilisuk, 1981). Many of the agencies serving ethnic minority populations began as alternative mental health clinics.

Besides the obvious strategy of placing more indigenous ethnic group members on agency boards, greater community control has been achieved by including former or current clients as board members and by selecting indigenous personnel for administrative positions. With respect to the former, one alternative clinic, El Centro de Salud Mental, considers all clients eligible for board nomination after their third visit. The inclusion of clients in board membership reflects a consumer orientation to which many community-based agencies purportedly subscribe. Thus it is surprising that only a few of these programs have adopted a concerted effort to enlist client participation in board activities. Such efforts require not only recruitment, but the preparation of the client for this decision-making role. Preparation may involve orientation to the larger mental health or health system to which the agency belongs, education in patient's rights and ethical principles, clarification of advisory board responsibilities, and training in problem-solving skills.

The employment of indigenous personnel to conduct a service program undoubtedly represents one of the most direct extensions of community control. Considering that conflicts over agency direction initially arose as a result of administrative resistance to meaningful participation by disadvantaged groups (Mann, 1978), the administration of a program by community individuals obviates many of these control issues. The problem has been to find indigenous personnel who have the requisite managerial skills and bureaucratic expertise to perform effectively as administrators. Recently, a program was developed to train ethnic minority mental health professionals for managerial positions (Wong, 1981). It is the first project of its kind designed to ameliorate the current shortage of qualified ethnic minority administrators in the mental health field.

Thus far this discussion has focused on ways to increase community involvement, with the assumption being that community participation will improve services. However, is this premise always valid? At times, it appears that community involvement hampers the design and implementation of innovative intervention approaches. Mann (1978) has observed that communities frequently oppose intervention programs with the same fervor that characterizes their opposition to research studies. While there is a tendency to consider this resistance as due to self-serving actions on the part of certain vested interests in the community, it should be made clear that this type of reaction is more the result of the inherent cyclical nature of the social change process operant in any community system.

Using Hegelian dialectics, Boulding (1970) has examined the social change phenomena. In his analysis a social innovation, or "thesis" (as it is referred to in dialectic terms), contains within itself a contradiction. This contradiction tends to produce an opposing reaction or antithesis as the thesis develops and peaks. Following this ascent of the thesis, the antithesis develops and gains dominance. Because the antithesis also contains a contradiction, it declines and is followed by a synthesis. Although the synthesis is essentially the restoration of the original thesis, it includes elements that integrate both thesis and antithesis. Probably due to this integrative process, the cycle does not return to its original baseline in social functioning. Rather, there is a gradual increase in the baseline of social functioning that reflects a cumulative process of development as a result of learning. In other words, social change involves two processes. The cyclical dialectic process is commonly referred to as "revolutionary" changes, while the cumulative process can be considered to consist of "evolutionary" changes. The total social change process can be seen graphically as a series of alternating peaks and valleys representing the more transitory revolutionary changes, with the cumulative effect of evolutionary changes gradually raising the baseline of the curve such that the resultant graph is tilted upward.

The history of the civil rights movement reflects the revolutionary and evolutionary aspects of social change. An atmosphere of political and social reform to establish equity between advantaged and disadvantaged groups in terms of political, social, and economic opportunities in the 1960s gave way to the reactionary conservatism of the 1970s. Despite the deemphasis on civil rights in that period, there was an increased sensitivity to ethnic minority concerns. Due to this and other related evolutionary changes, the political and social climate of the 1970s was only somewhat similar to that of its cyclical sister, the socially conservative 1950s.

The descriptive model of social change suggests that significant, consistent social progress develops more from evolutionary processes than from revolutionary changes. If this assumption is valid, it has important implications for the relationship between community control and social interventions. Responsive service delivery to ethnic communities is not simply a matter of designing culturally appropriate program content. Any intervention, regardless of the culturally relevant features that it possesses, may be opposed by the community if it is considered revolutionary in nature. The problem with innovative interventions is that they often are implemented in a revolutionary manner, which generates a reaction. The crucial question then becomes: How can innovative programs be introduced and operationalized such that they do not trigger a dialectical process? Boulding (1970, p. 61) underscores the utility of information in facilitating evolutionary processes: "It is ignorance, rather than knowledge which makes for dialectical processes. Once knowledge is achieved (disseminated and absorbed) the dialectical pattern disappears."

Viewed from this perspective, community involvement can be either an effective catalyst or a retarding influence on the development and implementation of innovative mental health approaches. The pivotal factor is the degree to which participants are knowledgeable about mental health in general and about the intervention program in particular. The value of having informed community input is not a new assertion. Its importance has been argued on the basis of common sense and the right of individuals and communities to determine their own destiny (the self-determination principle). Boulding's analysis reveals that, apart from social responsibility concerns, there are valid technical reasons for developing informed cooperative relationships with community members.

In order to contribute to evolutionary processes, programs must attend more to the actual process of keeping the community knowledgeable about its current operations and future plans. In practice, this translates to the design of specific procedures to disseminate information about the program to community members, particularly to those serving in advisory board capacities. Frequently, it has been assumed that the personal motivation of certain community individuals to stay apprised of a program's current activities through their regular attendance at board meetings was sufficient to maintain consistent information exchange between program and community. Chu and Trotter (1974) have questioned the adequacy of this practice. Additional procedures for knowledge dissemination are necessary.

Most ethnic community advisory boards still confine their primary functions to defining program policy and to making various fiscal decisions (such as budget approval). However, community control implies service accountability. It appears that the monitoring of the design and the results of program evaluation projects should become one of the primary responsibilities for community boards.

The inclusion of evaluation findings as a major focus of business in advisory board meetings would greatly increase the availability and accessibility of relevant and current information about program interventions. Such "on-call" evaluation indices as the number of clients seen, types of problems treated, mean length of waiting period (in days), mean Global Assessment Scale score, mean number of clients on waiting list per day, mean client satisfaction rating, mean number of program complaints, mean number of delinquent client accounts, number of sick and vacation days taken by staff, number of referrals made and received, and so on could be required information for presentation at each board meeting. The assumption of evaluation responsibilities by community boards can only serve to enhance community control over service programs. More important, the resultant gain in knowledge acquisition among both community members and program personnel should foster the cooperation and sense of community that Boulding (1970) associates more with evolutionary processes.

Knowledge Development and Utilization

At this point it has become exceedingly clear that there exist viable system models for the responsive delivery of mental health services to ethnic minority populations. Most of these programs have been described in professional journals or books. They have been recognized by both mental health personnel and community consumers as effective delivery systems. Yet, despite consensus concerning the value of such programs, they have had little impact on the mental health field. At this time it appears that the widespread adoption of innovative service delivery models has lagged far behind their original development. This situation constituted a major reason for the recommendation by the President's Commission on Mental Health (1978) to develop a new mental health system designed to serve ethnic minority populations and other disadvantaged groups appropriately.

The serious gap between knowledge development and its subsequent utilization involves two issues in the marketing of innovative programs. According to Shore (1974), problems in dissemination and problems related to the nature of the program itself can reduce its marketability. The optimal dissemination of research information has been prevented by the lack of data retrieval systems that can both keep pace with the rapid increase in mental health knowledge and provide relevant, current information for an agency's daily and long-range needs. The publication lag has exacerbated this difficulty in knowledge distribution. By the time information is printed, much of it is obsolete or is received too late to have any impact on important program decisions. The National Institute of Mental Health found that only 9 percent of the new developments in mental health services were stimulated by printed research findings. The HEW Task Force (1978) has proposed that the Alcohol, Drug Abuse, and Mental Health Administration (ADAMHA) establish an explicit policy and program initiatives to encourage research information dissemination. As yet, there are no plans in the near future for the development of a central data retrieval system for mental health practioners and administrators.

Even with adequate publicity, a program may not be adopted because of certain specific features it may possess. Many innovative approaches are not simple interventions. A complex design can be especially detrimental to marketability if the program is not well articulated in terms of a clear conceptual model. Well-conceptualized models allow for flexibility in the adoption of innovative programs. A model identifies operational principles that guide the replication of the program's essential features without preventing the consumer agency from changing certain aspects to accommodate the specific nuances of the ethnic community it serves.

Many innovative ethnic programs require a service delivery role that cuts across professional boundaries. In these systems, the service provider will alternate in the roles of counselor, agency advocate, educator, fiscal agent, employment advisor, and so on. Although this generalist orientation effectively responds to the multiple needs of minority clients, it clashes with the current service structure based on specialized mental health disciplines. Finally, a program may contest some basic values of the community in which the agency is embedded or of the larger society. This is particularly true of many social problem approaches that challenge traditional sources of authority in an effort to reduce the specific adverse social conditions that plague minority communities.

Given that the resistance to innovative programs may stem from the inflexible nature of service system structures, the adoption of these programs depends on the ability of minority interests to institute major organizational changes. Typically, major changes in service structures can only be achieved by effective political action. Again, the importance of collective action and community organization efforts becomes evident, this time in terms of facilitating the implementation of ethnically responsive service delivery systems. Scientific and social merit are insufficient in the promotion of appropriate intervention approaches. Such information must be integrated successfully into the political process to achieve maximum impact on program design.

Conclusions

A variety of service systems that operate from well-conceptualized, culturally relevant models have been designed and implemented successfully. The lack of coherent service delivery models can no longer be cited as a major reason for the mental health field's slow progress in effectively responding to the multiple needs of ethnic minority communities.

Despite these advances in theoretical and technical knowledge, certain gaps in service delivery still tend to exist. Inflexible catchment area boundaries and poor public awareness of services have limited attempts to make a wide range of services (particularly costly and/or highly specialized services) available and accessible to ethnic minority clientele. Few explicit assessment strategies have emerged to guide the incorporation of cultural knowledge into an integrated understanding of the minority client. Often the cost effectiveness value of an intervention is unclear due to the lack of an evaluation-controlled approach to service delivery. Most agencies have not adopted the potent therapeutic role of the client as healer into their treatment programs. There are no efficient data retrieval systems to keep mental health personnel apprised of recent innovative developments in service delivery. The lack of systematic attempts to keep the community informed of a program's progress has enhanced the development of dialectical processes that can often result in community rejection of an innovative proposal. A possible solution to this problem involves the reorganization of advisory board functions such that they emphasize program evaluation responsibilities.

However, it is the absence of programmatic approaches to organize the community to change organizational or social system conditions that constitutes the major gap in service delivery to ethnic minority communities. Effective collective action programs are vital because they can have important multiple influences on both the agency and the community. Besides working to ameliorate social problems, community organization efforts can advocate for the continued fiscal support of an agency and campaign for major structural changes in a system to facilitate the adoption of innovative service delivery approaches.

It is time that those in mental health move past elegant discussions of conceptual models and concentrate on the task of encouraging the widespread adoption of these models by agencies serving ethnic minority populations. A beginning step would involve the state agencies administering block grant funds. Such agencies could require applicant organizations to address the six principles discussed in terms of a service delivery model tailored to the specific needs of the ethnic community being served. The use of clear conceptual models to describe a program enables the sponsoring agency to determine how the program explicity relates cultural and community features to service delivery. This approach also facilitates the parsimonious evaluation of interventions in terms of their culturally relevant content and their therapeutic effectiveness.

References

Abad, V., Ramos, J., & Boyce, E. A model for delivery of mental health services to Spanish-speaking minorities. *American Journal of Orthopsychiatry*, 1974, 44, 584-595.

ADAMHA News. State directors look at federal mental health role. August 7, 1981, p. 2.

Aoki, B. *Role preparation of Asian American clients for psychotherapy*. Paper presented at the American Psychological Association Convention, Los Angeles, August 1981.

Atteneave, C. Medicine men and psychiatrists in the Indian Health Service. *Psychiatric Annals*, 1974, 4, 49-55.

Baker, F. From community mental health to human service ideology. *American Journal of Public Health*, 1974, 64, 576-581.

Bandura, A. Self-efficacy: Toward a unifying theory of behavioral change. *Psychological Review,* 1977, 84, 191-215.

Boulding, K. *A primer on social dynamics.* New York: Macmillan, 1970.

Brown, T., Stein, K., Huang, K., & Harris, D. Mental illness and the role of mental health facilities in Chinatown. In S. Sue & N. Wagner (Eds.), *Asian Americans: Psychological perspectives.* Palo Alto, CA: Science and Behavior Books, 1973.

Chan-sew, S. *Chinatown Child Development Center: A service delivery model.* Paper presented at the Conference on a Mental Health Delivery Model for Chinese American Children and Families, San Francisco, October 1980.

Christensen, A., Miller, W., & Muñoz, R. Paraprofessionals, partners, peers, paraphernalia, and print: Expanding mental health service delivery. *Professional Psychology,* 1978, 9, 249-270.

Chu, F., & Trotter, S. *The madness establishment: Ralph Nader's study group report on the National Institute of Mental Health.* New York: Grossman, 1974.

Cuellar, I. Application and service concerns in Hispanic psychology. *Hispanic Journal of Behavioral Sciences,* 1980, 2, 10-12.

Delgado, M. Hispanic foster parents program. *Child Welfare,* 1978, 57, 427-431.

Delgado, M., & Scott, J. Strategic intervention: A mental health program for the Hispanic community. *Journal of Community Psychology,* 1979, 7, 187-197.

Goldberg, C. Group counselor or group therapist: Be prepared. *Psychotherapy and Social Science Review,* 1972, 26, 24-27.

Goldberg, C., & Kane, J. A missing component in mental health services to urban poor: Services in-kind to others. In A. Goldstein & L. Krasner (Eds.), *Mental health issues and the urban poor.* Elmsford, NY: Pergamon, 1974.

Harwood, A. *Ethnicity and medical care.* Cambridge, MA: Harvard University Press, 1981.

Health, Education and Welfare Task Force. *Report of the HEW Task Force on implementation of the report to the president from the President's Commission on Mental Health.* Washington, DC: Government Printing Office, 1978.

Heller, K., Price, R., & Sher, K. Research and evaluation in primary prevention. In R. Price, R. Ketterer, B. Bader, & J. Monahan (Eds.), *Prevention in mental health: Research, policy, and practice.* Beverly Hills, CA: Sage, 1980.

Kahn, M., Williams, C., Galvez, E., Lejero, L., Conrad, R., & Goldstein, G. The Papago psychology service: A community mental health program on an American Indian reservation." *American Journal of Community Psychology,* 1975, 3, 81-97.

Karno, M., & Edgerton, R. Perception of mental illness in a Mexican American community. *Archives of General Psychiatry,* 1969, 20, 233-238.

Kim, S. *A conceptual analysis of the family systems approach as applied to Asian American families.* Paper presented at the Western Psychological Association Convention, Sacramento, April 1982.

King, L. *Serving black communities.* Paper presented at the Workshop on Instituting Changes to Improve Mental Health Services for Minority Communities, Los Angeles, March 1981.

Kleinman, A. *Patients and healers in the context of culture: An exploration of the borderline between anthropology, medicine, and psychiatry.* Los Angeles: University of California Press, 1980.

LaFollette, J., & Pilisuk, M. Changing models of community mental health services. *Journal of Community Psychology*, 1981, 9, 210-223.

Lawrence, M. Developing program models for the human services. In H. Schulberg & F. Baker (Eds.), *Developments in human services* (Vol. 2). New York: Behavioral Publications, 1975.

Lee, E. Mental health services for the Asian Americans: Problems and alternatives. In United States Commission on Civil Rights (Ed.), *Civil rights issues of Asian and Pacific Americans.* Washington, DC: Government Printing Office, 1979.

Lefley, H. Environmental interventions and therapeutic outcome. *Hospital and Community Psychiatry*, 1979, 30, 341-344.

Lefley, H., & Bestman, E. Community mental health and minorities: A multi-ethnic approach. In S. Sue & T. Moore (Eds.), *Community mental health in a pluralistic society.* New York: Human Sciences Press, 1982.

Leighton, D., Harding, J., Macklin, D., Macmillan, A., & Leighton, A. *The character of danger.* New York: Basic Books, 1963.

McFadden, J. Stylistic dimensions of counseling blacks. *Journal of Non-white Concerns*, 1976, 5, 23-28.

Mann, P. *Community psychology: Concepts and applications.* New York: Macmillan, 1978.

Miller, F. Mental health center versus community perceptions of mental health services. *Journal of Community Psychology*, 1981, 9, 204-209.

Mollica, R., Blum, J., & Redlich, F. Equity and the psychiatric care of the black patient, 1950 to 1975. *Journal of Nervous and Mental Disease*, 1980, 168, 279-286.

Morrison, J. An argument for mental patient and advisory boards. *Professional Psychology*, 1976, 7, 127-131.

Muñoz, R. A strategy for the prevention of psychological problems in Latinos: Emphasizing accessibility and effectiveness. In R. Valle & W. Vega (Eds.), *Hispanic nàtural support systems: Mental health promotion perspectives.* Sacramento: State of California Department of Mental Health, 1980.

Murase, K. Delivery of social services to Asian Americans. In National Association of Social Workers (Ed.), *The encyclopedia of social work.* New York: Author, 1977.

Murdock, S., & Schwartz, D. Family structure and the use of agency services: An examination of patterns among elderly Native Americans. *Gerontologist*, 1978, 18, 475-481.

Orne, M., & Wender, P. Anticipatory socialization for psychotherapy: Method and rationale. *American Journal of Psychiatry*, 1968, 124, 1202-1211.

Ostendorf, F., & Hammerslag, C. An Indian-controlled mental health program. *Hospital and Community Psychiatry*, 1977, 28, 682-685.

Padilla, A., Ruiz, R., & Alvarez, A. Community mental health services for the Spanish-speaking/surnamed population. *American Psychologist*, 1975, 30, 892-905.

Parsons, R. *The social system.* New York: Macmillan, 1951.

President's Commission on Mental Health (PCMH). *Report to the president of the President's Commission on Mental Health* (Vol. 1). Washington, DC: Government Printing Office, 1978.

Schulberg, H. Community mental health and human services. *Community Mental Health Review*, 1977, 2, 1-9.

Seligman, M. *Helplessness: On depression, development, and death*. San Francisco: Freeman, 1975.

Shore, M. Making innovative community mental health programs marketable. In A. Goldstein & L. Krasner (Eds.), *Mental health issues and the urban poor*. Elmsford, NY: Pergamon, 1974.

Silverman, W., & Mossman, B. Knowledge assessment of mental health advisory boards. *American Journal of Community Psychology*, 1978, 6, 91-95.

Snow, D., & Newton, P. Task, social structure, and social process in the community mental health center movement. *American Psychologist*, 1976, 31, 582-593.

Sue, S. Community mental health services to minority groups: Some optimism, some pessimism. *American Psychologist*, 1977, 32, 616-624.

Sue, S. *Mental health in a multiethnic society: The person-organization match*. Paper presented at the American Psychological Association Convention, Toronto, September 1978.

Torrey, E. Mental health services for American Indians and Eskimos. *Community Mental Health Journal*, 1970, 6, 455-463.

Tung, T. *Indochinese patients: Cultural aspects of the medical and psychiatric care of Indochinese refugees*. Washington, DC: Action for South East Asians, Inc., 1980.

Weidman, H. *Implications of the culture broker concept for the delivery of health care*. Paper presented at the annual meeting of the Southern Anthropological Society, Wrightsville Beach, North Carolina, March 1973.

Wong, H. *Middle managers development in mental health programs: A curriculum guide focusing on the minority administrator. Technical report*. Rockville, MD: Staff College, National Institute of Mental Health, 1981.

Yee, T., & Lee, R. Based on cultural strengths, a school primary prevention program for Asian American youth. *Community Mental Health Journal*, 1977, 13, 239-248.

Zane, N. *Rational restructuring with Asian American clients*. Paper presented at the American Psychological Association Convention, Los Angeles, August 1981.

Zane, N. *The provision and evaluation of mental health services for Chinese immigrant children and families*. Paper presented at the First Annual Conference on Ethnic Mental Health in the '80s, Pasadena, California, February 1982.

12

Indigenous Paraprofessionals in Mental Health

An Analysis and Critique

Yvette Gisele Flores-Ortiz

University of California, Berkeley

The widespread utilization of paraprofessionals has its origins in the social, political, and cultural awakening of the 1960s, a decade that also brought about the birth of community psychology and community mental health. Prior to that time, paraprofessionals were utilized in small numbers by a few mental health institutions around the country under the classification of aides, nonprofessionals, auxiliaries, or subprofessionals (Vidauer, 1969; Kobrin, 1969; Greenberg, 1967).

Several elements in particular from the general philosophy of community mental health prompted the widespread use of paraprofessionals. First was the limited availability of services from existing sources to those believed to be in most need, the poor and the ethnic minorities (Iscoe & Spielberger, 1970). Second was a massive shortage in human resources that not only exacerbated problems in current service delivery but threatened the provision of possibly more appropriate innovative services to these same groups (Albee, 1968a). Along with these factors were others related to the circumstances of potential paraprofessionals themselves. Recognized was a need for jobs unavailable in the private sector, particularly jobs that might take advantage of mental health-related skills of lesser trained individuals who were involved in and sensitive to their own communities. Since these people were locked out of the helping professions by traditional educational requirements and licensing mechanisms, paraprofessional status promised them access to roles otherwise unavailable.

On a policy level, the Economic Opportunity Act of 1964 provided a basis for the expansion of paraprofessional programs in its mandate that services to the poor be provided with maximum participation of those to be served. Also, the Career Opportunity Act of 1966 assured paraprofessional employment to low-income and ethnic minority persons.

Thus a concern for the poor and ethnic minority groups, and realization that they were unable to obtain either mental health services or training and general education motivated the ideology of the paraprofessional movement. This ideology was most clearly expressed by Pearl and Reissman (1965) in the New Careers concept, a series of precepts that may be seen as hypotheses about who is able to do human service work and with what impact (Cohen, 1976).

The New Careers philosophy suggested that talented people from nontraditional backgrounds, trained in focused, specialized ways, could perform traditional clinical work well, as well as carry out alternative work of innovative intervention models. Further, their very presence would challenge the status quo, breaking the vested interests of professionals, to democratize institutions and facilitate acceptance of new interventions. These goals may be seen at three levels: workers, programs, and mental health system (Cohen, 1976).

Workers. The paraprofessional movement would create a new type of worker, the previously under- or unemployed, the poor, the culturally different. It was expected that training, education, and employment would alter significantly the lives of these individuals: It would provide them jobs, enhance their self-esteem, and prevent the stresses of poverty. As a social movement, utilization of this work force was seen as a direct attack on poverty and its concomitant problems (Gartner & Reissman, 1974).

Programs. Paraprofessionals were expected to ameliorate the effects of human resources shortage by direct service delivery, as well as by providing assistance to overburdened professionals with those duties that required less training. As a result, additional mental health services would be available. In addition, paraprofessionals would provide the new services community psychology proposed: consultation, education, advocacy, information, and referral. Most important, these workers were expected to bridge the gap between mental health services and underserved communities.

The system. By their very existence paraprofessionals were expected to eventually change the mental health system away from service provision in hospital-like settings, by means almost exclusively of direct clinical interventions. Rather, it was presumed that given the presence of a nonelite work force, mental health services would become more inclined toward efforts at prevention and community-based interventions under the control of the community (Reiff, 1964).

In sum, the paraprofessional movement could be conceptualized in four ways: (1) as a vehicle for providing services to the underserved, (2) as a set of goals based on an ideal of service needs and service delivery, (3) as a social movement promising social reform, and (4) as a proposal of ways to meet the above.

In order to institutionalize the philosophy of New Careers, the United States Office of Education and the National Institute of Mental Health funded programs to select, train, and place these new workers. The main difference between New Careers and other paraprofessional programs was the New Careers commitment to persons from low-income communities and ethnic minorities in particular. To meet the task of serving the underserved, New Careers proposed to train paraprofessionals who would be particularly effective in those communities and to assure them within-agency promotions and movements up the career ladder. Consequently, New Careers focused primarily on training the poor and ethnic minorities.

The Indigenous Minority Paraprofessional

The notion of an indigenous worker was first introduced by Reiff (1964) who described a worker from the community who was presumed to have similar attitudes, beliefs, and communication styles as the potential clientele. These similarities were believed to arise out of a shared background and personal experience (Lorion & Cahill, 1980). It was expected that such a worker could become the link between the service providers (the professionals) and the underserved.

The available literature indicates certain role expectations for paraprofessionals (see Boyette, Pettaway, Bount, Jones, & Hill, 1978; Hallowitz & Reissman, 1967). Under one heading, "bridging the gap," indigenous workers were expected to be involved in: (1) case finding, which includes the identification of the prevalence and incidence of untreated psycho-pathology in the community; (2) identification of internal community resources utilized or potentially available to residents (such as community gatekeepers, faith healers, spiritualists); (3) referral and information, that is, matching client need and existing service, provide relevant information concerning fees, type of treatment, services, and so on; (4) community education, demystification of mental health services to promote utilization of existing resources; (5) in-house consultation, to help educate professionals as to needs and treatment strategies to utilize with underserved populations; (6) advocacy, using the worker to intercede for the client with social service agencies; and (7) mediation, since as a member of both the community and the mental health establishment, the worker could present mutual needs and concerns, thus facilitating communication and service delivery.

It is interesting to note that the functions indigenous workers were to perform are exactly those described by community psychology as ideal interventions (Heller & Monahan, 1977). Thus where traditional services had failed, these new strategies would reach the underserved ethnic minority client and prove effective.

A second function of indigenous workers, "assisting professionals," was not clearly defined. Later, Sobey (1970) found that agencies often classified ancillary services as filling out charts for doctors and other professionals, performing clerical duties, acting as receptionists, serving as interpreters, and working as janitors.

Finally, indigenous paraprofessionals were expected to serve as therapists for their own group. This was done as a means of more successfully engaging outgroups in psychotherapy since dominant-culture professionals had proven ineffective in reaching and treating these clients. Further, if indigenous workers were successful in their other tasks, and numbers of underserved people increased, the human resource shortage would worsen, making their psychotherapeutic services greatly needed.

Reiff (1964) proposed that by recruiting, selecting, training, and employing indigenous workers, the various goals and tasks of the paraprofessional movement would be met. The National Institute of Mental Health (NIMH) classified these indigenous workers along two dimensions: (1) similarity of problem or illness between staff and client groups, and (2) similarity of socioeconomic characteristics, living situation (ghetto or barrio), or ethnic group (Sobey, 1970). The present chapter is a review of paraprofessionals and underserved groups, focusing on Reiff's second group of paraprofessionals, indigenous workers, and their functions and accomplishments in ethnic minority communities during the past two decades.

The Indigenous Paraprofessional: An Evaluation

In judging the effectiveness of paraprofessionals, one is beset by myriad problems. Particularly serious is the absence of empirical studies, even descriptive ones, of these workers, despite the fact that their training and utilization were major goals of the movement.

Due to this lack of data with specific reference to indigenous workers, the information presented in this section has been distilled from evaluation and analysis of the movement in general. To date three major attempts have been made to evaluate the paraprofessional movement. The earliest was conducted in 1970 by Francine Sobey; it focused on 185 projects funded by NIMH that utilized over 10,000 paraprofessionals. The data obtained were derived from a survey consisting of a "comprehensive, 17 page questionnaire" (Sobey, 1970, p. 13). The findings are limited in that project directors were the sole source of information concerning their programs and their utilization of paraprofessionals. No paraprofessionals were interviewed, nor did they particpate otherwise. However, the data shed some light on the state of the movement in the early 1960s.

The second project was conducted by Cohen (1976), who evaluated the New Careers movement from 1965-1975. His data came primarily from reviewing extant literature, from direct experience and observation of New Careers programs from 1968 to 1976, from an original attitude question-naire administered to 45 novice and veteran paraprofessionals, from an open-ended telephone and written survey of 15 "experts" in the field of New Careers used to locate current information and provide presumably well-formed views of the status and impact of the movement, and, finally, from in-depth interviews with several experienced New Careerists, used to provide anecdotal material conveying a sense of the workers' experiences in the field of mental health.

Sobey's and Cohen's reports are not comparable due to their focus on two relatively different populations of workers. However, together they provide a comprehensive view of the state of the paraprofessional move-ment to the mid-1970s.

The most recent review (Lorion & Cahill, 1980) focused on the effec-tiveness of paraprofessionals in urban mental health settings. It evaluated the movement's promise of reducing the human resource crunch, providing employment for large numbers of the under- or unemployed, and pro-viding effective services in the field of mental health.

Cohen (1976) identifies several pitfalls in the assessment of the parapro-fessional movement and the New Careers program. The multiple goals of the movement must be evaluated separately and at the appropriate level of analysis. This is crucial since each level of assessment may require different series of questions and individually designed sets of measures, criteria, or indices. The paucity of empirical studies on the effectiveness of any aspect of the movement precludes any general conclusions. Furthermore, until the mid-1970s most of the data available were descriptive and were often compiled after a project had been terminated. As a result, Cohen (1976, p. 51) concludes that it would be misleading and inaccurate to pass global judgment claiming that "a vast multipurpose effort such as New Careers either succeeded or failed." Rather, he proposes specificity—targeting the aspect of the movement being evaluated in relation to the objective and population.

Cohen's (1976) proposed framework will be utilized in this review by looking at the impact of the paraprofessional movement on three levels— policies, workers, and programs—as well as at the interface of policies and goals of the movement as a whole.

Policies

No evaluation of the paraprofessional movement can be made without an analysis of the policies that created it as well as those that have affected its history over the past two decades. This is particularly true with regard to the movement's goal to radically change the basic structure and character of the human service delivery system away from a medical model identification and toward greater accessibility and community control.

New Careers obtained its initial impetus from Congress and the Community Mental Health Centers Act, so that from the outset the paraprofessional movement was affected by the ambiguities and contradictions of the community mental health movement. First, control of funds and planning were largely delegated to members of the psychiatric profession who had little experience with community service and a vested interest in maintaining the status quo. Second, the problems community mental health was to tackle were framed incorrectly—as a shortage of personpower rather than as a basic need for change in the mental health disciplines and in society (Snow & Newton, 1976). Third, there was a general lack of consensus regarding the major tasks and priorities of the community mental health movement. Two central tasks were proposed: development of a wide range of both direct patient services and indirect services. While there was considerable clarity and support for the first, the second task required great change from the medical model in organization, structure, and ideology, thus generating the most resistance (Snow & Newton, 1976). This situation resulted in uncertainties over who would provide indirect services, confusion over issues of selection, training, employment, and supervision of workers, as well as ambiguities regarding job descriptions and goal attainment. It is not surprising that the advent of the paraprofessional movement was seen as a potential panacea by those who considered indirect services a secondary and less critical task of community mental health; the paraprofessional could be delegated the duties and responsibilities that appeared less important and that had received little planning.

Thus the paraprofessional movement inherited the limitations and contradictions affecting the community mental health movement. Snow and Newton (1976) propose that it was the spirit of the times, not any real legislation, that created the illusion that radical change was to happen, since the policymakers were representatives of the medical profession. In effect the paraprofessional movement promised little more than the provision of old services in new settings (Reiff, 1964).

Given this sociohistorical context, it should come as no surprise that the services the paraprofessional was to provide were often seen as nonessential, hence largely at the mercy of the political climate of the Nixon and subsequent administrations, which played a part in the decline of financial support for paraprofessional programs in later years. For example, in 1970 the New Careers program was incorporated into Public Service Careers; however, the Labor Department discontinued its support for New Careers in 1974. In addition, the federal policies regarding employment moved away from federal dominance to a policy of decentralization and decategorization, which gave the state, county, and city sponsors freedom to choose in fitting the components of personpower services into existing personnel strategies and policies. Thus decisions about who and how people would be trained and employed were left to local agencies. This contributed to increased variation among training and employment agencies, and consequently to problems in evaluation of program effectiveness.

Furthermore, in 1973 the Comprehensive Employment and Training Act (CETA) provided grants to state and local government for the purpose of providing on-the-job training and employment opportunities for the unemployed and underemployed. Ironically, this resulted in another source of competition for New Careerists, who were often displaced from their jobs by the new CETA trainees (Cohen 1976).

Along with changes in federal policy, New Careers has suffered most from the state of the economy (Cohen, 1976). In general, the displacement of professionals from mental health programs has led to their employment in jobs that might otherwise have hired paraprofessionals. Also, attempts to curb inflation through budgetary cutbacks have resulted in unemployment for New Careerists.

Local issues also have contributed to the demise of New Careers programs. In particular, the lack of preparation or attention given to strategies for enhancing implementation, reducing resistance, and accounting for individual differences within specific agencies often resulted in resistance at the agency to institute New Careers programs or maintain them when the funds ran out. In many instances the required cooperation and flexibility at the agency level to assure success were not developed or fostered by program planners. In settings where effective administration, leadership, and adequate support services were provided, New Careers programs flourished. When this was not the case, programs were not able to meet their promise of improved service. Instead, the frustration accompanying these efforts sometimes resulted in a backlash that prevented future development of other programs (Cohen, 1976).

In spite of the evidence that for the most part program output was worth the expense of implementation (Sobey, 1970; Cohen, 1976) it was often difficult to convince funding sources to initiate or renew paraprofessional programs. Since New Careers required a relatively large output of dollars and time, often only the largest employers were able to participate; their standards often conflicted with the ideology of the planners. Other paraprofessional programs under the auspices of NIMH also have faced financial difficulties resulting from major cutbacks in mental health budgets. Consequently, the number of paraprofessional programs and workers has steadily decreased over the last ten years.

There is little evidence to show that New Careers or any other paraprofessional program fulfilled its social reform-institutional change objectives on a broad scale. The evidence does indicate that the movement had an impact on mental health, but one of limited magnitude and scope (Cohen, 1976). However, this goal of social reform so avidly promoted by the early supporters of the movement has been the most difficult to achieve, largely because it was never really intended to happen (Snow & Newton, 1976). However ill defined, this task was to fall primarily on the shoulders of New Careerists themselves. As Cohen (1976) has pointed out, it was naive to assume that a few low-status workers would be able to generate system-wide changes in fields that are relatively entrenched in their institutional structures and organizational styles.

While some policies have changed, NIMH has demonstrated continuing support and commitment to the utilization of paraprofessionals by developing the Manpower Development Branch in 1971 for the purpose of planning, implementing, training, and developing programs for paraprofessionals. In the last few years the branch has funded a number of programs around the country to tackle the various aspects of paraprofessional personpower development and evaluation of such programs. While each program has its own governing body and project director, each is directly responsible to NIMH, thus presumably centralizing resources and facilitating evaluation.

Unfortunately, some of the limitations and weaknesses of previous efforts are evident in these programs. For instance, few if any initially had paraprofessionals on their advisory boards, and fewer still have as a goal the study of paraprofessional effectiveness, training, and implementation for minority populations.

In summary, the policies that created New Careers and other paraprofessional programs have changed in the past two decades. Often later policies took away the funding provided by earlier ones. In the end, federal decentralization efforts, compounded by questionable approaches to improve a failing economy, unrealistic expectations of New Careerists' abilities to change institutions without having the power or training to do so, professional criticism of workers, and community and agency rejection of paraprofessionals, have led to a reduced potency of New Careers and the paraprofessional movement as a whole (Cohen, 1976).

Workers

To assess the impact of New Careers on indigenous paraprofessionals, three basic areas must be considered: human resources, career advancement, and personal development.

Human resources. The New Careers movement appears to have been successful in providing employment to large numbers of people who previously would not have been able to participate directly in the delivery of human service. How long this employment lasted and how rewarding it was are issues of contention (Pearl, 1974; Ruiz, 1976).

The exact number of paraprofessionals employed thus far in the history of the movement is estimated at hundreds of thousands (Lorion & Cahill, 1980). Precise statistics as to the number of indigenous minority workers are not available, but Sobey's (1970) evaluation yielded the following information. White personnel predominated in paid and volunteer positions; Blacks were the ethnic minority group most represented among paid workers. A total of 34 projects employed predominantly Black staff who were paid, and 56 projects employed a majority of White paid staff. Many projects that hired nursing and ward personnel, tutors, and case aides reported that their staff were predominantly Black.

Of all the projects in Sobey's study, one-fifth utilized paraprofessionals who had problems similar to the client group. One-sixth of the programs had volunteer workers with problems similar to the patient or client group.

In one-third of the projects paraprofessionals lived in the same area as the patient population or were of the same ethnic group. Only one-fifth of the projects, however, attempted to hire persons with similar work experience, age, culture, ethnic background, religious affiliation, or language spoken by the client group. Thus in spite of the stated goals of the movement, very little effort appears to have been made by agencies and organizations to hire indigenous minority paraprofessionals. Lorion and Cahill's (1980) review found that the majority of indigenous paraprofessionals were hired by inpatient services for primarily custodial roles.

The underrepresentation of minority individuals among the ranks of the employed paraprofessionals can be explained in part by the process of recruitment and selection utilized. In the early days of the movement this process was beset by two major problems: task ambiguity and insufficient knowledge of community needs. Thus those selecting people for training often did not know what functions the workers would serve nor how they would perform them.

Sobey (1970) contends that recruitment and selection methods discriminated against minority persons due to their reliance on formal searches and recommendations by professionals as well as the emphasis on structured interviews and utilization of standardized questionnaires that might "turn off" potential ethnic minority candidates not accustomed to such instruments or patterns of interaction. Cohen (1976) and Sobey (1970) recommend that to engage minority persons and the poor in training programs, specific recruitment techniques must be used that emphasize aggressive outreach into the community to identify community leaders as well as utilization of internal networks of communication such as local newsletters, churches, and word of mouth. In fact, even New Careers programs, which consciously attempted to recruit the poor and ethnic minorities, utilized internal resources almost exclusively to identify potential candidates.

The existing literature suggests that regardless of formal method of recruitment, screening, and selection, most programs looked for potential trainees who were personable (similar to and liked by the interviewers), handled a stressful situation well (the interview), had no significant personal problems, and appeared or were presumed to have some commonalities with the target population. In actuality, most training programs hired those applicants most liked by the interviewers and who were not too different from the rest of the staff with whom they would be working. Consequently, most of those selected tended to be middle-class, young Anglos with some level of education, often some college experience, even

B.A. and M.A. degrees in psychology and social work (Cohen, 1976). Thus through established recruitment and selection procedures the poor and the ethnic minorities for whom these programs were developed were once again excluded.

Those indigenous workers who were employed often received salaries only slightly higher than the poverty level. In addition, their jobs generally were tenuously held for a number of reasons: the move toward deinstitutionalization and shrinking dollars, being the last hired and the first fired when special funds expire or cuts are made, and the fact that they were providing services considered nonessential.

At the present time paraprofessional employment of truly indigenous personnel is made even more tenuous by the increase in associate-level training programs that produce accredited paraprofessional workers, who fill entry-level positions previously held by indigenous workers. There is ample evidence that the people for whom New Careers positions originally were established are holding a decreasing share of these jobs. A 1975 study of New Careers public employment (Cohen, 1976) found that only 18 percent of the participants could be considered disadvantaged on socio-economic lines and almost 75 percent had at least a high school education.

According to Alley and Blanton (1976), the picture in mental health programs is less bleak than elsewhere. They found that New Careerists in NIMH-funded programs were 2.8 percent Caucasian, 46.4 percent Black, 21.7 percent Latino (including Chicanos and Puerto Ricans), 3.7 percent Native American, and 2.8 percent Asian. Of these, however, 90 percent had finished high school and 50 percent had college educations. This suggests that many educated and trained minority persons were hired for low-paying and less promising jobs. In addition, it could be argued that these workers were not truly indigenous, since social class differences can override similarities in ethnicity or cultural background. Moreover, there is a definite trend toward the hiring of more highly educated (M.A. and B.A. level) candidates, thus displacing the population for whom New Careers programs were initially intended (Lorion & Cahill, 1980).

Career advancement. A related goal of the movement was to provide opportunities for mobility for workers. Early on, Pearl and Reissman (1965) and Leighton (1959) expressed concern that New Careers workers would end up in single-slot jobs with limited advancement opportunities. Their concerns appear to have been justified. On the basis of his investigation, Cohen (1976) found that opportunities for career mobility in most New Career and paraprofessional programs were severely limited or completely nonexistent. This finding was later corroborated by Lorion and Cahill (1980).

One reason for this failure was the flawed character of paraprofessional training. The crux of the New Careers concept was to train indigenous persons to assume entry-level positions in human service areas by providing a portfolio of specific skills (including reading and writing), developing the ability to relate positively to other members of the staff and clients, and by generating in the trainee a feeling of belonging to a team and a sense of competence. Presumably, career advancement would be made possible by such training experiences.

Reviews of training (Sobey, 1970; Cohen, 1976) have identified a number of inconsistencies that were symptomatic of larger problems within the movement. One major liability was role ambiguity, since it follows that unclear tasks preclude clear training guidelines. In addition, there was uncertainty as to the minimum requirements for effective human service work. The capabilities and potentialities of the paraprofessionals themselves were also at issue. Some argued that with sufficient training a paraprofessional could perform any task performed by a professional (Pearl & Reissman, 1965; Torrey, 1969); others opposed the role of paraprofessionals as anything other than liaisons or community workers (see Durlak, 1971, 1973). While recent investigations (Lorion & Cahill, 1980) find that paraprofessionals often do successfully perform a number of roles, including counseling and crisis intervention, the debate about paraprofessional limitations remains unresolved.

Major problems in training also pertained to the qualifications of the trainers and the issue of who would train the trainers, since many of the skills needed for successful community intervention were not practiced by the clinicians in the field who usually became the trainers. Consequently, most training programs emphasized "counseling" techniques, group process, and related clinical skills. Additional training concerns included confidentiality, overidentification with the institution and underidentification with community or clientele (cooptation), relationship of the paraprofessional to professionals both within and outside the organization, anxiety about job security and career advancement, becoming too involved in individual cases and feeling overwhelmed, and rejection of paraprofessionals by the community they were to serve.

This last problem was particularly troublesome. It involved the community's sense that the agency was coopting its best leaders, and threatened the workers' community identity and the community's trust of the agency.

Hardcastle (1971) in particular, has been concerned with the issues of paraprofessional cooptation. He has argued that training programs not culturally congruent tend to coopt the indigenous paraprofessional, forcing him or her to lose the very characteristics for which he or she was hired.

Moore (1974) proposes a training model that would prevent some of the difficulties outlined above. He identifies four tasks the professional trainer needs to perform: (1) assess the worker's beginning level so that task difficulty can be matched to level of competence; (2) teach the paraprofessional how to make use of supervision; (3) teach the worker the necessary skills for successful completion of the job by utilizing a behavioral model of successful approximations, role playing and immediate feedback, and in vivo supervision; and (4) help the paraprofessional identify and eliminate overextension. In addition to providing a blueprint for helping professionals work with paraprofessionals, Moore's recommendations emphasize the need for role clarity and precise job descriptions before effective training can occur.

Ruiz (1976), in one of the few studies available, conducted a 7-year follow-up of a training program in the Bronx that was designed to enable indigenous paraprofessionals to earn academic degrees as high as a master's degree in behavioral science while continuing to work at a mental health center. Of 91 eligible members of the staff, only 9 participated, and of those only a small number received academic status beyond the paraprofessional level. Several reasons were postulated for this, including resistance to participate in the program, conflicts with other commitments (family, work), length of travel to educational settings, and cultural and language barriers. These findings suggest that training programs, unless specifically designed for the worker, keeping cultural characteristics and ethnicity in mind as well as providing incentives that will override economic difficulties, may result in disappointment for trainers and trainees. It is apparent that some of the barriers keeping many of the indigenous paraprofessionals from finishing secondary education also kept them out of "alternative" educational opportunities.

Thus most evaluators agree that attempts to meet the goals of New Careers to provide career ladder and academic opportunity for the poor and ethnic minorities fell far short. Indigenous paraprofessionals found themselves primarily in low-status jobs with dim promise of advancement or security (Boyette et al., 1972).

Personal development. The impact of the movement on the workers as people has received some attention. The findings can be categorized as pertaining to worker satisfaction and to personal change. In Cohen's (1976, p. 63) opinion, "paraprofessionals have experienced personal changes as a result of their work experience, but the nature and direction of this impact have been determined primarily by the structure and quality of the particular setting in which they worked." He labeled this phenomenon of differential impact "setting variance."

With regard to worker satisfaction, Sobey (1970), Gartner and Reissman (1974), and Lorion and Cahill (1980) have concluded that paraprofessionals who were in well-planned and effectively implemented programs usually experienced positive feelings and increased self-esteem. On the other hand, paraprofessionals in impersonal settings conducive to feelings of marginality, and where task ambiguity prevailed, complained of low morale. The latter problems were more characteristic of large offices or impersonal mental health agencies (see Teare, in U.S. DHEW, 1974).

In addition to setting variance and marginality, the nature of the supervisory relationship surfaced as a critical indicator of worker satisfaction (Teare, in U.S. DHEW, 1974; Lorion & Cahill, 1980). When the supervisor was supportive and instructive the workers reported positive results; and when mutual respect was lacking, morale declined. Furthermore, relationships with other professionals also contributed to worker morale. Fishman, Mitchell, and Willenberg (1968) found that trainees in a New Careers demonstration project in Washington, D.C., experienced positive growth in psychosocial development, self-identity, and behavioral skills when staff were open and honest, sensitive to the needs and anxieties of the participants, and able to allow the trainees to build on their own strengths rather than pressure them into suppressing their own identities in order to conform to a new set of alien behaviors and attitudes.

Among the personal changes attributed to the paraprofessional work experience are the development of leadership and assertion exemplified most clearly by the development of alternative service centers or "storefront" sites from which services could be delivered. These centers were largely developed and run by paraprofessionals themselves. In addition it has been suggested that being in the midst of the community to facilitate rapport increased the workers' responsibility and leadership capabilities (Hallowitz & Reissman, 1967; Gottlieb & Schroeter, 1978).

Again, work focusing on indigenous paraprofessionals in particular, examining their experiences and growth, has not been forthcoming. A few reports (see Boyette et al., 1972) indicate that indigenous workers by and large experienced difficulties with supervision, feelings of marginality, poor salaries, lack of clear goals, and minimal career advancement, so that for many New Careers was yet another frustrating and unrewarding experience. Whether this was particularly prevalent among indigenous workers or was subject to setting variance and affected other workers is unclear from the available information.

Thus the impact of New Careers on all workers, indigenous ones included, appears to be mixed. On the positive side, many people were able to obtain significant employment; some workers had the opportunity to exercise leadership roles in their communities; and a few had occasion to pursue upward mobility for themselves and their families. Focusing specifically on indigenous workers, the results appear to be even more mixed. A few were involved in culturally relevant training programs and found employment in communities where they could share their expertise and be involved in social action. Others were able to attain education and subsequently found more remunerative situations. Some grew and gained self-confidence and were thus able to break out of the poverty cycle, others experienced additional frustration in their lives, and yet others may have been coopted. The vast majority appear to have regained their commitment to the communities from which they came, regardless of where their experience and training subsequently led them.

Programs

Most studies and demonstration programs have shown that paraprofessional workers make significant contributions in the delivery of human services. In Cohen's (1976) sample, paraprofessionals were found to be as "professional" in their work performance as workers who had four-year degrees. Both Sobey (1970) and Cohen (1976) found that program planners and supervisors generally considered the role and performance of paraprofessionals to have been effective, when effectiveness was determined on the basis of whether or not the agency would use the paraprofessional, and if so, for what roles; and in perceived and measured increase in service demand and client satisfaction.

Durlak's (1979) review of professional and paraprofessional psychotherapeutic effectiveness found that, out of 42 intervention modalities assessed, paraprofessionals were found to be judged as effective as professionals in 28 of them, more effective in 12, and less effective in only 2.

For New Careerists and indigenous workers combined, out of seven studies (six of individual and group counseling and one of crisis intervention), paraprofessionals were judged as effective as professionals in four studies and more effective in three. Other studies indicate that indigenous workers and other paraprofessionals can serve effectively as counselors and therapists for disturbed children and adults (Cowen, 1969; Thomas & Yates, 1974), and that the involvement of psychiatric aides as treatment personnel in hospital milieu programs enhances the rate of improvement and return of the chronic patients to the community (Goldstein, 1973).

Paraprofessionals also have been able to carry out effectively more innovative services, including early detection and treatment of emotional problems, crisis intervention, and family, school, and community outreach programs (Cowen, 1969; Pearl & Reissman, 1965, Zax & Specter, 1974; Brown, 1974; Gartner, 1969, Gordon; 1965; Alley & Blanton, 1976). Specific population groups successfully used as paraprofessionals have been college students (Cowen, Durr, Izzo, Madonia, & Troost, 1971), unemployed housewives (Edisofer & Golann, 1969), the clergy (Dworkin, 1974), and gays (Enright & Parsons, 1976).

Specific focus on indigenous paraprofessionals has reported using them as staff in community mental health centers, as "big brothers" to Black predelinquents (Taylor, Stewart, & Forman, 1973), as peer counselors to Chicano heroin addicts (Scott, Orzen, Murillo, & Cole, 1973), and as providers of ancillary services to Puerto Ricans in mainland cities (Abad, Ramos, & Boyce, 1974).

Assessment of the roles uniquely ascribed to indigenous workers suggests that paraprofessionals could and often did bridge the gap between agencies and their services and previously underserved communities. Data here come primarily from two sources: (1) reported reactions of consumers and (2) agency personnel and service utilization studies indicating consumer use before and after the introduction of paraprofessionals. The results available provide partial evidence that indigenous workers are capable of reaching the underserved (Ruiz & Langrod, 1976).

One successful program instituted in large part by indigenous workers was the neighborhood service center (NSC), where the paraprofessional's role was more that of a friend than a therapist or community worker (Hallowitz & Reissman, 1967). In these centers paraprofessionals performed a number of functions, including direct services such as counseling, crisis assistance and psychological support, community action and community education, social planning, coordinating, and organizing cultural events and celebrations. In these centers paraprofessionals appear to have carried out the various mandates of community mental health; the degrees of success, however, have not been measured.

According to some investigators (Hallowitz & Reissman, 1967; Wallace, 1970; Wade, Jordan, & Nyers, 1969) the introduction of indigenous minority workers often brought about radical change in community action and service utilization. In most cases the most effective and successful programs appear to have been those that were fairly independent from the traditional agency such as the NSC. In this sense paraprofessionals did not so much bridge the gap as create new services and agencies within the community. Assessing their contribution to established agencies, Sobey (1970) has argued that indigenous workers enabled services to be initiated and completed faster, and to reach more people, sometimes trying innovative approaches that have since been institutionalized.

Of particular interest to this writer is the dearth of literature on the impact of indigenous workers and paraprofessional programs in minority commuities. This reflects a pervasive lack of interest in minority populations among many service providers. The few articles in the literature do suggest that, in general, paraprofessionals were effective and provided significant services to minority communities (Scott et al., 1973; Taylor et al., 1973).

It appears then that the goals of the paraprofessional movement to provide services for the underserved and to offer new services where traditional ones had failed were left to be executed by indigenous workers. Nonminority and better-educated workers seem to have concentrated on developing their therapeutic skills, perhaps as a result of greater educational opportunity and career advancement, a desire to upgrade their conditions in life, or the choice of an orientation different from that which was important to their communities.

In summary, on the basis of available data one can tentatively conclude that in spite of the many problems they faced, paraprofessional programs and the workers themselves had a significant impact on the populations they served and on coworkers with whom they interacted; and, to a lesser degree, paraprofessionals seem to have had an impact on the agencies' policies toward them, needed services, and alternative service delivery approaches. Indigenous workers appear to have been most effective when they operated independently in the community through some type of outreach service. The key elements for paraprofessional success clearly are well-defined roles, adequate supervision, and respect from and for professionals.

Conclusion

This chapter has presented a review of the utilization and impact of indigenous minority workers in third-world communities. Several problems were identified, a major one being the viewing of paraprofessionals as vehicles for social change without any strategy to accomplish social change objectives. The expectation that a few partially trained, low-status workers could alter the mental health establishment was tremendously naive.

However, evidence does exist that paraprofessionals, by their efforts, did have an impact on the systems with which they interacted, although such efforts were modest and within the existing framework of relationships.

Over the last two decades a number of other issues have surfaced, including those pointing to careful selection and training of paraprofessionals. Moreover, tasks workers are to perform must be well defined, and goals and objectives clearly delineated, to promote greater success. At the federal level policies must reflect a commitment to the paraprofessional in terms of financial parity, possibilities for advancement, and assurance of long-term employment. Without these, low morale and poor satisfaction and performance are bound to continue.

The paraprofessional movement was catalyzed in part by a need to reach underserved communities. Yet efforts to recruit, select, train, and employ indigenous workers were half-hearted, at best. Further, the specific training needs of indigenous workers remain unresearched and undocumented.

The need to study the role and effectiveness of minority paraprofessionals is crucial in view of one major fear shared by proponents of the paraprofessional movement and minority professionals alike: that poorly trained paraprofessionals could become the major service providers for underserved communities. The concern was that by using paraprofessionals, professionals from the dominant culture would absolve themselves of any responsibility to learn about the needs of ethnic groups, and consign minority consumers to receiving services from lesser-trained individuals. Sue, McKinney, Allan, and Hall (1974) found this to be true, particularly for Blacks.

A related issue that must be considered by funding sources and service providers is the relevance of traditional clinical services to ethnic groups. Sue et al. (1974) found that even when good-quality traditional services were offered to ethnic minorities, the outcome was often unsatisfactory. Clearly more research is needed in this area to isolate the needs and the best treatment strategies for ethnic groups.

Similarly, the special needs and qualifications of indigenous workers must be acknowledged and their contributions must be recognized. As a bridge between the professional world and the community, the paraprofessional is in a strategic position to alleviate human suffering and misunderstanding of Third World peoples. Given adequate training, supervision, remuneration, authority, and respect, the indigenous paraprofessional can do much to translate the needs of the community into program realities within agencies.

The mental health needs of Third World peoples are many, while the number of people available to provide direct and preventive services is likely to remain limited. When adequately trained, indigenous paraprofessionals can do much to alleviate this shortage of services and human resources. A substantial number of paraprofessionals have been trained and employed in the last twenty years. By listening to their reports and assessing their needs and accomplishments, and by clarifying organizational structures, tasks, and outcomes of their contributions, their value can be recognized. The inclusion of representatives from this work force is crucial in planning, implementing, and evaluating future paraprofessional efforts. The evidence and technology currently exist to make the utilization of paraprofessionals a true community psychology paradigm.

References

Abad, V., Ramos, J., & Boyce, E. A model for delivery of mental health services to Spanish speaking minorities. *American Journal of Orthopsychiatry*, 1974, 44, 584-595.

Albee, G. W. Conceptual models and manpower requirements in psychology. *American Psychologist*, 1968, 23(5), 317-320. (a)

Albee, G. W. Models, myths and manpower. *Mental Hygiene*, 1968, 52(2), 168-180. (b)

Alley, R. S., & Blanton, J. A study of paraprofessionals in mental health. *Community Mental Health*, 1976, 12(2), 151-160.

Alley, R. S., Blanton, J., Feldman, R. E., Hunter, G. D., & Rolfson, M. *Paraprofessionals in mental health: Twelve effective programs*. Berkeley, CA: Social Action Research Center, 1977.

Boyette, R., Pettaway, K., Bount, W., Jones, E., & Hill, S. A bright horizon overshadowed by a dark cloud. *American Journal of Orthopsychiatry*, 1972, 42(21), 596-602.

Brown, B. M., & Stockdill, J. W. The politics of mental health. In C. Eisdorfer & S. E. Golann (Eds.), *Handbook of community mental health*. New York: Appleton-Century-Crofts, 1972.

Brown, W. F. Effectiveness of paraprofessionals: The evidence. *Personnel and Guidance Journal*, 1974, 2, 87-93.

Christensen, M., Miller, W. R., & Munoz, R. F. Paraprofessionals, partners, peers, paraphernalia, and print: Expanding mental health service delivery. *Professional Psychology*, 1978, 9, 249-270.

Cohen, R. *New Careers grows older: A perspective on the paraprofessional experience, 1965-1977*. Baltimore: Johns Hopkins University Press, 1976.

Cowen, E. L. Combined graduate and undergraduate training in community mental health. *Professional Psychology*, 1969, 1(1), 72-73.

Cowen, E. L., Door, D., Izzo, L. Vl, Madonia, A., & Troost, M. A. The Primary Mental Health Project: A new way to conceptualize and deliver school mental health services. *Psychology in the Schools*, 1971, 8(3), 216-225.

D'Augelli, A. R., & Danish, S. J. Evaluating training programs for paraprofessionals and nonprofessionals. *Journal of Community Psychology*, 1976, 23(3), 247-253.

Durlak, J. A. *The use of nonprofessionals as therapeutic agents: Research issues and implications.* Unpublished doctoral dissertation, 1971.

Durlak, J. A. Myths concerning the nonprofessional therapist. *Professional Psychology*, 1973, 4(3), 300-304.

Durlak, J. A. Comparative effectiveness of paraprofessional and professional helpers. *Psychological Bulletin*, 1979, 86(1), 80-92.

Dworkin, E. P. Implications and evaluation of a clergy in-service training program in personal counseling. *American Journal of Community Psychology*, 1974, 2(3) 232-237.

Eisdorfer, C., & Golann, S. E. Principles for the training of "new professionals" in mental health. *Community Mental Health*, 1969, 5(5), 349-357.

Enright, M. F., & Parsons, N. B. Training crisis intervention specialists and peer group counselors as therapeutic agents in gay communities. *Community Mental Health Journal*, 1976, 12(4), 383-397.

Fishman, N., Mitchell, L. V., Willenberg, C. Baker's dozen: A program of training young people as mental health aides. *Mental Health Program Reports*, 1968, 2, 11-24.

Gartner, A. The use of the paraprofessional and new directions for the social service agency. *Public Welfare*, 1969, 27(2), 111-115.

Gartner, A. *Paraprofessionals and their performance: A survey of education, health and social service programs.* New York: Praeger, 1971.

Gartner, A., & Reissman, F. The paraprofessional movement in perspective. *Personnel and Guidance Journal*, 1974, 53(4), 253-256.

Goldstein, A. P. *Structured learning therapy: Toward a psychotherapy for the poor.* New York: Academic, 1973.

Gordon, J. E. Project Cause: The federal antipoverty program and some implications for subprofessional training. *American Psychologist*, 1965, 20, 334-343.

Gottlieb, B. H., & Schroeter, C. Collaboration and resource exchange between professionals and natural support systems. *Professional Psychology*, 1978, 9, 614-622.

Greenberg, B. *Review of the literature related to the use of paraprofessionals in education (1942-1967).* New York: University Press, New Careers Development Center, 1967.

Hallowitz, E., & Reissman, F. The role of the indigenous non-professional in a community mental health neighborhood service center program. *American Journal of Orthopsychiatry*, 1967, 37(4), 776-778.

Hardcastle, D. A. The indigenous nonprofessional in the social service bureaucracy: A critical examination. *Social Work*, 1971, 16(2), 56-63.

Heller, K., Monahan, J. Alternative institutions and new careers. In K. Heller & J. Monahan (Eds.), *Psychology and community change.* Homewood, IL: Irwin, 1977.

Iscoe, H., & Speilberger, C. *Community psychology: Perspectives in training and research.* New York: Appleton-Century-Crofts, 1970.

Kobrin, S. The Chicago Area Project: A 25 year assessment. *Annals of the American Academy of Political and Social Science,* 1972, 322.

Leighton, A. *My name is Legion.* New York: Basic Books, 1959.

Lorion, R. P. Socioeconomic status and traditional treatment approaches reconsidered. *Psychological Bulletin,* 1973, 79, 263-270.

Lorion, R. P., & Cahill, J. Paraprofessional effectiveness in mental health: Issues and outcomes. *Paraprofessional Journal,* 1980, 1 (1), 12-38.

Moore, M. Training professionals to work with paraprofessionals. *Personnel and Guidance Journal,* 1974, 53(4), 308-312.

Pearl, A. Paraprofessionals and social change. *Personnel and Guidance Journal,* 1974, 53(4), 264-268.

Pearl, A., & Reissman, F. *New careers for the poor: The nonprofessional in human service.* New York: Macmillan, 1965.

Reiff, R. *The use of nonprofessionals in community mental health.* Paper presented at a conference on New Careers for Disadvantaged Youth, Howard University, Washington, D.C., 1964.

Ruiz, R. A seven year evaluation of a career-escalating training program for indigenous nonprofessionals. *Hospital and Community Psychiatry,* 1976, 27(4), 253-257.

Ruiz, R., & Langrod, L. The role of folk healers in community mental health services. *Community Mental Health Journal,* 1976, 12(4), 392-398.

Scott, M., Orzen, W., Murillo, C., & Cole, P. Methodone in the southwest: A three-year follow-up of Chicano heroin addicts. *American Journal of Orthopsychiatry,* 1973, 43(3), 355-361.

Snow, D. L., & Newton, P. M. Task, social structure, and social process in the community mental health movement. *American Psychologist,* 1976, 31, 582-593.

Sobey, F. *The nonprofessional revolution in mental health.* New York: Columbia University Press, 1970.

Sue, S., McKinney, H., Allan, D. C., & Hall, J. Delivery of community mental health services to black and white clients. *Journal of Consulting and Clinical Psychology,* 1974, 42, 794-801.

Taber, R. A system approach to the delivery of mental health services to black ghettos. *American Journal of Orthopsychiatry,* 1969, 39, 702-709.

Taylor, G., Stewart, R. J., & Forman, M. A. The Black Brother Program: An innovative approach to mental health care delivery. *American Journal of Orthopsychiatry,* 1973, 43(2), 215-216.

Teevan, K. G., & Gabel, H. Evaluation of modeling role-playing and lecture-discussion training techniques for college student mental health paraprofessionals. *Journal of Counseling Psychology,* 1978, 25(2), 169-171.

Thomas, L. E., & Yates, R. I. Paraprofessionals in minority programs. *Personnel and Guidance Journal,* 1974, 53(4), 245-288.

Torrey, E. F. The case for the indigenous therapist. *Archives of General Psychiatry,* 1969, 20, 365-373.

U.S. Department of Health, Education and Welfare. *National Study of social welfare and rehabilitation of workers: Overview study of employment of paraprofessionals.* Washington, DC: Government Printing Office, 1974.

Vidauer, R. M. The mental health technician: Maryland's design for a mental health career. *American Journal of Psychiatry,* 1969, 125(8), 1013-1023.

Wade, R., Jordan, G., & Nyers, G. The view of the paraprofessional. *American Journal of Orthopsychiatry,* 1969, 39(4), 677-683.

Wallace, H. The paraprofessional mental health worker: What we are all about. *American Journal of Orthopsychiatry,* 1970, 40(2), 296-297.

Zax, M., & Specter, G. *An introduction to community psychology.* New York: John Wiley, 1974.

13

Help Seeking and Underservice

Lonnie R. Snowden
William B. Collinge
M. Cecilia Runkle
University of California, Berkeley

The fundamental concern within the problem area of underservice has been that certain population groups are not entering the service delivery system at the rates expected. How are we to understand this low participation? The literature on this problem tends to focus on barriers to specific groups with regard to service delivery systems. In this vein, reforms have been recommended urging administrators to set fees in relation to income, to recruit staff who match clients demographically and ethnically, to locate clinics within easy reach, to advertise to inform clients and dispose them more favorably toward service utilization, and to reorganize service institutions to create units and procedures more compatible with client lifestyles and values. Measures such as these are just and valuable; however, they are usually recommended in general terms and fail to address the true basis of any particular case of underservice in any certain or systematic manner.

The question of why potential clients do not become actual clients is considerably more complicated than is often recognized. Behind any potential episode of professional help is a background of perceptions, judgments, and actions, all moving the person toward or away from contact with services. To focus on a factor or set of factors in isolation from the total context of action is to risk a mistaken understanding of the problem. Distortions and oversights of true reasons for underservice have important practical implications: We may overlook valuable opportunities for its elimination, or we may take well-intended but meddlesome actions that ultimately prove detrimental.

The purpose of this chapter is to examine underservice from the point of view of underserved people themselves, looking at their behavior in response to potentially threatening experiences of the kind that are usually labeled psychosocial problems. How are such experiences interpreted? What actions are taken toward solutions if such experiences are labeled as problems? From this broader view centered on individual behavior in social context, entry into the mental health system is but one option among many coming into focus after a series of prior decisions.

To illustrate the process of continuing attempts to clarify a problem and find relief, consider the following case described by Warner (1977). A woman in Denver, a Chicana, is brought to a community mental health center. She claims that "my family, they are all corpses. They have lost their souls. . . . I am a corpse too. This side of my body (pointing to her right breast) is dirt. I see white film over it and a green film on this side (pointing to her left side)" (Warner, 1977, p. 686).

The case history reveals a series of attempts to deal with this problem before it is taken to the community mental health center. Warner (1977, pp. 687-688) reviews the woman's actions in the following description:

> Mrs. Gonzalez described herself as a Pentacostalist, but she did not go to a church for help because her husband, a Catholic, would not let her. A sister-in-law brought an Anglo-Catholic Priest to see her. He told her she was not evil, but he did not return for follow-up visits.
>
> With another sister-in-law Mrs. Gonzalez visited an Anglo fortune teller who impressed her by telling her a lot about her situation and background. The fortune teller offered to get in touch with Mrs. Gonzalez' dead mother to ask her if her daughter had reached heaven yet. However, because of her husband's objections, Mrs. Gonzalez postponed her returning to the fortune teller. By the time she decided to ignore her husband and returned, the fortune teller had died.
>
> Mrs. Gonzalez also wanted to consult a Chicana indigenous therapist, the old lady across the tracks. She called the woman an Albolaria and said she used herbs and prayers to heal. In the Denver area the term Albolaria is apparently used interchangeably with, and more frequently than, Curandera. In other parts of the country, the former term would refer to an herbalist, the latter to a religious healer, and both would be distinguished from a Senora, an elderly neighborhood lady who was an expert in home remedies. Just what

the old lady over the tracks would have done is unknown, for Mrs. Gonzalez, without the help of her family, was unable to locate her.

As can be seen from this example, movement into formal service systems may be represented within a larger field of choice or decision points, each presenting the person with alternative interpretations of what has been experienced, and logical courses of action in response. By linking these various points we can construct pathways, and find formal services represented at the end of some pathways, but not others. Of course, it is possible to examine choice points occurring after service contact has been made, by extending pathways through alternatives encountered after formal intervention. However, to do so would exceed the scope of this chapter. These issues are usually discussed under the rubrics of treatment dropout, the "revolving door," and relapse versus maintenance of behavior change.

As may also be apparent, the help seeker navigating decisional pathways does not do so in isolation but is subject to the influence of significant individuals and groups in his or her life. The influence of Mrs. Gonzalez's family, particularly her spouse and two sisters-in-law, is shown in their suggesting and supporting her involvement with particular resources. These relatives expressed beliefs and standards that were personal and that carried the values of the social reference group. In general, the web of relationships that define the help seeker's social world affects the directions taken in pursuit of understanding and relief, as part of the larger process by which social forces influence behavior.

Finally, there are cultural elements of help-seeking revealed by this example. The help seeker turns to religious and folk sources of help and is presented with certain interpretations of her predicament. The nature of what she is told, and her ability to accept it, have significance within a larger world view, with its own customs and traditions. These lie partly outside the societal mainstream and are associated with a distinctive cultural orientation.

These reference-group-related elements are readily identified as cultural because of differences in language and national origin associated with them. However, such trappings are not essential in order to define important features characteristic of reference groups affecting help seeking; common expectations and standards for illness and health may be shared by persons similar in age, religion, or social standing. It is in this sense that the term "culture" (Weaver's [1977] "communities of interest," and

Brislin & Pedersen's [1976] "roles as cultures") is used throughout the present chapter.

Use of Health Services: Orientations and Findings

In a discussion of approaches to the study of health service utilization, McKinlay (1972) identified six models for explaining health-related behavior in general. Each model corresponds with certain reported attempts to rectify underuse of mental health services. Together these models form a useful basis for analysis.

The "economic approach" addresses the impact of financial barriers on client use of services. The importance of ability to pay to the utilization of services was officially recognized in the Community Mental Health Centers Act of 1963, in its provision to minimize this factor by means of sliding fee schedules. Recently the relationship between fees and service use has been acknowledged by those concerned with limiting the use of medical services. In the opinion of some, federally supported health care has become too easy to obtain, and should require more consumer payment. Clearly, economic factors matter. Even when cost barriers are eliminated, however, there still exist wide variations based on income and ethnicity, and the poor still tend to underutilize services (McKinlay, 1972).

The "sociodemographic approach" examines the behavior of population groups who share certain characteristics, usually demographic. For example, studies show a higher utilization rate for females over males, and for Whites over non-Whites; and correlations with age, income, and education (McKinlay, 1972). Research of this kind is the most common conducted on the problem of underservice. Its value is self-evident in identifying underserved groups and may focus on the variables that are of the greatest power in predicting utilization rates (Windle, 1980). Specific findings and interpretations from this research will be considered later. However, it must be borne in mind that the resulting statements are descriptive, not explanatory.

The "geographic approach" focuses on relationships between the physical environment—usually distance—and utilization of health services. With regard to the variable of proximity, it is known that its effects are important at the relatively great distances found in rural areas; however, no clear evidence exists on its effects within the shorter distances of the metropolis. Here, factors such as convenience to major lines of transportation and receptivity of the neighborhood to persons like those seeking help may outweigh sheer physical distance, or combine with it in complex ways to create a variable, "perceived access," that is important to service utilization. Perceived access has received some attention as a factor related to use of general community resources among the chronically mentally ill (Segal & Aviram, 1978).

The "organizational delivery system approach" emphasizes the study of how the elements of the system may foster or impede utilization of services. One variable within this approach is widely known because of affirmative action policies and minority representation among staff, one aspect of staff characteristics that may encourage or thwart utilization. In an empirical study of the relationship between minority staff presence and minority client utilization, Wu and Windle (1980) found that the two were indeed related among Blacks, Hispanics, Asian Americans, and Native Americans. In another study examining a wide range of community mental health center characteristics, Windle (1980) found that these character-istics were associated with relative utilization by a general category of non-Whites. However, the relationships for organizational variables tended to be weaker than those for demographic variables describing the catch-ment area. It must be noted that structural characteristics of the delivery system and their impact on underserved groups are only beginning to be considered (see Sue, 1977). Those concerned with underservice would be well advised to consider a full range of variables describing internal organization and functioning, as well as external relationships with other service units. It has been discovered by some that in matters of service distribution and equity, organizational variables outpredict sociodemo-graphic ones (Lineberry, 1977).

Finally, two other approaches have been identified—the "sociocultural approach" and the "sociopsychological approach"—that apply to much of the remaining discussion of this chapter. In understanding the use of mental health services, the former term refers to factors such as group norms, values, and lifestyles, while the latter term refers to beliefs, percep-tions, and motivations. With their capacities to go beyond labels of general social status, these orientations may help begin to specify the actual dimensions of experience leading toward, or away from, mental health service systems.

Help Seeking

The study of how institutions of health care become more or less attractive options to people has been carried out under the rubric of "help seeking." As used by Gourash (1978), help seeking refers to any communication about a problem or troublesome event that is directed toward obtaining support, advice, or assistance in times of distress. The help seeking literature includes variables discussed in the previous section, but ranges over a broader scope, bringing into consideration aid from informal sources that may precede or substitute for contact with formally designated mental health services.

At a conceptual level, Veroff, Kulka, and Douvan (1981) have replaced the gross dichotomy of use versus nonuse of services (as a dependent variable), with a subtler, dispositional dimension termed "readiness for self-referral." In their view, actual use of professional help is seen as lying at one end of a continuum. Other points defining decreasing levels of readiness for self-referral include: having faced a problem for which professional help was seen as relevant; not having faced such a problem, but allowing that one could arise at some time; denying that the need for mental health services might arise; and, at the pole opposite from having used services, feeling able to always manage one's own problems, rely on self-help, and never seek professional assistance.

There are three decision points, according to Veroff et al., related to one's standing on readiness for self-referral. The options at each point involve: (1) defining a problem in mental health versus other terms; (2) seeking help versus not seeking help; and (3) choosing among alternative potential sources of help. Further, factors influencing the making of these choices are characterized as either "psychological" or "facilitating or hindering." The latter categories are primarily social, making the distinction between categories that is roughly parallel to that between person variables ("perception, cognition, and health benefits") and environmental variables ("environmental resources") developed in the present chapter.

The help-seeking literature as reviewed by Gourash (1978) focuses on three major themes: the people who seek help, the role of social networks, and outcomes of help-seeking interactions. The primary focus, however, has usually been on demographic characteristics. Gourash reports that nonseekers tend to be differentiated by age and race; that is, help seeking declines as age increases, and is less among Blacks. Other writings tend to support this conclusion, although confirmation has not been universal. For example, Asser (1978) found no evidence of an age or race effect.

Veroff et al. (1981) extended and clarified these general findings on help seeking in an extensive study of mental health beliefs and practices. In 1976 they surveyed a representative sample of Americans, repeating an earlier survey conducted in 1957. They included a comprehensive representation of variables, statistical controls to account for overlapping relationships, and representative samples from the two historical periods. Among their major findings were the following: "Although a number of exceptions are apparent, there is considerable stability in these relationships over the nineteen year interval between the two surveys. Women, young people, and the higher educated are consistently high in readiness for self referral; and, net of these three factors, urban and suburban residents, people who grew up or live in the Pacific states, Jews, high church attenders, children of professionals, adult children of divorce, and those divorced themselves are all relatively open to accepting professional help" (Veroff et al., 1981, p. 111).

The network of natural social relationships of the help seeker also plays an important role in dictating his or her behavior. It can be concluded that most people who experience troublesome life events tend to seek help first from their natural support systems and turn to formal organizations as a last resort (Gourash, 1978). Further consideration will be given to social ties and help seeking in the section of this chapter on environmental resources.

The consequences of having sought help, and their variation across alternative resources, are also vital to a complete understanding. Much has been written about the impact of formal mental health services, particularly psychotherapy, indicating a definite, if quite modest, degree of improvement (Smith & Glass, 1977). However, little is known about the fate of groups of primary interest from the vantage point of help seeking— the broad categories of those seeking professional services; those seeking informal help; and those seeking no help, but who are self-reliant instead. In one of the few studies in this area, Lieberman and Mullan (1978) found that after several confounding demographic and psychological differences had been statistically controlled, groups going to professionals, using their social networks, and seeking help from no one could not be distinguished in adaptation. Although hardly definitive, such a finding presents a challenge to the assumption that we must always encourage persons in need to follow our ideas about what will help them.

Thus, a tradition has evolved in the form of examining use of professional services not as a discrete act, dictated by the form of service organization, but as an ongoing process grounded in personal attitudes and social experiences. We now turn to consideration of one formal attempt from the sociopsychological perspective to account for these various influences on help seeking.

The Health Belief Model

The Health Belief Model (HBM) was drawn most directly from Kurt Lewin's theory emphasizing the subjective world of the individual in seeking help, as he or she interacts in a field of social events and influences. It offers a perspective of analysis on the constructed reality of the help seeker. In essence, the model proposes that the likelihood of a person taking action to relieve distress is a function of the interaction between two variables: perceived threat and perceived benefit.

Stone (1979) describes the original version of the HBM as having four elements. The first, called "readiness," considers the person's perceptions of susceptibility to, and the seriousness of, a health threat. Readiness is seen as influenced by the person's understanding of the situation. The second element, "beliefs about the benefits of action," incorporates the person's perception of barriers to taking action. Thus the above two elements taken together result in "likelihood to act." The third element, "cues to action," refers to internal and external experiences that "trigger" action. These may include somatic or cognitive experiences, or input from the support system such as advice or confrontation. The final element, "modifying factors," refers to any factors that could qualify or interact with any of the three elements above, such as demographic variables (age, sex, ethnicity), social and psychological variables (personality dynamics, class, reference groups), structural variables, or knowledge about the disease or prior contact with it.

In summary, perceived threat is a function of perceived susceptibility (a subjective probability) and perceived seriousness (a value decision). Perceived benefit of seeking help relates to the probability that threat will be reduced (by some amount) minus the perceived cost of action. Thus the process makes relative predictions in choosing whether, and how, to act.

Perception, Cognition, and Health Beliefs

It should be apparent that perception and cognition—part of the psychological factors referred to by Veroff et al.—take on a central role in using the HBM as a framework to understand help seeking. A great deal of additional work has been carried out on social perception and cognition, increasing in what has been described as a "cognitive revolution" (Sampson, 1981). Although easy to overstate, a role for cognitive factors exists in help seeking, particularly at the level of interpreting symptoms. An examination of cognitive theory and research may enlarge and clarify our understanding of psychological processes in help seeking, as well as demonstrate a relationship to a larger body of knowledge.

A headache, feelings of confusion, and angry outbursts at a child, or any other events from the wide array that may be potentially characterized in mental health terms, are notoriously ambiguous. It is this uncertainty about meaning that lets a far greater proportion of mental health sufferers into medical clinics than into psychological clinics (Kiesler, 1980). From a broader perspective, recognition of the slippage between event and interpretive label is only to reaffirm the widely studied phenomenon wherein a given stimulus is open to various cognitive responses. In his theory of stress and coping, Lazarus (Lazarus & Launier, 1979) has emphasized the discrepancy between "stress as stimulus" and "stress as response." The latter of these is a function of the person's reaction to the original stimulus, which is not inherently upsetting but may become so if interpreted in a specified fashion. Even stimulus events that would seem to be relatively clear-cut in prompting a given physiological reaction are subject to transformation through cognitive processing. Janis and Rodin (1979, p. 489) state that there is "considerable evidence that the degree of pain and the level of distress that people experience depend in large part on the labels and cognitions applied to the physical state and are not intrinsic properties of the state itself. These labels can in turn further influence perceptions regarding both the source and the level of arousal."

With specific reference to symptoms, ambiguity is a widely recognized problem. Issues of reliability and validity haunt professional diagnosis and assessment. Mechanic (1972) and Zola (1973) suggest that one source of difficulty is that stimuli capable of being interpreted as symptoms of ill health occur much of the time in almost everyone. In some people, and at some times, such stimuli are discriminated and labeled as personal problems; the process by which this occurs is a subject for further study. Similarly, Janis and Rodin (1979) conclude that help-seeking behavior is largely based on an individual's perception of a bodily state rather than on the body's true physical condition. In explaining this view they point out that people do not normally monitor their physiological processes consciously when everything is working well. When a disturbance is felt, however, a cause/effect explanation is sought, which may implicate peripheral factors going on for some time, but only noticed in a heightened state of vigilance.

Thus to understand how people judge themselves to have mental health problems, we cannot restrict ourselves to examining direct stimulus-and-response linkages. How is raw experience transformed into cognitive perceptual representation within the realm of health-related behavior? To understand this transformation we must consider a system of beliefs, organized in a hierarchy, through which stimulus events are processed.

Belief systems regarding health phenomena may be visualized as consisting of levels. At the lowest level lies the immediate task of problem recognition and identification of possible solutions. There are judgments to be made at this level, but they are relatively concrete and tied to immediate experience: "Am I dizzy, or just tired? Should I take vitamins, herbs, or bed rest?" Such are the issues of immediate concern that are in need of clarification to the potential help seeker.

At another level are found more general styles and dispositions toward health-related information. One such issue is "health locus of control" (Wallston, Wallston, Kaplan, & Maides, 1976), a special application of the ubiquitous personality-related distinction. This variable reflects a point of view with regard to whether health outcomes in one's life are subject to personal control or are at the mercy of fate, chance, or powerful others. It is concerned with the sense of personal efficacy as applied to matters concerning health.

The dimensions discussed thus far are applied primarily to the study of individuals. However, certain aspects of cognitive structure are held in common with certain reference groups, and important distinctions here are differences between groups. Membership in these groups, which are often ethnic and cultural, includes socialization in a particular cognitive template—a perspective on the world serving as one basis for affiliation, solidarity, and familiarity in interaction.

The study of these commonly held cognitive structures has been carried out within a tradition called the analysis of subjective culture (Triandis, 1972). There are two general areas of inquiry within the study of subjective culture: categorization and evaluation. Categorization is concerned with understanding the formation of abstract classes from concrete experiences, while clarifying relationships among these classes. For example, one class distinction describing people is that between the in-group and the out-group. Studies have found differences across national boundaries in the membership of in-groups and out-groups: Greeks, for example, include visitors from other nations within their in-group, while Americans relegate such persons to the out-group.

The other area of inquiry, evaluation, is often approached by means of the semantic differential. From this orientation concepts are judged on what have been repeatedly confirmed as fundamental underlying dimensions of evaluative judgment: evaluation (that is, good versus bad), potency, and activity. Applied to the study of subjective culture, knowledge is gained of a type that clarifies basic contrasts in cultural world views. The concepts "world" and "future," for example, are judged active in rich countries but passive in poor ones; the concepts "tradition" and "past" are judged passive in rich countries, but active in poor ones.

The application of subjective culture as an orientation to understanding problems of mental health and illness is an important priority for future research. Cross-cultural studies of such problems suggest that no disorder is immune to at least some variation among cultures in its expression, particularly at the level of specific symptoms (Draguns, 1980). Also, patterns of manifestation of psychopathology often reflect themes and conflicts characteristic of a culture in exaggerated form. Thus, by clarifying the subjective culture of psychopathology presented by international groups, we achieve not only a deep and systematic knowledge of a vital link in the chain of events leading to help seeking, but also a window into the world view and life circumstances of a particular cultural group.

But what reason is there to believe that psychopathology is different, even in part, from mainstream conceptions for ethnic and regional groups within the United States? And can the application of methods for studying subjective culture, as outlined above, capture any differences that might exist? Reason to expect an affirmative answer to both of these questions may be found in literature on racial differences in psychopathology; consider, for example, the controversy over the validity of widely used clinical instruments such as the MMPI.

Research on Black-White differences on the MMPI has revealed several important facts. Various studies have found that: (1) Black normals, psychiatric patients, and inmates score higher than their White counterparts on both validity and clinical scales; (2) Blacks and Whites respond differentially on 39 percent and possibly more of MMPI items (Jones, 1978); and (3) some differentiating items have different meaning to Blacks than to Whites, as indicated by social desirability (Gynther, 1972) and Semantic Differential ratings (Witt & Gynther, 1975).

Perhaps the most interesting of these findings, certainly for our present purposes, are the last. They imply that evaluation, an area of study for subjective culture measured with the Semantic Differential, reveals clear differences between racial groups within the United States on the most widely used structured inventory of psychopathology. Application of subjective culture as a framework for identifying and interpreting group-related differences in the expression of symptoms will contribute to a deeper understanding of how people first recognize their suffering.

Environmental Resources

Existing apart from the potential help seeker's personal view of what is wrong and what might be done is an array of social situations and structures, embodying rules that strongly influence his or her options. These events have an independent reality that exists apart from the subjective reality of the individual. Cognitive factors of a kind outlined in the previous section are seductive as a complete explanation for social behavior (see Sampson, 1981). However, they provide only one piece of the puzzle.

The aggregate of significant personal relationships—the social network—is increasing in importance as a unit of focus. Well-functioning social networks have been shown effective in helping those under various stresses to cope successfully and maintain psychological and physical health (Gottlieb, 1981). In addition, social network relationships are probably the first line of assistance that is sought when a problem is recognized. Gourash (1981) cites several investigations, converging on the conclusion that in the face of trouble, relatives and friends are the pivotal figures in the decision to seek intervention from formal services. Another work (Friedson, 1961) describes a more specialized lay referral network, consisting of people with expert knowledge about various distressing conditions.

It may well be social networks that are the medium through which demographic descriptors related to help seeking are translated into actual ongoing behavior. People of higher education or those who attend church regularly, for example, are likely to have similarly disposed persons within their networks, who transmit and enforce group expectations about the seeking of help. It has been argued that, in a similar way, professionals socialize each other and take on a common perspective that may be termed cultural (Green, 1982); one element of professional belief is a willingness to seek the services of fellow mental health professionals (Veroff et al., 1981). Clearly, practices such as these of selective association and mutual influence apply with the underserved, sustaining beliefs and actions in the seeking of help.

Informal social entities that guide and shape help seeking may be termed social networks from one point of view, but are also effectively considered "mediating structures." The brokering and buffering functions implied in this label place them between the large, impersonal institutions of society, and the single person. They are the family and religious and neighborhood groups that form social surroundings more intimate than the massive bureaucracies dominating human affairs. Their increasing emphasis in community mental health has been noted (Price & Monahan, 1980) and, on a grander scale, their importance has been demonstrated as an element in a pervasive system of hidden health care (Levin & Idler, 1981).

Perhaps the most immediate and enveloping of these mediating structures is the family. Traditionally the major source of diagnostic and treatment efforts, the family was relieved of many such responsibilities with the rise of modern medicine, and the "medicalization" of an ever-increasing range of life functions (sometimes, as in the case of childbirth, with arguable benefits). Despite the decline of indigenous responsibility for health, a major share of problems continues to be handled by sufferers themselves. As reported in Levin and Idler (1981), a study in Britain found that even with national health insurance 79 percent of problems were handled without professional intervention. Another study suggests that ties to immediate family are the resource of first resort (Horowitz, 1977). The actual process by which problems are defined and solutions proposed within families remains unknown. With increasing attention to support, self-help, and other informal features of problem solving, the future may yield a greater fund of answers to such questions.

Although no direct evidence is available, there are data to suggest that help-seeking influences exerted by families may vary with ethnicity, in line with established family-related structural and functional differences. One study (Mindell, 1980) found that an extended family structure providing ready instrumental aid was particularly characteristic of Mexican-American families. Other work (Martin & Martin, 1978) suggests a similar degree of active mutual responsibility among Blacks, but from a fairly distinctive extended family structure. Considered in conjunction with traditions, national heritage, religion, and local customs, such cultural variations in family patterning are likely to mediate some degree of divergence in when and how advice is given, and with what consequences for future action. A task for future research is to clarify consistencies and deviations not only in what is conveyed about problems and help, but also how it is conveyed.

The fundamental mechanisms by which these mediating structures exert their influence are probably related to usual processes of socialization, commitment, and identification. Levin and Idler (1981, p. 28) describe this process in the following terms: "Mediating structures assist individuals not only in making decisions, but also in carrying out the consequent actions. They help interpret situations according to traditional moral, religious, or other criteria and encourage individual action in harmony with the groups's values and goals." In connection with help seeking, the situations to be interpreted and the actions to be taken will be states of physical and mental distress and potential courses of remedial action.

One study that contributes to our understanding of social processes surrounding help seeking was carried out by Schreiber and Glidewell (1978). With a large survey sample, these investigators asked about rules governing reciprocity in the provision of tangible and emotional supports; about *rights* to emotional support, advice, money, goods, and services; and about *duties* to participate, cooperate, and contribute money, time, and trouble. Various patterns of rights and obligations were discovered, but the most striking finding was the general result indicating that only 55 percent of the sample felt themselves having any right to receive support from their families.

There are other promising concepts not yet applied to the process of help seeking. From general medical sociology comes the study of the sick role and processes of normalizing or discounting the pathological implications of deviant behavior (Kasl & Cobb, 1966). Questions related to the assumption of the formal status of being sick in one way or another, the choice of sickness labels applied, and withholding of such labels may be extended from their operation in formal institutions of health and sickness to informal aggregates and reference groups.

Mediating structures are by no means self-contained, and views from the larger society toward health, illness, and cure are represented to a varying (often large) degree. A category of societal attitudes of particular concern to those interested in problems of underservice are stereotypes based on ethnicity and social status. Block (1981) has described how judgments concerning the capacity of Blacks to profit from any but the most coercive forms of intervention inspired a tradition of shunning mental health services. Segal and Aviram (1978) have shown that differences in community acceptance affect prospects for social integration among the chronically mentally ill.

One institution with wide-ranging potential for affecting help-seeking patterns is that of the mass media. For example, in one project a large public information campaign was mounted to promote recognition of heart disease risk and the making of salubrius lifestyle choices (Alexander & Maccoby, 1979). Thus communication processes at the microsocial level are often held to be partly translations of signals from the larger society, as efforts to promote more constructive social attitudes may filter down to enhance help-seeking patterns.

Help Seeking Among the Underserved: Implications for Program Planning

Referral by self or others to the mental health system is a function of complex social and psychological processes. Moreover, these processes are more likely to result in something other than an episode of formal service, particularly for some societal groups. These outcomes include ignoring the problem or trying to manage and live with it, trying home remedies or those suggested by peers, or seeking out indigenous practitioners. These events are so natural and pervasive as to almost seem inevitable. With mental health program staff, they may inspire either of two somewhat opposite reactions: complacency or missionary zeal. The former reaction has its roots in the view that those who might be served, but fail to appear at the agency, may be best taken care of without uninvited assistance. The latter reaction originates in the view that help-seeking processes afford an unsurpassed opportunity for effective "marketing" of services, reaching the largest possible audience with the greatest range of possible mental health problems. Both reactions are mistaken.

An appropriate stance for mental health planners is to understand help seeking as it occurs among their constituents. This will involve developing detailed inventories of personal problems recognized in a particular community, including standards for deviance and attributions of cause; clarifying the norms that govern what will be disclosed to significant others; and charting the pathways among sanctioned healing practices and practitioners. Assessment such as this is not entirely without precedent. Higginbotham (1976) has proposed related methods for designing mental health services that are culturally sensitive.

From a basis such as this, the planner may then contemplate deployment of formal mental health services as a resource that is complementary to naturally unfolding patterns of health-related interaction. Some problems may be best left alone or to the ministrations of self-help or indigenous healers. This "neglect" may even need to be carefully maintained—a danger exists of creating or exacerbating a problem, by "psychologizing" what had previously been experienced as normal or temporarily inconvenient. Another kind of service response is to seek enhancement of ongoing healing practices and processes through mental health education, consultation, or partnership with indigenous healers. This latter arrangement, although not without its pitfalls and hazards, is receiving increasing attention worldwide (see Draguns, 1980).

A comprehensive system of coordinated care may result, of a kind taking place with more physically based medicine in certain regions of Africa, where "an individual who breaks his or her leg frequently goes to a Western clinic to get it repaired. The individual then consults a medicine man to determine the cause for the calamity and for a prescription (figuratively) to alleviate the problem (sorcery or spirit)" (Rappaport & Rappaport, 1981, p. 780).

Finally, there will be instances in which the direct services of a mental health clinic—psychodiagnostic assessment, and psychological or biological therapy—are the most productive courses of action. In these cases the task of planners for services is to make this help known and available at a strategic point in the help-seeking process, in a manner that makes it understood, accepted, and likely to be acted upon.

As mentioned earlier, there is an increasing interest in international and cross-cultural mental health in reconciling indigenous sources and designated mental health sources of healing. In the United States a similar trend began with community-oriented mental health, and its attention to gate-keepers and peer help. Its continuation would be constructive, particularly for consideration of folk institutions of healing, the day-to-day experiences of people in discriminating and labeling troublesome events and using themselves and their social relationships to find relief. Bridging the gap between mental health agencies and underserved people would, if done in this fashion, be more challenging and uncomfortable for mental health professionals, but more palatable and useful to underserved people.

References

Alexander, J., & Maccoby, N. Reducing heart disease risk using the mass media: Comparing the effects on three communities. In R. F. Munoz, L. R. Snowden, & J. G. Kelley (Eds.), *Social and psychological research in community settings.* San Francisco: Jossey-Bass, 1979.

Asser, E. S. Social class and help-seeking behavior. *American Journal of Community Psychology*, 1978, 6, 465-475.

Block, C. B. Black Americans and the cross-cultural counseling experience. In A. J. Marsella & P. J. Pedersen (Eds.), *Cross-cultural counseling and psychotherapy.* Elmsford, NY: Pergamon, 1981.

Brislin, R. W., & Pedersen, P. J. *Cross cultural orientation program.* New York: Gardner, 1976.

Draguns, J. G. Psychological disorders of clinical severity. In A. C. Triandis & J. G. Draguns (Eds.), *Handbook of cross-cultural psychology* (Vol. 6). Boston: Allyn & Bacon, 1980.

Friedson, E. *Patients' views of medical practice.* New York: Russell Sage Foundation, 1961.

Gottlieb, B. H. *Social networks and social support.* Beverly Hills, CA: Sage, 1981.

Gourash, N. Help-seeking: A review of the literature. *American Journal of Community Psychology*, 1978, 6(5), 413-424.

Green, J. W. *Cultural awareness in the human services.* Englewood Cliffs, NJ: Prentice-Hall, 1982.

Gynther, M. D. White norms and the MMPI: A prescription for discrimination? *Psychological Bulletin*, 1972, 78, 386-402.

Higginbotham, H. N. A conceptual model for the delivery of psychological services. In R. W. Brislin (Ed.), *Topics in cultural learning* (Vol. 4). Honolulu: East-West Center, 1976.

Horowitz, A. The pathways into psychiatric treatment: Some differences between women and men. *Journal of Health and Social Behavior*, 1977, 18, 169-178.

Janis, I., & Rodin, J. Attribution, control, and decision making: Social psychology and health care. In G. C. Stone, F. Cohen, & N. Adler (Eds.), *Health psychology.* San Francisco: Jossey-Bass, 1979.

Jones, E. E. Black-white personality differences: Another look. *Journal of Personality Assessment,* 1978, 42, 244-252.

Kasl, S. W., & Cobb, S. Health behavior, illness behavior, and sick role behavior. *Archives of Environmental Health,* 1966, 12, 246-266.

Kiesler, C. A. Mental health policy as a field of inquiry for psychology. *American Psychologist,* 1980, 35(12), 1066-1080.

Lazarus, R. S., & Launier, R. Stress related transactions between persons and environments. In L. A. Pervin & M. Lewis (Eds.), *Internal and external determinants of behavior.* New York: Plenum, 1979.

Leavitt, F. The health belief model and utilization of ambulatory care services. *Social Science and Medicine,* 1979, 13A(2), 105-112.

Levin, L. S., & Idler, E. L. *The hidden health care system: Mediating structures and medicine.* Cambridge, MA: Ballinger, 1981.

Lieberman, M. A., & Mullan, J. T. Does help help? The adaptive consequences of obtaining help from professionals and social networks. *American Journal of Community Psychology,* 1978, 6(5), 499-517.

Lineberry, R. *Equality and urban policy: The distribution of municipal services.* Beverly Hills, CA: Sage, 1977.

McKinlay, J. Some approaches and problems in the study of the use of services: An overview. *Journal of Health and Social Behavior,* 1972, 13, 115-151.

Martin, E. P., & Martin, J. M. *The Black extended family.* Chicago: University of Chicago Press, 1978.

Mechanic, D. Social psychologic factors affecting the presentation of bodily complaints. *New England Journal of Medicine,* 1972, 20,6, 1132-1139.

Mindell, C. H. Extended familialism among urban Mexican-Americans, Anglos, and Blacks. *Hispanic Journal of Behavioral Sciences,* 1980, 2(11), 21-34.

Price, R. H., & Monahan, J. Preface. In R. H. Price, R. F. Ketterer, B. C. Bader, & J. Monahan (Eds.), *Prevention in mental health.* Beverly Hills, CA: Sage, 1980.

Rappaport, H., & Rappaport, M. The integration of scientific and traditional healing: A proposed mode. *American Psychologist,* 1981, 36(7), 774-781.

Sampson, E. E. Cognitive psychology as ideology. *American Psychologist,* 1981, 36(7), 730-743.

Schreiber, S. T., & Glidewell, J. C. Social norms and helping in a community of limited liability. *American Journal of Community Psychology,* 1978, 6(5), 441-453.

Segal, S. P., & Aviram, U. *The mentally ill in community-based sheltered care.* New York: John Wiley, 1978.

Smith, M. L., & Glass, G. V. Meta-analysis of psychotherapy outcome studies. *American Psychologist,* 1977, 32, 752-760.

Stone, G. C. Psychology and the health system. In G. C. Stone, F. Cohen, & N. Adler (Eds.), *Health psychology.* San Francisco: Jossey-Bass, 1979.

Sue, S. Community mental health services to minority groups: Some optimism, some pessimism. *American Psychologist,* 1977, 32(8), 616-624.

Triandis, H. C. *The analysis of subjective culture.* New York: John Wiley, 1972.

Veroff, J., Kulka, R. A., & Douvan, E. *Mental health in America: Patterns of help-seeking from 1957-1976.* New York: Basic Books, 1981.

Wallston, B. S., Wallston, K. A., Kaplan, G. D., & Maides, S. A. Development and validation of the health locus of control scale. *Journal of Consulting and Clinical Psychology*, 1976, 44(4), 580-585.

Warner, R. Witchcraft and soul loss: Implications for community psychiatry. *Hospital and Community Psychiatry*, 1977, 28(2), 686-690.

Weaver, J. L. *National health policy and the underserved.* St. Louis: C. V. Mosby, 1977.

Windle, C. Correlates of community mental health center underservice to non-Whites. *Journal of Community Psychology*, 1980, 8(2), 140-156.

Witt, P., & Gynther, M. Another explanation for Black-White MMPI differences. *Journal of Clinical Psychology*, 1975, 31, 69-70.

Wu, I., & Windle, C. Ethnic specificity in the relation of minority use and staffing of community mental health centers. *Community Mental Health Journal*, 1980, 16(2), 156-168.

Zola, I. Pathways to the doctor: From person to patient. *Social Science and Medicine*, 1973, 7 677-689.

About the Contributors

Manuel Barrera, Jr., is currently an Assistant Professor in the Department of Psychology at Arizona State University. He received his Ph.D. in psychology (clinical) from the University of Oregon in 1977. In addition to his interest in the mental health of Mexican Americans, he has conducted outcome research on the treatment of fear and depression. He is currently engaged in studying the relationship of social support to psychological well-being.

Jim Baumohl is a Field Research Specialist in the Mental Health and Social Welfare Research Group of the School of Social Welfare, University of California, Berkeley. He was formerly a member of the Community Alcoholism Services Review Committee of the National Institute on Alcoholism and Alcohol Abuse, Department of Health and Human Services. He is a founder and the first director of Berkeley Support Services, an agency that has provided casework services and emergency shelter to chronic mental patients and street people since 1971.

Richard G. Blouch holds the rank of Professor of Counseling and Human Development at Millersville State College, Millersville, Pennsylvania. His interest in rural mental health services derives from his rural background and his work as a teacher of agriculture. Following his work in agriculture, he earned his Ed.D. from the University of Florida (1969) and came to Millersville as an Associate Professor of Psychology. He has served as a counseling psychologist since 1970 and as Director of Counseling Services for six years.

Felipe G. Castro is Assistant Professor of Psychology at the University of California, Los Angeles. He received his master's degree in social work from UCLA in 1976 and his Ph.D. in clinical psychology from the University of Washington in 1981. He has worked with the Hispanic community in Los Angeles and is currently a member of the UCLA Spanish Speaking Psychosocial Clinic. His research interests are in the areas of cardiac rehabilitation and the promotion of culturally appropriate lifestyle changes to enhance health for ethnic minority communities.

William B. Collinge, ACSW, was Instructor and Program Associate in Community Mental Health and the Underserved, School of Social Welfare, the University of Kansas. He has practiced in several community mental health settings, and is currently pursuing a doctorate in social welfare at the University of California, Berkeley.

Barbara J. Felton is Associate Professor of Psychology at New York University. She received her Ph.D. in social work and psychology from the University of Michigan in 1975. Most of her research has focused on environmental factors in late-life adjustment. Her work on the social relationships of elderly urbanites has included studies of elderly ex-mental patients in residential hotels and research on the role of the larger social context in defining the value of social relationships. She is currently working on a study of the role of coping responses in older people's adjustment to chronic illness.

Yvette Gisele Flores-Ortiz recently completed her Ph.D. in clinical psychology at the University of California, Berkeley. Her research has included the development of a scale to measure acculturation. She has also conducted research on patterns of stress and coping within Mexican American families. She is interested in these and other topics related to Raza mental health.

William George is a Clinical Psychology Intern at the University of Washington School of Medicine and is completing his Ph.D. in clinical psychology at the University of Washington. His clinical and research interests include anger arousal and management, the role of alcohol use in sexual violence, ethnic minority issues in psychotherapy, and cognitive-behavioral models of addiction.

Enrico E. Jones is Associate Professor of Psychology at the University of California, Berkeley. He has written and published extensively in the areas of cross-cultural psychology and clinical intervention. In addition, he has conducted several psychotherapy research studies focusing on the impact of social-class status, race, gender, and other cultural and social psychological factors on treatment processes and outcome. He has served as research consultant to the National Institutes of Mental Health and as consulting editor to a number of journals.

Spero M. Manson, Ph.D., is currently an Assistant Professor in the Department of Psychiatry at the Oregon Health Sciences University in Portland, Oregon. He is an anthropologist and, until recently, served as the Research Director of the National Center for American Indian and Alaska Native Mental Health Research. He currently coordinates community and trans-cultural research within the OHSU Department of Psychiatry. His research interests fall within the broad domain of mental health, specifically, prevention/promotion, epidemiology, clinical services, program evaluation, mental health law, and health care professional education. He works in a variety of populations, including over 40 tribal groups, as well as Black and Southeast Asian refugee communities. He has been the principal investigator/project director on 8 major federally supported research projects and has published extensively on these and related efforts.

David R. Matsumoto is a graduate student in the Doctoral Program in Clinical Psychology at the University of California, Berkeley. He received his B.A. from the University of Michigan, and is currently involved with research on the expression of emotions and psychotherapy process.

Thom Moore is Coordinator of Outreach and Consultation Services at the Psychological and Counseling Center at the University of Illinois. He received his degree in psychology from West Virginia University. His major interests are in community psychology and the impact of social intervention on the quality of life.

Sheila Namir is a Ph.D. candidate in clinical psychology at the University of California, Berkeley. She has a master's degree from California State University, Northridge, in community/clinical psychology. She has been involved in planning, implementing, and evaluating community services for mentally disabled individuals, chemically dependent women, and school-aged children. She has also conducted research on the prevention and treatment of drug abuse in youth. Currently, she is studying risk-taking motives and decisions across the life span.

M. Cecilia Runkle, ACSW, MPH, has practiced medical social work in several health care settings. She is a health education consultant for Kaiser-Permanente Medical Program, and is pursuing a doctorate in social welfare at the University of California, Berkeley.

Steven P. Segal is an Associate Professor and Director of the Mental Health and Social Welfare Research Group of the School of Social Welfare, University of California, Berkeley, where he has practiced as a psychiatric social worker and has chaired the direct services and community mental health training programs. He is currently a member of the Epidemiology and Mental Health Services Research Review Committee of the National Institute of Mental Health, Department of Health and Human Services.

Lonnie R. Snowden is Associate Professor in the School of Social Welfare at the University of California, Berkeley. He received his Ph.D. in clinical psychology from Wayne State University in 1975, and has been Assistant Professor of Psychology at the University of Oregon and Visiting Professor of Psychology at UC Berkeley. He has published articles on program evaluation and substance abuse, has contributed chapters to books on minority mental health, and has written on other topics related to social and community approaches to mental health. Among his works are the book *Social and Psychological Research in Community Settings,* with Ricardo F. Muñoz and James G. Kelly, and two chapters in the *Annual Review of Psychology.* He has served on committees of the National Institute of Mental Health and the National Institute of Alcohol Abuse and Alcoholism, and as consulting editor to several journals. He is currently investigating problems related to cross-cultural patterns of coping, and to social integration among the chronically mentally ill.

Stanley Sue is Professor of Psychology at the University of California, Los Angeles. He previously served as Director of Clinical and Community Psychology Training at the National Asian American Psychology Training Center in San Francisco. His research interests are in the areas of mental health service delivery systems and mental health of ethnic minority groups. He recently completed a book entitled *Asian American Mental Health: Knowledge and Directions,* with James Morishima.

Joseph E. Trimble is an Associate Professor of Psychology at Western Washington University, Bellingham, Washington. He received his B.A. in psychology from Waynesburg College (1961) and his Ph.D. in social psychology from the University of Oklahoma (1969). His research interests include the study of adaptive strategies of culturally diverse groups to life-threatening events and mental health intervention and prevention efforts with American Indians and Alaska Natives. His current research efforts involve an examination of the response patterns of Black and American Indian elderly to problematic life events.

Rhona S. Weinstein is Associate Professor of Psychology at the University of California, Berkeley, as well as a staff member of the Psychology Clinic there. She completed an undergraduate degree in psychology at McGill University and a Ph.D. in clinical and community psychology at Yale. Her research is concerned with the self-fulfilling prophecy in the classroom and she is currently principal investigator of an NIE and NIMH-funded study of children's perceptions of the communication of expectations in the classroom. She has also been involved in developing consultation services for schools, in providing consultation training, and in implementing and evaluating paraprofessional resources in a wide variety of human service settings.

Herbert Z. Wong is the Executive Director of the Richmond Area Multi-Services, Inc. (RAMS) and the Richmond Maxi-Center (District V CMHC). He is also the Principal Investigator/Program Director of the National Asian American Psychology Training Center and of the Bay Area Indochinese Mental Health Project. His clinical, training, and research interests are in the areas of mental health services, system design, and human resource development for ethnic minority groups, with particular focus on Asian and Pacific Americans.

Nolan Zane is Research Associate for the Pacific Asian Mental Health Research Project in San Francisco and is completing his Ph.D. in clinical psychology at the University of Washington. His research interests include alternative treatment and assessment strategies for Asian Americans, the role of acculturation in ethnic minority relationships, the cognitive treatment of disorders of behavioral excess, and nonspecific effects in therapy.